Clinical Psychopharmacology for Neurologists

George T. Grossberg • Laurence J. Kinsella

Editors

Clinical Psychopharmacology for Neurologists

A Practical Guide

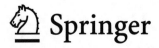
Springer

Editors
George T. Grossberg, MD
Professor & Director
Division of Geriatric Psychiatry
Department of Psychiatry & Behavioral
Neuroscience
St. Louis University School of Medicine
St. Louis, MO, USA

Laurence J. Kinsella, MD
Co-Director of Neurology
SSM Neuroscience Institute
St. Louis, MO, USA

Adjunct Professor of Neurology
St. Louis University School of Medicine
St. Louis, MO, USA

ISBN 978-3-030-09033-3   ISBN 978-3-319-74604-3   (eBook)
https://doi.org/10.1007/978-3-319-74604-3

Printed on acid-free paper

This Springer imprint is published by the registered company Springer International Publishing AG
part of Springer Nature.
The registered company address is: Gewerbestrasse 11, 6330 Cham, Switzerland

Foreword

Neurology and psychiatry grew up together. A century ago, most doctors interested in the nervous system were neuropsychiatrists and practiced both disciplines. With the rise of analytical psychiatry in the mid-twentieth century, the two fields drifted apart. Even though there was a common Board of Neurology and Psychiatry, they, in reality, became two distinct specialties with their own residencies, fellowships, board certification examinations, and funds of knowledge. Over time, this resulted in less training in psychiatry by neurology residents and vice versa. In the second half of the twentieth century, useful treatments for both psychiatric and neurological diseases began to emerge, putting the lie to the old saw that nervous system diseases were complex and interesting but largely untreatable. Then modern neuroscience was impacted by structural and functional imaging, molecular biology, neuroimmunology, and genetics. This revolution led to the animation of brain science which addressed such vital questions as the nature of consciousness, drives, emotions, and behaviors. Among these changes was the emergence of an enormous new field of psychopharmacology. Most modern medical centers now have Divisions of Cognitive and Behavioral Neurology and Neuropsychiatry where physicians are trained in the interface between these two fields. Despite the ubiquity of these pharmacological treatments for many human ailments, the modern neurologist is no longer facile with managing behavioral disorders and knowing the uses and side effects of the panoply of drugs that are now available and widely used.

For all these reasons, *Clinical Psychopharmacology for Neurologists: A Practical Guide* is a very timely book. The coeditor, Dr. George T. Grossberg, a skilled psychiatrist with special expertise in geriatric psychiatry, writes an introductory chapter on the general principles of psychopharmacology, a knowledge of which is critical to understanding the wide array of therapies that are utilized in practice. Dr. Grossberg also adds a chapter on the special issues surrounding the use of psychoactive drugs in the elderly. Following these are chapters on various classes of drugs, including antidepressants, anxiolytics, sedatives, mood stabilizers, antipsychotics, and cognitive enhancers. There is a special chapter on the important but vexing problem of treating behavioral symptoms in the context of dementia. Finally, the other coeditor, Laurence J. Kinsella, a skilled and experienced clinical neurologist,

contributes a chapter on psychiatric side effects and interactions, covering nonpsy-
chiatric medications and the ubiquitous class of over-the-counter medications,
including herbs and supplements.

All neurologists, neurology residents, neuropsychiatrists, neuropsychologists,
and psychiatrists in training will find this practical guide invaluable on the wards of
the general hospital, in chronic care facilities, and in the ambulatory setting. Like
Humpty Dumpty, neuropsychiatry had come apart into many pieces. Drs. Grossberg
and Kinsella have successfully put them back together again.

Martin A. Samuels, MD
Miriam Sydney Joseph Professor of Neurology
Harvard Medical School
Chair, Department of Neurology
Brigham and Women's Hospital
Boston, MA, USA

Contents

Contributors

Christine L. Beck, RN, BSN, FNP Maryville University, St. Louis, MO, USA

David A. Beck, MD Departments of Psychiatry and Behavioral Neuroscience and Internal Medicine, Saint Louis University School of Medicine, St. Louis, MO, USA

Alexander Chen, MD Department of Psychiatry and Behavioral Neuroscience, Saint Louis University School of Medicine, St. Louis, MO, USA

William James Deardorff, MD Department of Psychiatry and Behavioral Neuroscience, Saint Louis University School of Medicine, St. Louis, MO, USA

George T. Grossberg, MD Division of Geriatric Psychiatry, Department of Psychiatry & Behavioral Neuroscience, St. Louis University School of Medicine, St. Louis, MO, USA

Leigh Jennings, MD Department of Psychiatry, Methodist Healthcare Systems, San Antonio, TX, USA

Laurence J. Kinsella, MD Department of Neurology, SSM Neuroscience Institute, St. Louis, MO, USA

Department of Neurology, St. Louis University School of Medicine, St. Louis, MO, USA

Henry A. Nasrallah, MD Department of Psychiatry and Behavioral Neuroscience, SSM Health Saint Louis University Hospital, St. Louis, MO, USA

Brianne M. Newman, MD Adult Psychiatry Training Program, Department of Psychiatry and Behavioral Neuroscience, Saint Louis University School of Medicine, St. Louis, MO, USA

William J. Newman, MD Department of Psychiatry and Behavioral Neuroscience, Saint Louis University School of Medicine, St. Louis, MO, USA

Neha Prakash, MD Department of Neurology, Northwestern University Feinberg School of Medicine, Chicago, IL, USA

William Maurice Redden, MD Department of Psychiatry and Behavioral Neuroscience, Saint Louis University School of Medicine, St. Louis, MO, USA

James M. Williams, MD St. Louis University School of Medicine, St. Louis, MO, USA

Chapter 1
Psychopharmacology for Neurologists

Laurence J. Kinsella and George T. Grossberg

Clinical Vignette

In your office, a long-term patient with dementia and her daughter wish to discuss recent behavioral disturbances. She is 85 years old with a 5-year history of progressive memory loss and a recent impairment in language. Despite this, she has remained fairly functional. She is able to perform most activities of daily living and continues to walk independently, but stopped paying bills and cooking. She reluctantly stopped driving 2 years earlier at the family's request due to several near accidents and getting lost. She has been able to remain in her home, largely due to the efforts of her daughter, who pays the bills and provides the cooking and shopping. The daughter notes that hallucinations are becoming more frequent, especially at night. The patient frequently sees small children in the home. She has become increasingly agitated and has walked out of the house "looking for the police," only to be brought back by a neighbor when she couldn't find her way home. The daughter has since moved in with her mother and is frequently awakened by her vocal outbursts. The patient has been accusing her of stealing checks. This has led to her daughter's exhaustion, depression, anger, and resentment.

On examination, her performance on the St. Louis University Mental Status (SLUMS) Exam has remained stable at 14/30, demonstrating deficits in orientation, word fluency, visuospatial orientation, and short-term recall with relative preservation of language.

L. J. Kinsella, MD (✉)
Department of Neurology, SSM Neuroscience Institute, St. Louis, MO, USA

Department of Neurology, St. Louis University School of Medicine, St. Louis, MO, USA
e-mail: Laurence.Kinsella@ssmhealth.com

G. T. Grossberg, MD
Division of Geriatric Psychiatry, Department of Psychiatry & Behavioral Neuroscience,
St. Louis University School of Medicine, St. Louis, MO, USA

© Springer International Publishing AG, part of Springer Nature 2018
G. T. Grossberg, L. J. Kinsella (eds.), *Clinical Psychopharmacology for Neurologists*, https://doi.org/10.1007/978-3-319-74604-3_1

1

Discussion

This scenario is common in the clinical practice of neurology. The patient's agitation and behavioral outbursts threaten her desire for dignity and independence in her own home. The behavior has also led to caregiver burnout in the daughter. Behavioral disturbances are a common reason for nursing home admission in patients with neurocognitive dysfunction [1, 2].

What are the reasons for the behavior? Although agitation and hallucinations are common in advancing dementia, one needs to consider a wide range of other causes. This could include poor vision and hearing loss leading to sensory-deprivation psychosis. Other considerations include urinary tract infection, sleep aid toxicity from diphenhydramine, electrolyte disturbances, and dehydration. Once these have been excluded, non-pharmacologic strategies such as better lighting to reduce shadows, new glasses, etc. may be tried. Once these options are exhausted, however, the neurologist may consider a sedative medication to control these behaviors. Atypical antipsychotics have been effective and widely prescribed for behavioral and psychiatric disturbances of dementia but have been associated with increased cardiovascular mortality [3]. Despite the risks, atypical antipsychotic use remains common both at home and in nursing homes.

Neurologists frequently encounter patients with psychiatric conditions, either primary or as a complication of neurologic disease. All neurologists see patients with mood disorders, and many are comfortable prescribing a first-line agent such as an SSRI. In fact, a majority of mood disorders are treated by non-psychiatrists [4]. Newer data shows the high prevalence of mood disorders in neurologic disease, such as Parkinson disease, stroke, and dementia. Depression occurs in a third of survivors of stroke [5] and is associated with higher mortality [6]. Depression has also been noted to increase the likelihood of later dementia [7–9].

Patients taking psychiatric medications are prone to drug interactions. Most are metabolized by P450 enzymes, the principal mechanism of drug-drug and drug-diet interactions. These medications may act as inhibitors or inducers of P450 enzymes, resulting in toxicity or reduced efficacy of other drugs. Some medications, such as codeine, may be inhibited in the inactive, prodrug state by potent inhibitors of 2D6 such as fluoxetine, leading to lack of efficacy (i.e., inability to convert to morphine).

Inhibitors and substrates of P450 enzymes are commonly coprescribed, increasing the likelihood of a clinically relevant drug interaction [10, 11].

Anticholinergic use is common among the elderly and has been linked to increased prevalence of dementia [12].

It is important that all neurologists be comfortable with these medications. Indications, side effects, diagnosis, treatment, and potential drug interactions are a principal focus of this book.

Scope of this Book

Most chapters in this book begin with a case that allows an explanation of psychopharmacology, with emphasis on six teaching points:

1. Choosing an agent, including what you need to know about the history
2. Therapeutic dose and length of time needed for efficacy
3. Switching if not effective
4. Common side effects and withdrawal symptoms
5. Neurological scenarios
6. How to monitor response

The chapters conclude with clinical pearls, summarizing the main take-home points.

It is our hope that this book will lead to greater recognition and treatment of psychiatric manifestations of neurologic disease. This book may serve as a resource regarding drug metabolism and indications, improving the prescriber's level of comfort, and provide a public service to reduce the burden of psychiatric illness in the community.

References

1. Cohen-Mansfield J, Wirtz PW. The reasons for nursing home entry in an adult day care population: caregiver reports versus regression results. J Geriatr Psychiatry Neurol. 2009;22(4):274–81.
2. de Vugt ME, Stevens F, Aalten P, et al. A prospective study of the effects of behavioral symptoms on the institutionalization of patients with dementia. Int Psychogeriatr. 2005;17:577–89.
3. Ballard C, Creese B, Aarsland D. Atypical antipsychotics for the treatment of behavioural and psychological symptoms of dementia with a particular focus on longer term outcomes and mortality. Expert Opin Drug Saf. 2011;10:35–43.
4. Trends in elderly patients' office visits for the treatment of depression according to physician specialty: 1985–1999. J Behav Health Serv Res. 2003;30(3):332–41.
5. Hackett ML, Yapa C, Parag V, Anderson CS. Frequency of depression after stroke: a systematic review of observational studies. Stroke J Cereb Circ. 2005;36:1330–40.
6. Ayerbe L, Ayis S, Crichton SL, Rudd AG, Wolfe CD. Explanatory factors for the increased mortality of stroke patients with depression. Neurology. 2014;83:2007–12.
7. Richard E, Reitz C, Honig LH, et al. Late-life depression, mild cognitive impairment, and dementia. JAMA Neurol. 2013;70(3):383–9. https://doi.org/10.1001/jamaneurol.2013.603.
8. Verdelho A, et al. Depressive symptoms predict cognitive decline and dementia in older people independently of cerebral white matter changes. J Neurol Neurosurg Psychiatry. 2013;84(11):1250–4.
9. Yaffe K, Hoang TD, Byers AL, Barnes DE, Friedl KE. Lifestyle and health-related risk factors and risk of cognitive aging among older veterans. Alzheimers Dement. 2014;10:S111–21.
10. Molden E, Garcia BH, Braathen P, Eggen AE. Co-prescription of cytochrome P450 2D6/3A4 inhibitor-substrate pairs in clinical practice. A retrospective analysis of data from Norwegian primary pharmacies. Eur J Clin Pharmacol. 2005;61(2):119–25.

11. Preskorn, Shah R, Neff M, Golbeck AL, Choi J. The potential for clinically significant drug-drug interactions involving the CYP 2D6 system: effects with fluoxetine and paroxetine versus sertraline. J Psychiatr Pract. 2007;13(1):5–12.
12. Mate KE, Kerr KP, Pond D, et al. Impact of multiple low-level anticholinergic medications on anticholinergic load of community-dwelling elderly with and without dementia. Drugs Aging. 2015;32:159-67.

Chapter 2
General Principles of Psychopharmacology

James M. Williams and George T. Grossberg

Advances in neurobiology over the past several decades have revolutionized psychiatry and the related discipline of psychopharmacology. While once predominantly psychoanalytical, modern psychiatry embraced the neurobiological-altering power of psychopharmacology. With this embrace came a seemingly daunting obsession with efficacies, toxicities, indications, contraindications, drug-to-drug interactions, and ever refined clinical studies. Although our knowledge of psychopharmacology has inevitably widened, there are many fundamental properties of pharmacology that can be used to prescribe psychotropic agents more accurately and effectively. All clinicians who are exposed to patients with mental illness will benefit from a basic understanding of the kinetics and dynamics of pharmacology, as well as the uses and considerations of common agents. This chapter details some of the overarching principles of psychopharmacology in an attempt to lay the groundwork for many of the specific details regarding psychotropic classes. When prescribing psychotropic agents, details can be recalled through an understanding of a drug's inherent properties, what it works on, and what the body does to the drug. Rather than memorizing every detail of a drug's side effects, it is manageable to recall the neurotransmitter systems impacted, and how this interaction can lead to side effects. This chapter also focuses briefly on the process of drug development and marketing. Awareness of an agent's conception to widespread use will answer some of the hesitations physicians may have such when encountering psychotropics with black box warnings or prescribing an agent during pregnancy. Finally, some of the most common side effects and lab monitoring considerations that neurologists will likely encounter are reviewed.

J. M. Williams, MD (✉)
St. Louis University School of Medicine, St. Louis, MO, USA
e-mail: jamesmwilliams@slu.edu

G. T. Grossberg, MD
Division of Geriatric Psychiatry, Department of Psychiatry & Behavioral Neuroscience,
St. Louis University School of Medicine, St. Louis, MO, USA

© Springer International Publishing AG, part of Springer Nature 2018
G. T. Grossberg, L. J. Kinsella (eds.), *Clinical Psychopharmacology for Neurologists*, https://doi.org/10.1007/978-3-319-74604-3_2

Pharmacokinetics Vs. Pharmacodynamics

Individualized drug regimens in psychopharmacology herald from variability in both pharmacokinetics and pharmacodynamics. Pharmacokinetics, broadly interpreted as the body's physiologic interactions with a drug, describes processes related to how an individual incorporates, modifies, and releases a drug. Variability in polymorphic genes, anatomy, and organ function fundamentally alters the way each body processes a drug and, in turn, can influence the efficacy of a prescribed agent. A cirrhotic liver patient on chlordiazepoxide, for instance, may show signs of increased sedation due to the loss of phase I metabolism in dysfunctional liver cells, whereas lorazepam and oxazepam levels are not greatly affected by diminished liver metabolism [1]. Similarly, pharmacodynamics, or the physiologic processes a drug does to the body, varies from individual to individual due to differences in target tissues, receptors, and channels. A firm understanding of these processes is instrumental for understanding the dosage variability of psychopharmaceuticals. Furthermore, the decreasing costs of genetic testing may make personalized dosing based on pharmacokinetic and pharmacodynamic principles attractive for improving future psychotropic prescribing [2].

Pharmacokinetics

Efficacious plasma drug concentrations for patients can be achieved through an understanding of the pharmacokinetics. The balance between efficacy and toxicity of a given agent usually depends on its concentration in the body. A given psychotrope may only be therapeutic at specific blood levels, and those levels are directly dependent on how the body incorporates, modifies, and releases the agent. Physicians use therapeutic drug monitoring (TDM), or plasma concentration measurements, to adjust dosages for steady-state concentrations of antidepressants such as nortriptyline, mood stabilizers like lithium, and some anticonvulsant mood stabilizers such as divalproex [3]. Pharmacokinetics specifically describes a drug's absorption, distribution, metabolism, and evacuation out of the body.

Absorption refers to the shift of a chemical into the bloodstream after administration. Oral absorption usually indicates drugs that are taken by mouth and absorbed by the GI tract. Oral preparations can be modified for quick or slow release. Bioavailability, a subcategory of absorption, is a measurable value defined as the fraction of unaltered drug that reaches systemic circulation by any route. Intravenous administration of a drug has 100% bioavailability in systemic circulation. In contrast, oral administration has an incomplete bioavailability that is influenced by factors such as presence of food, capsule dissolution, gastric pH, small intestinal surface area, permeability of membranes, and blood flow. For oral preparations of drugs like ziprasidone, food is crucial to ensure adequate absorption, bioavailability, and reliable blood levels [4]. The absorption of drugs administered intramuscularly or subcutaneously is limited primarily by regional blood flow. Solutions that change capsule dissolution rates or modify the transepithelial physiology of the small bowel can be used to both slow and enhance oral absorption. Lipid emulsifiers like bile salts, for example, inhibit drug efflux transporters like gut CYP450 and P-gp [5] and increase absorption by other mechanisms.

Oral drugs may be degraded by enzymes from bacteria, gut cells, or the liver. Oral bioavailability is also influenced by physiological and physicochemical factors, such as solubility and permeability. Foods like grapefruit juice inhibit CYP3A4, an important metabolic enzyme in the gut and liver, leading to increased blood levels of some drugs. Medications that pass into the GI tract are delivered to the liver by the portal vein before they reach systemic circulation. Most commonly, an amount of drug is metabolized by liver enzymes and inactivated in a process called hepatic first-pass effect. This process limits the total amount of drug absorbed systemically, thereby decreasing bioavailability. The extent of loss of bioavailability by hepatic first pass is drug specific. Drugs like the opioid reversal agent naloxone are almost completely metabolized by hepatic first pass and are thus not routinely used orally [6].

The distribution of a drug is the amount of agent delivered to the body's tissues after reaching the bloodstream. The rate of distribution to tissues influences drug efficacy. Blood flow, plasma protein binding, regional pH, membrane permeability, and tissue-specific binding all influence the amount of drug that reaches a given tissue. Highly vascularized tissues like the liver, kidney, and heart receive a large distribution of a drug quickly. Distribution is also affected by partitions (e.g., the blood-brain barrier does not readily allow polar compounds or large-molecular-size drugs free passage) and regional blood flow, which may restrict certain chemicals from distributing to a given tissue. The volume of distribution (V_d) is a theoretical dilutional space that would contain the dose administered of a drug to match the plasma concentration of the drug. For example, if 100 mg of a drug is administered and the plasma concentration is 1 mg/L, then you would need to disperse that same 100 mg of drugs in 100 L, the V_d, to match the plasma concentration. The volume of distribution is inversely related to the plasma concentration of an agent and is influenced by lipophilicity, plasma protein binding, and dissociation characteristics in body fluids. A highly tissue-bound drug will have a high V_d and a low plasma concentration. Many psychotropic drugs favor plasma protein binding, and in patients with protein-restricted plasma due to diseases like renal or hepatic failure, it would be expected that higher free levels of psychotropes may cause increased effects. Yet, compensation by elimination of free drug makes protein-binding alterations a less significant cause of distribution variability [7]. Currently lack of studies permits large conclusions to be drawn about the clinical significance of protein-binding distribution variability.

The body prefers lipophilic compounds for absorption and favors polarity during excretion. Metabolism, in a pharmacokinetic sense, refers to the hepatic transformation of lipid soluble molecules into excretion-favored water-soluble molecules. Metabolism occurs in two phases. Phase I refers to chemical reactions (e.g., oxidation, reduction, hydrolysis) that usually inactivate a compound and prepare the subsequent product for phase II reactions. Although most compounds are inactivated prior to phase II, there are some chemicals that may have enhanced activity after a phase I reaction. The most common phase I reaction is an oxidation reaction in the smooth endoplasmic reticulum of hepatocytes. This reaction utilizes isoenzymes of the cytochrome P450 system. In phase II, metabolites of phase I are conjugated with a charged chemical species (e.g., glucuronic acid, glutathione, glycine, or sulfate) by transferase enzymes to create a water-soluble compound that can be subsequently excreted in urine.

The cytochrome P450 system is important when considering the pharmacokinetics of psychopharmaceuticals. CYP1, CYP2, and CYP3 are the three gene families of cytochrome P450 known to be involved in drug metabolism, specifically phase I reactions. The large variation in individual drug metabolism primarily comes from genetic differences and varying levels of both expression and catalytic activity. Pharmacogenetic studies can be used to predict the activity of individual enzymes and their relative effects compared to other genetic variants in the cytochrome P450 system. Consequently, unusual drug responses occasionally occur in related family members [8]. A working knowledge of an enzyme's interaction with a substrate can be used to predict potential drug interactions. The CYP450 family of enzymes is both inhibited and induced by a wide variety of medications, foods, and herbs. Inhibition of a given CYP enzyme can result in increased levels of chemicals normally broken down by the inhibited enzyme. Selective serotonin reuptake inhibitors (SSRIs) are a commonly prescribed class of drugs that have the potential to cause dangerous interactions through cytochrome-P450 inhibition. Fluoxetine can cause persistent CYP450-2D6 inhibition for weeks, which could in turn cause the buildup of dangerous levels of other antidepressants, anxiolytics, calcium channel blockers, and more. Drugs like rifampin, ritonavir, and phenytoin can induce CYP450 enzymes leading to increased degradation of other medications. It is important to consider all medications, not just psychotropes, that may inhibit or induce the CYP450 system to avoid potentially dangerous interactions [9].

The clearance of a drug refers to the rate of elimination relative to plasma concentration. Clearance is reported as a unit of plasma volume from which drug is removed per unit of time. The body eliminates drugs through renal excretion or by liver biotransformation. For many drugs, the clearance is proportional to plasma concentration. Higher plasma concentrations in the bloodstream allow for more elimination by the liver or kidneys. Because an IV administered drug has 100% bioavailability, clearance is the main consideration when determining average drug concentration after IV doses. Variations in IV clearance stem from individual dysfunction in the kidneys or liver. For instance, an agent's effective concentration may linger in the bloodstream for longer than anticipated if a patient with kidney failure cannot excrete a compound normally. Drugs with significant elimination by an organ should have a clearance similar to organ blood flow. Many psychiatric drugs have clearance values close to 1500 ml/min, or total hepatic blood flow, indicating that a substantial amount of the drug is cleared before it ever reaches target tissues. Zaleplon, a sedative hypnotic, has a systemic availability of only 30% due to significant presystemic elimination [10]. Therefore, patients with liver dysfunction may be exposed to dangerous levels of many psychiatric drugs which normally have large presystemic clearance.

Drug accumulation refers to the addition of a second, or subsequent dose of a drug before the previous dose has been eliminated. When treating psychiatric illness, a steady level of a drug may be necessary. Drugs that follow first-order elimination are inactivated at a steady rate that is proportional to the amount of drug available. After many doses, a drug may enter a *steady state* which describes the point at which the amount of drug entering the body is equivalent to the amount leaving the body. In reality, drug concentrations vary constantly due to pharmacokinetic properties, but *steady state* is a useful estimate of drug concentration that is determined by dose and clearance. The steady-state concentration resides in between the peak and trough concentrations that occur with each dosing interval. Clinicians can modify the amount of drug administered and the dosing frequency to adjust peaks, troughs, and *steady-state* concentrations [3]. The antipsychotic clozapine has a half-life that would be suitable for once-daily dosing every 24 h, yet the peak concentrations cause toxicity at this dose. Clozapine is dosed two or three times daily to retain efficacious steady state while avoiding seizure provoking toxicity.

Pharmacodynamics

The study of the biochemical and physiologic effects of drugs, through receptor binding and chemical reaction, is referred to as pharmacodynamics. A drug's effect in the body can be influenced by numerous factors including the amount of drug available, the drug stability, individual receptor variability, and tolerance. Both the concentration at which a drug has effect and the effect magnitude at constant concentration vary widely among individuals. In pharmacology, the site of action refers to the specific mechanism by which a drug has an effect. Generally, site of action refers to a receptor or enzyme that, when stimulated, produces a cellular effect. Yet, drugs may bind multiple receptors and can have intended as well as unintended effects or side effects. These unintended effects may have pharmacodynamic parameters that are dissimilar to a drug's main effect. Low doses of quetiapine can cause increases in weight gain and triglyceride levels, an unintended effect, even in patients who are not responding to the intended effect of the antipsychotic [11]. Importantly, normal physiological processes such as aging can effect the pharmacodynamics of a psychotropic medication. Drugs that effect the CNS should be used cautiously in the elderly [12].

Although the plasma concentration of a drug and a drug's effect are correlated, they are not always linearly correlated. A dose-response curve (a dose or dose function plotted on the x-axis and a measured dose response plotted on the y-axis) can be used to graphically represent the response of a drug at given doses. A hypothetical example of such a sigmoidal graph is shown in Fig. 2.1. As concentration of a drug increases, the effect increases until a maximal value is established. The potency of a drug is described as the location along the x-axis. More potent drugs show

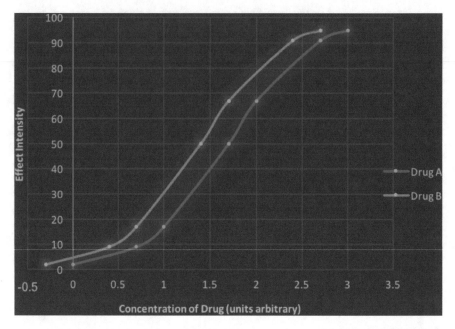

Fig. 2.1 Dose-response curves for two hypothetical drugs. Drug B is more potent (left shifted) than drug A

biologic response at lower (more left-shifted) doses on the x-axis (i.e., drug B in Fig. 2.1). The slope of the graph or the change in effect per unit dose has practical applications in psychopharmacology. Dose adjustments at low concentrations can be liberal to achieve maximal response, whereas adjustments toward the higher end of the curve need minimal increases to achieve maximal response. In contrast, dose adjustments at linear parts of the curve should result in directly proportional increases in drug effect. This phenomenon is due to concentration dependent saturation of enzymes, explained through each drugs site of action [3].

One of the major considerations in pharmacodynamics is drug safety versus efficacy. The effective dose (ED50) is the dose that produces the intended effect in 50% of test subjects. In contrast, the lethal dose (LD50) is the drug dose that is lethal for 50% of test subjects. The therapeutic index is the ratio of the lethal dose to the effective dose. A low ratio indicates a drug with low safety, or low LD50 relative to ED50. A drug with a narrow therapeutic index (e.g., those drugs with similar effective and lethal dosages) has a higher likelihood of causing toxicity when dosages are increased. TDM is recommended with some psychotropics such as clozapine, tricyclic antidepressants, and lithium due to narrow therapeutic indices [13]. TDM can prevent dangerous toxicities from psychotropes from minimal changes in blood concentration.

Tolerance refers to a decrease in the maximal effect or potency of a drug due to prior exposure to the drug. Mechanistically, tolerance occurs through adaptive changes in a receptor or receptor binding, and through biological thwarting of the effect that binding induces. Cells can upregulate and downregulate receptors due to prior drug exposure. Alcohol tolerance occurs both through desensitization of GABA-ergic receptors in the CNS and through changes in the firing rate of individual neurons. GABA-ergic receptors are upregulated with chronic alcohol use, and higher alcohol requirements are necessary to obtain the same effect. When an alcoholic stops drinking, these upregulated GABA receptors are not potentiated and have a decreased responsiveness in the brain, leading to alcohol withdrawal. Stimulants like methamphetamine, an agonist of adrenergic receptors, cause downregulation of target receptors over time. When the stimulant is stopped, there are a fewer total number of adrenergic receptors than before stimulant use, leading to withdrawal side effects such as lethargy and depression. Tolerance and withdrawal may lead to drug dependence, or the state by which one only functions normally in the presence of the drug (i.e., an alcoholic who gets seizures and tremors without regular use of alcohol). Clinicians should take tolerance, withdrawal, and dependence into account as they are not necessarily long-term consequences of a drug. Patients on benzodiazepines for 3–4 weeks will likely have some withdrawal after abrupt stoppage, and yet the quantity of these meds per prescription indicates that they are still widely overused [14].

Drug Interactions

Drug-drug interactions occur via the effects of a drug modifying the effects of another drug. Interactions are not limited to prescription psychotropic medications but encompass the effects of supplements, herbal medications, and other over-the-counter compounds. These interactions can be explained by both pharmacokinetic and pharmacodynamic processes. As briefly mentioned above, the major pharmacokinetic process for drug interaction occurs via induction or inhibition of the cytochrome P450 enzymes. Naringin, found in grapefruit juice and other citric juice chemicals, inhibits CYP3A4 causing increased intestinal absorption of many medications. Numerous psychotropic drugs and supplements influence the cytochrome P450 system, with most acting as inhibitors. Phenytoin, phenobarbital, and carbamazepine, however, will induce cytochrome P450 enzymes and should be used with caution when co-prescribed with drugs metabolized by these induced enzymes. Interactions can also occur at other important pharmacokinetic steps. Questran and Colestid (cholesterol-binding resins) have been shown to decrease intestinal absorption of acidic drugs like thiazide diuretics by up to 85% [15]. Regarding excretion, NSAIDs and some diuretics inhibit the renal elimination of lithium, which can lead to toxic buildup of this mood stabilizer.

Pharmacodynamic drug interactions occur via end-target synergism or antagonism (i.e., a medication increasing or decreasing the effects of another drug). The combination of MAOIs and other antidepressants can lead to excess amounts of CNS serotonin and cause agitation, high core body temperature, tremors, dilated pupils, increased reflexes, and possible death due to "serotonin syndrome."

Over-the-counter supplements like Saint John's wort, a natural supplement used for mood, also increase serotonin in the brain and have the same risks when combined with serotonergic antidepressants. Benzodiazepines and alcohol, both GABA potentiators, act synergistically to cause occasionally fatal respiratory depression and sedation. Some antagonistic interactions can occur, especially in populations of patients on numerous medications. Elderly patients on cholinesterase inhibitors may be prescribed anticholinergic medications such as oxybutynin or diphenhydramine that block cholinergic receptors and lead to conflicting effects.

FDA Drug Approval

Few drugs make it through the process of drug approval and onto the market. Candidate drugs are conceived in a preclinical phase that usually consists of 6–7 years of basic science research into the pathophysiology of a disease and the multitude of chemicals that may modify a disease. Countless compounds are tested in the laboratory before a potential candidate drug emerges. Before new drugs can be administered in humans, they are tested in other living animals such as rodents to give an estimate of the overall safety of the new agent. Only around 5 out of 5000 compounds tested show enough promise to move past the preclinical testing phase. If the drug is deemed safe at predicted effective dosages, an investigational new drug (IND) application may be submitted to the FDA to start the process of drug approval.

Phase 1 of the FDA approval process is usually a 1–2-year process concerned with the safety of the drug in humans. Generally, 20–100 healthy volunteers undergo low dosing of the compound with subsequent monitoring. Overall, 70% of new drugs make it past phase 1 safety testing. Phase 2 focuses on the efficacy of the new compound with ongoing safety monitoring. Up to 300 patients with the disease in question are given the new agent and monitored for effectiveness and toxicity. Researchers may modify the routes of administration, dosing intervals, and other parameters based on data from phase 2. Controlled phase 2 trials may compare the effectiveness of the new agent to a placebo or other commonly used drug in patients with the disease in question. Few drugs make it past phase 2 due to ineffectiveness or intolerable side effects. If a drug continues to look promising in phase 2, manufacturers meet with the FDA to set plans for continued testing as well as the drug design process [16].

If a drug is found to be effective, larger phase 3 studies are conducted to explore effective dosages, variability in populations, and interactions with other agents. Phase 3 studies generally consist of drug administration to thousands of patients and can last up to 10 years. Around 10% of drugs fail during phase 3 trials. Postmarketing studies are agreed upon by drug sponsors and the FDA for continual monitoring of a drug's safety and efficacy once the drug has made it to the market. The agents that survive phase 3 are summarized in a new drug application (NDA) that is submitted to the FDA. Review of the NDA can take up to 2 years. The NDA contains all the information on how a drug behaves in human and animal studies, as well as how the drug is manufactured. Post-market studies are conducted after a drug finishes approval to further characterize long-term information about the agent. A drug can be removed from the market at any point in time if serious adverse effects are reported.

Off-Label Use

Despite the arduous process of drug approval, drugs only receive FDA approval for specific indications and dosages when they make it to the market. Off-label drug use is defined as the medical use of a drug for an indication or at a dosage that has not been approved by the FDA. Off-label drug use (OLDU) occurs broadly in medicine and most commonly in populations that may not be included in clinical trials such as children, the elderly, and pregnant women. With such prevalence, it is surprising that physicians oftentimes struggle with its meaning and application. The controversies surrounding the term come from many major lawsuits and settlements caused by pharmaceutical promotion and harm from OLDU [17]. Although controversial at times, OLDU may constitute up to 21% of prescriptions [18]. Drug manufacturers cannot advertise for off-label indications, but the FDA does not regulate a doctor's ability to prescribe based on his or her clinical judgment. OLDU by clinical judgment can even become standard of care for certain conditions. Aspirin, for instance, is recommended by the American Heart Association guidelines for coronary artery disease prevention in diabetics [19] yet is not FDA approved for this purpose. Cases like these reveal the power of clinical evidence in prescribing off-label drugs but do not encompass all OLDU. Many drugs prescribed off label are done so with little to no clinical evidence, increasing the risk of harm for patients [18]. A practical approach based on available evidence gives doctors the freedom to prescribe off label only when indications are in the best interest of an individual patient and based on the highest amount of evidence. Because populations such as the elderly, children, pregnant women, and psychiatric patients are often excluded from many trials, OLDU is common and effective in some circumstances [20].

DEA Schedules of Drugs

The controlled substance act of 1970 regulates the creation, importation, use, and possession of substances in the United States. Those who manufacture, distribute, and dispense controlled substances must register with the Drug Enforcement Administration (DEA). The DEA enforces the controlled substance act federally. Controlled substances are divided into five schedule categories based on the potential for medical use versus the potential for addictive or otherwise harmful effects [21]. Table 2.1 summarizes the DEA schedules of drugs.

Table 2.1 Description of DEA schedule of drugs with common examples

Schedule	Description	Common examples
I	No currently accepted medical use and have a high potential for abuse with limited safety profiles	LSD, heroin, ecstasy, and marijuana
	These drugs cannot legally be prescribed in many states	
II	Includes drugs with some medical benefit	Morphine, opium, codeine, hydromorphone, oxycodone, fentanyl, and nonnarcotics such as amphetamine and amobarbital
	Have a high potential for abuse with dependence (physical or psychological)	
III	Have abuse potential less than schedule I or II	Vicodin, Tylenol with codeine, and nonnarcotics like ketamine and anabolic steroids
	Have moderate physical and high psychological addiction potential	
IV	Have lower abuse potential than drugs in III but more abuse potential than V	Alprazolam, clonazepam, and lorazepam
V	Lowest abuse potential of controlled substances	Robitussin AC, Phenergan with codeine
	Generally consist of preparations with limited amounts of opiates	

Common Side Effects of Psychotropic Drugs and How to Manage Them

Neurotransmitter Systems

Almost all psychotropes work in the brain by stimulating or inhibiting neurotransmitter systems. Agonists bind to receptors to activate a response, while antagonists inactivate or dampen a receptor's response. Some psychotropes inhibit enzymes or pumps that allow for more neurotransmitters to remain in a synaptic cleft and bind to their receptor. Understanding the mechanism of influence each drug has over a given neurotransmitter system provides a framework by which many psychotropic drug effects can be understood.

Acetylcholine (Ach) is the principal neurotransmitter in cholinergic neurotransmission and is dispersed throughout the body as part of the autonomic nervous system. Mesopontine cholinergic fibers transverse the substantia nigra and striatum as well as other parts of the thalamus and brainstem. Cholinergic neurons in the forebrain, specifically the nucleus basalis, are affected in Alzheimer's disease. Limiting cholinergic transmission in the basal ganglia is behind the antiparkinsonian effects (reduced tremor) seen with some anticholinergics. Atypical antipsychotics have varied degrees of anticholinergic activity, but in general result in less movement disorder, or extrapyramidal symptoms (EPS), and reduced tardive dyskinesia relative to the weakly anticholinergic traditional antipsychotics [22]. In cholinergic nerve terminals, acetyl coenzyme A and choline are combined by the enzyme acetyltransferase to form Ach. After synthesis, Ach is sequestered in secretory vesicles by vesicle acetylcholine transporters. Upon release, Ach can interact with muscarinic, g-coupled protein receptors and nicotinic, ion channel-coupled receptors. Cholinergic transmission is terminated by the degradation of Ach by the enzymes acetylcholinesterase and butyrylcholinesterase. Muscarinic receptors, classified as M1-M5, are the main receptors stimulated by Ach release by postganglionic neurons of the parasympathetic nervous system. These receptors produce effects either through a second messenger or by regulating an ion channel. Muscarinic receptors, in the presence of Ach, produce a variety of tissue effects including salivary and stomach secretion (M1, M3), reduced heart rate (M2), smooth muscle contraction, bronchoconstriction, eye accommodation, and vasodilation (M3). Many psychotropic drugs block Ach's interaction with muscarinic receptors causing an anticholinergic effect. Predictably, anticholinergic symptoms include dry mouth, decreased sweating, blurry vision, constipation, confusion, sedation, hallucinations, and difficulty urinating. Nicotinic receptors consist of a variety of subunits including those in neurons and those in skeletal muscle. Neural nicotinic receptors are involved in cognition, memory, and alertness, whereas skeletal muscle nicotinic receptors are the targets for muscle relaxers. Blockade of nicotinic receptors by anticholinergic medications may cause memory problems, cognitive difficulties, agitation, and disorientation. Nicotine dependence results from stimulation of nicotinic receptors in the dopamine reward pathways of the mesolimbic system. Freedman et al. [23] showed linkage data that suggests an auditory defect in schizophrenia may be linked to the 7 nicotinic receptor gene which could lend support to notion that high rates of cigarette smoking among schizophrenic patients may represent a chance to slightly improve some physiologic aspects of the disease.

Noradrenergic neurons stem from the locus ceruleus and lateral tegmental nuclei and, alongside sympathetic nerves and ganglia, are involved in stress responses, alertness, and arousal. Dopamine-B-hydroxylase forms norepinephrine from dopamine and a hydroxyl group. Adrenergic receptors, stimulated by norepinephrine and epinephrine, are G protein-coupled receptors that activate the sympathetic nervous system. Noradrenergic transmission in the locus ceruleus is related to stressful stimuli and behavioral adaptation to challenges or barriers. Adrenergic receptors are of the alpha or beta subtype and have numerous effects including smooth muscle contraction; vasoconstriction (alpha 1); platelet activation (alpha 2); positive chronotropic, inotropic, and dromotropic effects (beta 1); and relaxation of the detrusor muscle (beta 3). The vasoconstriction by alpha 1 stimulation is relevant to psychotropic medications as hypotension is common in medications with alpha 1 blockade. Alpha 2 receptors are also involved in norepinephrine release and may be involved in the adrenergic dysregulation seen in depression [24]. Norepinephrine is degraded by MAO-A and COMT, two enzymes that are targeted by other psychotropic medications.

The cell bodies of histamine neurons in the posterior hypothalamus project broadly throughout the cortex and promote wakefulness and alertness. Psychotropes with antihistaminergic properties cause sedation. New antihistaminergic drugs which do not cross the blood-brain barrier do not cause drowsiness like the older, first-generation medications.

Dopamine is both a precursor to catecholamines and an important neurotransmitter. Once in the neuron, l-tyrosine is converted to dopamine through the intermediate l-dopa, a successful medication for those with dopaminergic depletion in Parkinson's disease. Dopaminergic neurons form circuits in the nigrostriatal, mesolimbic, tuberohypophyseal, and tuberoinfundibular regions of the brain. The neurons in the nigrostriatal circuits are important for normal motor control and have been identified as pivotal in the brain's reward response during learning tasks [25]. Destruction of dopaminergic neurons in the basal ganglia is attributed to movement disorders, and many strategies exist for increasing CNS dopamine levels in patients with diseases such as Parkinson's disease. As mentioned above, anticholinergics have some efficacy in treating the resting tremor of Parkinson's disease, but the mainstay of Parkinson's treatment is dopamine replacement therapy. Antipsychotics and some other psychotropic medications block dopamine receptors and cause abnormal stimulation of the nigrostriatal pathways, leading to movement abnormalities. This blockade can cause a variety of movement disorders referred to as EPS. These side effects can be broken down into dystonia (spasms and contractions), akathisia (unnerving inability to stay still), bradykinesia (slowed movements), tardive dyskinesia (jerky movements of mouth and tongue), and parkinsonism (tremor, rigidity, mask-like face). The smaller incidence of EPS with atypical antipsychotics has made them the mainstay of psychotic disorder treatment.

The primary excitatory pathway of the CNS is the glutamatergic system modulated by the neurotransmitters glutamate and aspartate. Glutamate, the most prominent neurotransmitter, is involved in memory and learning, and glutamate receptors are present throughout the nervous system in neurons and glia. Glutamate is also the precursor for GABA, the main inhibitory neurotransmitter in the brain. The glutamate receptors are classified as ionotropic or metabotropic based on whether the receptors are ligand gated or activated by indirect second messengers, respectively. The major known function of glutamate receptors is the regulation of synaptic plasticity, but these receptors are also involved in glial cell cycles and excitatory/inhibitory CNS balance. NMDA receptors, the target of PCP and ketamine, stimulate neuronal plasticity and have been linked to improved cognition and antidepressant effects when stimulated by agonists. Glutamate is cycled between neurons and glial cells via the glutamate-glutamine pathway, and precise extracellular regulation is required for normal CNS activity. Glutamate receptor activation can cause neurodegeneration by excitotoxicity in cases of trauma, chemical exposure, neurodegenerative diseases, and aging. Furthermore, glutamate receptors have an association with numerous diseases such as autism, ADHD, Parkinson's, and Huntington's, but their overall role in disease pathophysiology is not currently known. The diversity of glutamate receptors has made the modification of glutaminergic transmission difficult to isolate and predict. As our understanding of glutamate and glutamate receptors increases, it is presumed that its role in numerous mood disorders and neurodegenerative disorders will expand.

Specific Side Effects of Newer Psychotropic Drugs

Weight Gain

Excessive weight gain after the introduction of a psychotropic medication is a common clinical problem. Numerous psychiatric disorders and medications have been associated with higher rates of obesity. Studies have correlated a higher incidence of metabolic syndrome in patients with schizophrenia and other serious mental illnesses. Antipsychotic drugs, particularly olanzapine, clozapine, quetiapine, and risperidone, are commonly the cause of high amounts of weight gain during treatment. Among antidepressants, mirtazapine and paroxetine seem to cause the greatest weight gain, but MAOIs and TCAs also are linked with increasing weight. Mood stabilizers like lithium have been known to cause weight gain since they were first administered and have been shown to increase weight by 10 kg in 20% of patients [26]. With some medications, it is unclear whether mental illness predisposes to weight gain or if it is entirely an effect of the medication. However antipsychotics are directly correlated with increased weight and metabolic syndrome. For antipsychotics, evidence suggests that most weight gain occurs during the acute phase of treatment, specifically during the first 2 years. Aripiprazole and ziprasidone are antipsychotic alternatives when concerns for metabolic syndrome and subsequent complications are present in patients. Clinicians should monitor weight, check relevant labs, and be proactive when treating patients with psychotropic medications that cause weight gain.

Sexual Dysfunction

Although the pathophysiology of psychotropic-induced sexual dysfunction (SD) is not well understood, SD is a common complaint and deterrent to medication adherence. Sexual dysfunction is defined as problems with desire, arousal, or orgasm. Sexual dysfunction is among the top complaints of psychotropic therapy and a major indicator of poor quality of life. Meta-analysis studies indicated that among antidepressants, serotonergic drugs such as SSRIs have the highest rates of reported sexual dysfunction. The most widely accepted hypothesis hinges on disruption of dopaminergic neurons in the mesolimbic pathways by interference with serotonin receptors. Both traditional and new antipsychotics have also been associated with sexual dysfunction. Olanzapine and risperidone are the most likely antipsychotics to cause sexual dysfunction. Risperidone, in particular, may cause some form of sexual dysfunction in 60–70% of patients. Clozapine and quetiapine also cause sexual dysfunction, but, in general, the rates of SD are lower than for olanzapine and risperidone. The current treatment strategies for treating SD are primarily based on studies with antidepressants. Recommendations include switching to another agent in the hopes of encountering less SD or adding a phosphodiesterase inhibitor such as sildenafil. Sildenafil is widely used for this indication with moderate success. Bupropion has shown mixed results at curtailing SD from antidepressant use [27].

Movement Disorders

Extrapyramidal symptoms (EPS) are acute or tardive symptoms primarily caused by the blockade of dopamine D2 receptors. With the use of newer antipsychotics, incidences of EPS have declined, but are still important in clinical practice. Although once seen as an indicator of therapeutic dose, EPS has since become an important side effect that can negatively influence compliance and overall health outcomes. Tardive dyskinesia has generally been irreversible and debilitating, but with the FDA's recent approval of valbenazine, a drug targeting tardive dyskinesia, promising therapies are on the horizon. Currently, EPS is encountered most frequently in those who were previously exposed to high-potency traditional antipsychotics. EPS can occur with second-generation antipsychotics, but the risk is much lower. Clozapine and quetiapine are the least likely to induce EPS. Recent studies indicate that rather than promoting the dichotomy of typical versus atypical antipsychotics and their relative risk of EPS, it is more accurate to consider individual drugs and their binding affinities for dopamine receptors to predict the development of EPS [28]. If caused by an antipsychotic, EPS symptoms can be reduced or eliminated by switching to a different antipsychotic (usually a second generation). Neuroleptic-induced EPS can be treated with anticholinergics. Other options include dopamine agonists such as pramipexole.

Cardiovascular

Antipsychotics and antidepressants have a known association with delayed ventricular repolarization, which is a risk factor for the development of dangerous reentrant tachycardia such as torsades de pointes (Tdp). Although torsades can lead to sudden cardiac death, it is unclear how many fatalities result from complications of Qtc prolongation. Tdp is most commonly associated with haloperidol (in high IV doses), ziprasidone, and thioridazine, but has occasionally been associated with second-generation antipsychotics such as amisulpride and quetiapine. In terms of antidepressants, Tdp has been reported with use of most tricyclic and tetracyclic antidepressants and MAOIs. Paroxetine, fluoxetine, venlafaxine, and citalopram are the most notable [29]. The FDA has recently issued ceiling dose recommendations for citalopram and escitalopram secondary to risk of QTc prolongation and arrhythmias. The ceiling dose of escitalopram is 10 mg/d for the elderly and 20 mg/d for younger patients. The ceiling dose of citalopram is 20 mg daily for the elderly and 40 mg/d for younger patients. Qtc prolongation with or without Tdp usually occurs in patients with other cardiovascular risk factors, electrolyte imbalances, or on other predisposing medications. Qtc prolongation is normally encountered in patients over 65, females, patients with previous heart disease, and those with hypokalemia.

Before and after prescribing these medications, clinicians should monitor ECG and electrolytes, and assess the risk factors for cardiac abnormalities versus medication benefits.

Weight Loss

Although many antidepressants are associated with weight gain, individual patients may experience weight loss on virtually any antidepressant medication. Weight loss in this setting is usually attributed to behavioral changes in the depressed patient, but bupropion has been associated with weight loss over a placebo at 8 weeks of treatment [30]. There is also a well-known association between stimulant use and weight loss. Phentermine and lisdexamfetamine dimesylate, specifically, have been approved as weight loss drugs. In patients with ADHD, weight loss is also concurrent with slower growth rates during early childhood, but this delay is reversed by achievement of normal growth ratios in later childhood.

Hyponatremia

SSRIs, antiepileptics, and antipsychotics have been associated with the potentially dangerous side effect of hyponatremia. A systematic review of literature on antipsychotics and hyponatremia yielded no correlations between doses, serum sodium, and time of onset of hyponatremia. Hyponatremia can occur with both first- and second-generation antipsychotics, but risk factors and correlations with specific drugs and dosages are not currently known. A review of SSRIs and hyponatremia indicated that this adverse effect occurs in anywhere from 0.5% to 32% of patients on SSRIs. Risk factors identified were low baseline sodium, older age, female sex, low body weight, and concomitant use of diuretics. When hyponatremia is caused by an SSRI, it is thought to occur primarily as the development of SIADH. In general, treatment involves water restriction and possible diuresis with a loop diuretic [31]. The risk is highest in citalopram and lowest with mirtazapine, venlafaxine, and duloxetine [32].

Cognitive Impairment

Finding associations between psychotropic drugs and cognitive impairment can be difficult when treating diseases that can independently cause changes in mental functioning. Depression and anxiety, for instance, have an independent effect on cognitive functioning, but antidepressants and anxiolytics have conflicting data about whether they cause some cognitive impairment. The MMSE scores of individuals with depression or OCD obtained over consecutive weeks following SSRI treatment indicate that the acute phase of SSRI use is associated with some cognitive impairment that generally resolves within a few weeks [33]. The effects on cognition from antipsychotics are also debated; some studies have shown that neither first- nor second-generation antipsychotics have a clinically relevant effect on cognition in patients with schizophrenia [34]. Others argue that antipsychotic use in high doses is associated with some verbal and memory impairment in schizophrenics. In the elderly, cognitive impairment is a large concern with the higher rates of polypharmacy. It is also important to remember that the cognitive impairment reported from relatively safe drugs like SSRIs may be more pronounced in the elderly, and should justify an attempt to start this population on low doses of medications. From a psychopharmaceutical standpoint, current recommendations include avoiding anticholinergic agents, benzodiazepines, non-benzodiazepine hypnotics (i.e., zolpidem), first- and second-generation antipsychotics (increased stroke and mortality risk in those with dementia), tertiary TCAs, first-generation antihistamines, and alpha-1 blockers. As always, clinicians should weigh the risk benefit ratio of psychotropes before prescribing.

Serum Glucose Alterations

Along with weight gain, second-generation antipsychotics are associated with hyperglycemia, diabetes mellitus, and dyslipidemia. Large studies have shown that clozapine and olanzapine are most often implicated with these metabolic derangements. Risperidone is associated with a small risk of diabetes and dyslipidemia, but conflicting data in large studies makes this association questionable. Quetiapine is not associated with these risks, but little data is available currently. There is no evidence to indicate that ziprasidone and aripiprazole increase risk of diabetes mellitus or dyslipidemia. It is assumed that agents with a high risk of weight gain also confer risk of insulin resistance, hyperglycemia, and dyslipidemia. In this setting, clinicians should remember the risk of weight gain and blood sugar changes conferred by clozapine and olanzapine, and screen for changes when using other second-generation antipsychotics [35].

Gastrointestinal Issues

GI issues are common both in psychiatric disease, and as a side effect of psychiatric medications. Constipation is a common side effect of antipsychotic drugs, particularly clozapine. Bowel obstruction and death from antipsychotic caused constipation is not unheard of, and while the risk is well documented, there have been no randomized controlled trials assessing the efficacy of routine interventions. Osmotic laxatives have been effective in many cases, but whether they are actually superior to other common interventions is unknown. Tricyclic antidepressants can cause constipation through acetylcholine blockade. Constipation is less likely with SSRIs but is still reported. Patients who struggle with frequent constipation from psychotropes may benefit from fiber supplements, stool softeners, exercise, and other lifestyle modifications. Rarely, patients taking clozapine may need to discontinue the medication due to severe constipation and long-term fecal impaction. Dyspepsia, diarrhea, and loose stools are among the most common side effects reported with SSRI use. These side effects are almost always self-limiting but do sometimes contribute to early discontinuation of a drug. Interestingly, SSRIs have become an option for treatment of irritable bowel syndrome as serotonin is the main neurotransmitter involved in the gut-brain axis. The modification of serotonin by SSRIs likely plays a role in GI changes and disturbances, but most resolve within a few weeks of treatment. The long-term benefits of SSRI treatment on the GI tract have made these drugs a new option for patients with IBS and other motility disorders; however, their efficacy is seen inconsistently in current studies [36].

Rash

Drug-induced skin reactions can range from mild exanthems to dangerous, life-threatening reactions like Stevens-Johnson syndrome (SJS). Skin reactions with psychotropes may be twice as frequent as those caused by other medications. Antidepressants and antiepileptics used as mood stabilizers are the most common causes of skin reactions encountered with psychotropes. Allergic skin reactions to medications like antidepressants should warrant a switch in medication to a different class of drug. TCAs cause more examples of skin reactions, but SSRIs have been implicated in rare cases of similar reactions. When skin changes occur during acute treatment with an antidepressant, clinicians should be suspicious about possible antidepressant side effects. Lamotrigine, an antiepileptic and mood stabilizer, has been reported in very rare cases of the SJS, but confers a higher risk of this effect when coadministered with valproic acid [37]. Valproic acid may interfere with lamotrigine metabolism causing elevated lamotrigine blood levels. The scope of skin changes will not be covered here, but clinicians should be cautious in children and those over the age of 65, as they confer the highest risk of severe skin reactions [38].

What Is a Black Box Warning and Which Psychotropes Have One?

A black box warning (BBW) is the highest level of warning for a medication that the FDA issues. The name comes from the warning itself that is surrounded by a black box and printed on the medication package insert. The FDA issues a black box warning if a medication is associated with a life-threatening or otherwise serious side effect. This warning is prominent so that physicians do not miss considering the effects when prescribing a particular drug. Interestingly, most psychotropic medications carry a black box warning. Table 2.2 shows the current black box warnings printed by the FDA for psychotropic medications. Complexity arises when considering how physicians should respond to black box warnings in a field where the

Table 2.2 Current FDA black box warnings for psychotropic drugs

Black box warning/risk	Psychotrope
Suicidality and neuropsychiatric symptoms	Bupropion and varenicline (reduced from black box warning to warning FDA 2016)
Increased suicidality risk (thinking and behavior) in young adults, adolescents, and children with major depressive disorder	SSRIs: paroxetine, fluvoxamine, fluoxetine, citalopram, escitalopram, sertraline, vilasidone
	TCAs and heterocyclic antidepressants: nortriptyline, amitriptyline, desipramine, clomipramine, doxepin, trazodone, imipramine
	MAOIs: tranylcypromine, selegiline, phenelzine, isocarboxazid
	Atypical agents: aripiprazole, quetiapine, olanzapine/fluoxetine, lurasidone, brexpiprazole
	Other: bupropion Hcl, bupropion hydrobromide, duloxetine, venlafaxine, desvenlafaxine, mirtazapine, nefazodone, atomoxetine
Hepatic failure/potential for life-threatening or severe liver injury	Valproate/valproic acid, nefazodone, atomoxetine, duloxetine
Dermatological reactions such as Stevens-Johnson syndrome, toxic epidermal necrolysis, or others	Lamotrigine and carbamazepine
High risk for abuse and dependence	All formulations of psychostimulant medications
Risk with concomitant opioid drug use	All benzodiazepine medications
Pancreatitis, teratogenicity/fetal risk	Valproate/valproic acid
Orthostatic hypotension, syncope, bradycardia, neutropenia, myocarditis, cardiomyopathy, mitral valve incompetence, and seizures	Clozapine
Agranulocytosis and aplastic anemia	Clozapine and carbamazepine
Increased mortality risk in elderly with dementia related psychosis	All typical first-generation and atypical second-/third-generation antipsychotics

Adapted from US Food and Drug Administration, 2017

majority of medications carry one or more of the warnings. The FDA issues a black box warning after collecting post-marketing surveillance data, but the intricacies of how the process works are unclear. The highest percentage of black box issues are for the identification of high-risk populations or for harmful drug interactions and dosing considerations. While these warnings are effective ways to communicate post-market side effects and risks, they should not be seen as a complete hindrance to prescribing an effective drug for a patient. In a field like psychiatry, where almost every medication is stamped with a BBW, a clinician should weigh the risks and benefits of the medication to a specific patient.

Drug Withdrawal/Discontinuation

The pharmacology of a psychotropic drug reveals the drug's effect as well as side effects experienced from discontinuation. Effects experienced from abrupt changes in medication can be a cause of significant anxiety and medical morbidity for a patient. Studies have shown that tapering medications, especially antidepressant medications, provides a more favorable outcome for patients with lower rates of recurrence [39]. When considering discontinuation effects, it is important to keep in mind the specific neurotransmitters affected by each drug. If a drug with an anticholinergic effect is abruptly stopped, the resulting cholinergic rebound can cause sweating, increased urination, and nausea which are in contrast to anticholinergic effects. Similarly, quick discontinuation of a drug with an antiadrenergic effect may cause hypertension, irritability, anxiety, and heart palpitations. Predictably, stopping antihistaminergic drugs can result in wakefulness. In general, discontinuation effects of most psychotropic medications are not serious, with some important exceptions. Withdrawal from abrupt discontinuation of alcohol or benzodiazepines in a tolerant patient, for instance, can lead to seizures, brain damage, or death if not properly managed. In this section we review the effects of abrupt discontinuation of common classes of psychotropic medications as well as some of the withdrawal symptoms that may affect a medication tolerant patient.

Abruptly stopping antidepressant medications (SSRIs, MAOIs, TCAs, and SNRIs) has been associated with higher rates of anxiety and depression recurrence compared to gradual taper. The specifics of discontinuation symptoms can be understood by considering the neurologic effects of each individual medication. TCAs, for example, have a strong anticholinergic and antiadrenergic effect and, consequently, can cause cholinergic and adrenergic rebound. Abrupt discontinuation of SSRIs can cause lethargy, insomnia, dizziness, headaches, nausea, as well as tactile sensations. SNRIs can cause a similar discontinuation syndrome. MAOIs can occasionally be associated with a distinct flu-like illness with delirium, restlessness, body aches, and depressive states. MAOIs continue to inhibit enzymes for weeks after treatment and may interact with medications prescribed during this window.

Other psychotropes can result in severe illness rebound when stopped abruptly. For mood stabilizers like lithium or anticonvulsants, rapid discontinuation can lead to mood instability and relapse. Schizophrenic patients that abruptly discontinue antipsychotics often have earlier, more severe illness than seen with a gradual taper. Interestingly, abrupt antipsychotic discontinuation can also result in abnormal motor syndromes such as neuroleptic malignant syndrome, parkinsonian features, dystonias, and dyskinesias. Clinicians should gradually taper many psychotropes to avoid adverse effects and withdrawal symptoms [40, 41].

Pregnant and Nursing Women: Special Considerations

An estimated 86% of women with mental illness are not treated with medication during pregnancy due to fears about harm to the developing fetus. However, recent reviews of clinical data indicate that many psychotropic drugs are safe during pregnancy and that the risk of harm to mother and the fetus due to psychiatric illness often outweighs the risk of a psychiatric medication [42]. Nevertheless, the risk of spontaneous abortion, premature labor, and teratogenicity are feared complications of some psychotropic medications, and, while information regarding the actual risks to the fetus is scarce, many physicians are unwilling to prescribe psychotropic drugs during pregnancy. Clinicians should be aware of both the risks of a medication and the risk of not treating a psychiatric illness to make a decision that is in the best interest of the mother and developing fetus. This section reviews the considerations clinicians must explore when treating women with mental illness during pregnancy and breastfeeding.

As of June 2015, the FDA issued new labeling subsections for pregnancy, lactation, and reproductive potential that will include data summaries, clinical considerations, and risk summaries for each drug. Since 1979, the FDA has categorized medications in groups A, B, C, D, and X in order of amount of evidence for safety in humans and human-like animals (Table 2.3). Consequently, medications may have been in separate categories not from varied risk in harm during pregnancy but because of differences in amount of evidence available. This system, although in replacement, is still widely used and summarized in the table below. The category system has been replaced by narrative sections that focus on pregnancy, lactation, and risk to male and female reproductive potential.

Although some evidence is lacking about their use in pregnancy, first-generation antipsychotics like haloperidol and chlorpromazine are used frequently in pregnancy. A controlled cohort study investigating penfluridol and haloperidol revealed higher rates of preterm birth, elective terminations, low birth rate, and two confirmed cases of limb abnormalities, but the sample size was insufficient for solid conclusions [43]. A more recent study confirmed that first-generation antipsychotics confer higher rates of postnatal disorders, low birth weight, and preterm labor [42]. Malformations of the atria and ventricular septum have been associated with atypical antipsychotic use during pregnancy, but these findings are not yet statistically

Table 2.3 FDA pregnancy categories and descriptions

Category	Description
A	No risk to fetus found in controlled studies in humans
B	No risk to fetus in animal controlled studies but no controlled studies conducted in humans
C	No controlled studies have been performed in humans or animals
D	Some evidence of harm to the fetus has been shown, but circumstances may warrant medication use if benefits outweigh risk
X	Risk outweighs all benefit. Fetal harm shown in human and animal controlled studies

significant. Grouping first- and second-generation antipsychotics together, there is some data that these medications increase the risk of low birth weight, gestational diabetes, cesarean section, and premature birth [44]. No teratogenic risk was seen with haloperidol, chlorpromazine, perphenazine, trifluoperazine, loxapine, thioridazine, flupenthixol, fluphenazine, or promethazine in one comprehensive review of studies [45]. Many of these studies have numerous confounding factors such as the use of concomitant medications and smoking. Furthermore, there is an absence of individual drug studies. Most studies group first- and second-generation antipsychotics. Further, there is not enough data on newer agents to make conclusions about their safety profile in pregnancy. Currently, women on antipsychotics during pregnancy represent a high-risk pregnancy with increased risk of preterm labor, low birth weight, congenital malformation, and elective terminations [46].

Clozapine is contraindicated during lactation due to reports of somnolence, agranulocytosis, and high infant serum levels [47]. In contrast, olanzapine and risperidone achieve low infant plasma levels, but the lack of data on risperidone during lactation keeps it from being first line. Olanzapine has not been shown to affect the infant in a few studies when used during lactation. Drugs like aripiprazole and ziprasidone have scarce data during lactation [42].

Antidepressants are the most commonly prescribed psychotropic medication during pregnancy. Pooled patient analysis of patients on TCAs and fluoxetine has demonstrated the relative safety of these agents as none have been associated with major teratogenicity or behavioral teratogenicity. However, TCAs are usually avoided in pregnancy due to prominent maternal side effects. Paroxetine confers the highest pregnancy risk among SSRIs, with data showing increased instances of heart defects when used in pregnancy [48]. Bupropion may also cause heart malformations when used in the first trimester, but there is limited data regarding this association. Other less used SSRIs like nefazodone and venlafaxine are considered relatively safe during pregnancy but only with very few studies. Despite their relative safety, SSRI exposure during the third trimester has been associated with increased risk of persistent pulmonary hypertension for the infant as well as slowed growth and low birth weight [42]. Other transient perinatal symptoms have been documented from maternal SSRI use but are generally mild and not totally associated with SSRI use directly. Limited data exists on MAOIs and pregnancy, and these agents are not currently recommended [49].

In general, SSRIs can be used safely during breastfeeding; however, fluoxetine has a long half-life and an unknown side effect profile during lactation. Similarly there is no data on the use of escitalopram during pregnancy. When using an SSRI during lactation, paroxetine, citalopram, and sertraline have been shown to be safe at recommended doses. The lack of data on other antidepressants usually limits their use during lactation.

Among anxiolytics, benzodiazepines have shown an increased risk of orofacial clefts in the past, but more recent studies indicate no teratogenic risk [50]. However low birth weight and preterm labor are associated with benzodiazepine use in the second and third trimesters. There is currently no data on buspirone use during pregnancy.

For mood stabilizers, the knee-jerk association between lithium in the first trimester and Ebstein's anomaly is not supported by recent studies. However, the past association should provoke discretion especially during the first trimester. Valproic acid and carbamazepine are teratogenic and contraindicated during pregnancy. Lamotrigine is the first-line mood stabilizer during pregnancy as it does not increase the risk of congenital malformation of perinatal complications.

Lithium is transferred to breast milk and is therefore contraindicated during lactation. Other mood stabilizers are generally best avoided during lactation, but limited data exists on whether these drugs, even when transferred to breast milk, have effect on the infant. Topiramate, for instance, is transferred to infants in significant levels during breastfeeding but has not shown effects in infants.

Overall, there are large gaps in data concerning many of the psychotropic medications and their use in pregnancy and lactation. Aside from the clearly defined toxicities, many physicians must weigh the risks of harm of no treatment versus the risks of complications when prescribing a psychotropic medication, especially with those where current data does not confer conclusions. Even with limits in data, there are first-line agents for most psychiatric conditions shown to be relatively safe in pregnancy that should subside some of the fear associated with treating psychiatric conditions. Lactation data is similarly sparse, but some agents exist, especially antidepressants and antipsychotics with evidence indicating their relative safety during breastfeeding.

Hepatic/Renal Insufficiency: Impact on Dosing

Renal Insufficiency

Suboptimal renal function (SRF) can affect both the pharmacokinetics and pharmacodynamics of a psychotropic medication. Specifically, impaired renal function creates variability in the absorption, distribution, and metabolism, and excretion of a drug, while generally increasing the risk of adverse effects. Doses of psychotropic medications must be individualized for each patient, with care given to those drugs eliminated by the kidneys. In most cases, avoidance of kidney-eliminated drugs in kidney failure patients may be the safest route for clinicians. If kidney-eliminated psychotropes are used in renal insufficiency, significant dose alterations may be necessary.

Although SRF creates variability in the pharmacokinetics of psychotropes, it is difficult to predict with certainty how individual parameters may be altered. It has been shown that patients with renal insufficiency have altered bioavailability of oral medications. The uremia seen in renal insufficiency is thought to reduce gastrin levels and impair gastric absorption by causing chronic gastric alkalinity. This process may explain the decreased bioavailability of some oral psychotropes in the setting of SRF. However, in some cases, absorption can be increased due to reduced functional capacity of gastrointestinal CYP450 enzymes as well as decreased expression of drug efflux transporters.

Renal insufficiency affects the two primary variables of distribution: drug-protein binding and the volume of distribution. Most psychotropic medications are highly protein bound, and SRF alters protein-binding variables in the blood. Renal insufficiency causes proteinuria, hypoalbuminemia, and congregation of uremic toxins that prevent drug-protein binding. Consequently, the free, active drug in the bloodstream may increase. However, in patients undergoing dialysis, the amount of alkaline-binding protein alpha 1 acid protein may increase causing a decrease in free, active drug.

With respect to pharmacodynamics, renal insufficiency has been linked to increased side effects of psychotropic medications. While the mechanisms are not entirely clear, there is some evidence to suggest that the buildup of uremic toxins may increase the adverse effects of medications as well as increased permeability of the blood-brain barrier to psychotropic medications.

When available, physicians should consult guides for prescribing individual medications in patients with SRF. Many of these guides make dosage recommendations based on level of kidney dysfunction in each individual patient. There are no widely accepted contraindications of use for psychotropic drugs in patients with SRF. When possible, drugs that are renally eliminated should be adjusted or avoided in patients with SRF.

Hepatic Insufficiency

Psychotropic drugs, like most other substances, are primarily metabolized by the liver. Hepatic insufficiency can result in numerous pharmacokinetic changes that can affect how the body metabolizes these drugs. The primary alterations concern drugs like tricyclic antidepressants that experience significant—more than 50%—first-pass metabolism, as well as highly protein-bound drugs and drugs dependent on phase I metabolism.

The distribution of some medications depends on first-pass metabolism. End-stage liver disease results in significant blood flow alterations, with much of the portal vein contents bypassing the liver completely. With this bypass, many drugs that are largely metabolized by first-pass liver metabolism will have significant increases in blood concentration compared to concentrations in patients with normal liver function.

Much like in SRF, a cirrhotic patient produces lower levels of proteins like albumin, alpha 1 glycoprotein, and lipoproteins. In general this decrease in carrier proteins causes an increase in active drug concentrations for psychotropic medications. This is especially important with drugs such as diazepam which is 99% bound to plasma proteins normally. Significant liver dysfunction can elevate diazepam blood levels and magnifying symptoms like sedation and respiratory depression.

When considering phase I and phase II liver metabolism in patients with liver disease, it is important to remember that glucuronidation, a phase II reaction, is relatively preserved in circumstances where phase I metabolism may be significantly decreased. Clinically, drugs like lorazepam, oxazepam, and temazepam should be used in place of drugs that require a phase I deactivation step from the liver.

Considering these pharmacokinetic alterations, clinicians should avoid drugs with significant first-pass metabolism, phase I metabolism, and highly protein-bound psychotropes [51]. Before prescribing a psychotropic medication, LFTs and ALT are recommended to get a baseline liver assessment. Care should then be made to avoid high-risk psychotropic drugs, as well as those with significant liver metabolism. Routine labs should be used to follow progression of liver disease, and dose adjustments may be required for some medications.

Laboratory Monitoring

Therapeutic drug monitoring can prevent toxicity, expose drug effectiveness, isolate individual genetic variability, and influence patient adherence. Many psychotropic drug levels are routinely tested in patients to optimize drug treatment. Some psychotropic medications can have serious side effects that can be minimized or prevented by following laboratory work. In this section we will discuss routine laboratory monitoring for psychotropes.

Lithium Serum Levels

The efficacy of lithium, the gold standard for treatment of bipolar disorder, is dependent on a narrow range of serum concentrations. The trough serum concentration should range from 0.8 to 1.2 mmol/L to ensure effective treatment. However, a serum level above this range can lead to dangerous toxicity. The narrow therapeutic index has led most clinicians to test serum lithium 12 h after once-a-day (OD) dosing to determine trough concentrations. Some studies have suggested that measuring trough dose at 24 h after OD dosing gives a more accurate trough, as the 12 h trough is 1.3 times higher than the 24 h trough [52]. After stabilization of levels and resolution of an acute episode, a prophylactic dose of lithium should be monitored every 6 months or sooner [13].

WBC for Clozapine and Carbamazepine

Despite its effectiveness in patients with schizophrenia, clozapine is an underutilized medication primarily due to its adverse effects such as agranulocytosis, QTc prolongation, diabetes mellitus, gastroparesis, and myocarditis. At an incidence of 1–2%, agranulocytosis is one of the most feared side effects of clozapine therapy.

Although the incidence of agranulocytosis decreases after 6 months of treatment, it is required to monitor white blood cell counts after 6 months of therapy as late-onset agranulocytosis has been reported. The Clozapine Risk Evaluation and Mitigation Strategy [REMS] program requires clinicians to register patients in a program that ensures monitoring of absolute neutrophil count (ANC). Monitoring is performed weekly for the first 6 months of clozapine treatment, every other week for the subsequent 6 months, and every 4 weeks after a year of treatment. Guidelines are intermittently updated, but currently ANC under 1500/μL should be repeated and closely monitored. ANC less than 500/μL should result in immediate discontinuation of clozapine. Those numbers in between generally necessitate therapy interruption with subsequent continuation when ANC is above 1000/μL.

Carbamazepine is a broad antiepileptic with activity for focal and generalized seizures, mood disorders, and chronic pain syndromes. Like clozapine, carbamazepine can be associated with severe side effects, but they occur less frequently. Leukopenia, when it occurs, typically is seen in the first 3 months of treatment and should be monitored in patients who start carbamazepine with low WBC counts. Pancytopenia is a rare but life-threatening side effect of carbamazepine that also can occur most frequently in the first few months of initiations of therapy. Routine monitoring for pancytopenia is not currently recommended, although clinicians should educate patients about signs and symptoms. Some physicians opt to monitor WBC counts of certain groups of patients (high-risk individuals, those with predisposing blood disorders) during the first 3 months of therapy.

TCAs for Depression

Tricyclic antidepressants, much less benign compared to their counterpart SSRIs, are nevertheless very effective for a variety of psychiatric conditions. Cyclic antidepressants have been associated with a variety of cardiac, sexual, anticholinergic, antihistaminic, and seizure disorders. Determining the right dose for a patient requires close therapeutic drug monitoring (TDM). Research shows that considerable side effects occur more frequently in patients who do not have routine drug monitoring when taking TCAs. Generally, patients are started on a low-dose TCA and titrated up slowly to avoid side effects. When prescribing high doses in patients who have not responded to lower doses, it is important to routinely check serum TCA levels and make dose adjustments. One should also keep in mind that these drugs are highly anticholinergic and potentially fatal in overdose.

Antipsychotics

Clinicians should take into account the risks and benefits associated with each individual antipsychotic drug. Metabolic syndrome, characterized by increases in weight, dyslipidemia, and diabetes, can occur in both first- and second-generation antipsychotics. Patients with preexisting metabolic dysfunction are at increased risk of presenting with metabolic syndrome during antipsychotics treatment. Currently, there are recommendations for metabolic monitoring of weight, glucose, lipid profiles, blood pressure, and changes in weight circumference to follow development of metabolic syndrome.

QT prolongation by antipsychotic drugs has been linked to sudden death in rare cases. The FDA recommends avoiding thioridazine as first line for psychosis as it has the greatest risk for QT prolongation. Before prescribing thioridazine, IV haloperidol, ziprasidone, and pimozide, patients should get an ECG and serum potassium level. Patients on these medications should continue to have yearly ECGs, and doses should be adjusted or discontinued based on cardiac status. Patients with baseline QT intervals greater than 450 ms should not be started on these medications. For other antipsychotics such as chlorpromazine, fluphenazine, perphenazine, loxapine, thiothixene, and trifluoperazine, cardiac monitoring is only recommended in patients with cardiac history as these drugs show only slight QT prolongation or lack the evidence to make confident recommendations [53].

Conclusion

Much of psychopharmacology started as simple observations of chemical-induced improvement in psychotic and affective disorders. Once early antidepressants, antipsychotics, and mood stabilizers were discovered to have efficacy in the 1950s, considerable efforts were taken to describe the pharmacology and neurobiology behind both the psychiatric conditions and medications. With the exponential increase in knowledge of psychotropes, clinicians have had trouble sifting through the pharmacokinetics, pharmacodynamics, indications, contraindications, side effects, interactions, dosages, and special indications for individual drugs and classes of these drugs. Despite the breadth, a basic understanding of psychotropes is necessary so that patients receive the most effective treatment while avoiding treatment-associated complications. A basic understanding of some of the fundamentals of psychopharmacology will make drug navigation less of a task of memorization and more of an exercise in concept practice. When encountering complex patients on multiple medications, it can be comforting to consult a clinical guide for reminders of important issues such as hepatic P450 metabolic route and need for laboratory monitoring. Rather than mulling over every side effect of each individual drug, it's helpful to remember its mechanism of action and predictable side effects which may arise from impacting altering a neurotransmitter pathway such as adrenergic, serotonergic, cholinergic, or histaminergic neurotransmission. General knowledge of the principles of psychopharmacology presents a framework for the details of individual drugs described in later chapters.

References

1. Peppers MP. Benzodiazepines for alcohol withdrawal in the elderly and in patients with liver disease. Pharmacotherapy. 1996;16(1):49–57.
2. Eap CB. Personalized prescribing: a new medical model for clinical implementation of psychotropic drugs. Dialogues Clin Neurosci. 2016;18(3):313–22.
3. Schatzberg AF, Nemeroff CB. The American psychiatric publishing textbook of psychopharmacology. 4th ed. Arlington: American Psychiatric Publishing; 2009.
4. Miceli JJ, Glue P, Alderman J, Wilner K. The effect of food on the absorption of oral ziprasidone. Psychopharmacol Bull. 2007;40(3):58–68.
5. Holm R, Müllertz A, Mu H. Bile salts and their importance for drug absorption. Int J Pharm. 2013;453(1):44–55. https://doi.org/10.1016/j.ijpharm.2013.04.003.
6. Meissner W, Leyendecker P, Mueller-Lissner S, et al. A randomised controlled trial with prolonged-release oral oxycodone and naloxone to prevent and reverse opioid-induced constipation. Eur J Pain. 2009;13(1):56–64.
7. DeVane CL. Clinical significance of drug binding, protein binding, and binding displacement drug interactions. Psychopharmacol Bull. 2002;36:5–21.
8. Mrazek DA. Psychiatric pharmacogenomic testing in clinical practice. Dialogues Clin Neurosci. 2010;12(1):69–76.
9. Zhou SF. Drugs behave as substrates, inhibitors and inducers of human cytochrome P450 3A4. Curr Drug Metab. 2008;9:310–22. https://doi.org/10.2174/138920008784220664.
10. Aronson JK. Meyler's side effects of psychiatric drugs. 1st ed. Amsterdam: Elsevier Science; 2009.
11. Zhornitsky S, Potvin S, Moteshafi H, et al. Dose-response and comparative efficacy and tolerability of quetiapine across psychiatric disorders: a systematic review of the placebo-controlled monotherapy and add-on trials. Int Clin Psychopharmacol. 2011;26:183–92.
12. Aymanns C, Keller F, Maus S, Hartmann B, Czock D. Review on pharmacokinetics and pharmacodynamics and the aging kidney. Clin J Am Soc Nephrol. 2010;5(2):314–27.
13. Mitchell PB. Therapeutic drug monitoring of psychotropic medications. Br J Clin Pharmacol. 2000;49(4):303–12. https://doi.org/10.1046/j.1365-2125.2000.00174.x.
14. Brett J, Murnion B. Management of benzodiazepine misuse and dependence. Aust Prescr. 2015;38(5):152–5. https://doi.org/10.18773/austprescr.2015.055.
15. Neuvonen PJ, Kivistö K, Hirvisalo EL. Effects of resins and activated charcoal on the absorption of digoxin, carbamazepine and frusemide. Br J Clin Pharmacol. 1988;25(2):229–33.
16. Ciociola AA, Cohen LB, Kulkarni P, Gastroenterology FD-RMCotACo. How drugs are developed and approved by the FDA: current process and future directions. Am J Gastroenterol. 2014;109(5):620–3. https://doi.org/10.1038/ajg.2013.407.
17. Ratner M. Pfizer settles largest ever fraud suit for off-label promotion. Nat Biotechnol. 2009;27(11):961–2.
18. Radley DC, Finkelstein SN, Stafford RS. Off-label prescribing among off-based physicians. Arch Intern Med. 2006;166(9):1021–6. https://doi.org/10.1001/archinte.166.9.1021.
19. Stafford RS. Regulating off-label drug use – rethinking the role of the FDA. N Engl J Med. 2008;358:1427–9.
20. Wittich CM, Burkle CM, Lanier WL. Ten common questions (and their answers) about off-label drug use. Mayo Clin Proc. 2012;87(10):982–90. https://doi.org/10.1016/j.mayocp.2012.04.017.
21. Gabay M. The federal controlled substances act: schedules and pharmacy registration. Hosp Pharm. 2013;48(6):473–4. https://doi.org/10.1310/hpj4806-473.
22. Lieberman JA. Managing anticholinergic side effects. Prim Care Companion J Clin Psychiatry. 2004;6(suppl 2):20–3.
23. Freedman R, Coon H, Myles-Worsley M, Orr-Urtreger A, Olincy A, Davis A, et al. Linkage of a neurophysiological deficit in schizophrenia to a chromosome 15 locus. Proc Natl Acad Sci USA. 1997;94(2):587–92.

24. Cottingham C, Wang Q. α2 adrenergic receptor dysregulation in depressive disorders: implications for the neurobiology of depression and antidepressant therapy. Neurosci Biobehav Rev. 2012;36:2214–25.
25. Pessiglione M, Seymour B, Flandin G, et al. Dopamine-dependent prediction errors underpin reward-seeking behaviour in humans. Nature. 2006;442(7106):1042–5.
26. Livingstone C, Rampes H. Lithium: a review of its metabolic adverse effects. J Psychopharmacol. 2006;20(3):347–55.
27. Bella AJ, Shamloul R. Psychotropics and sexual dysfunction. Cent Eur J Urol. 2013;66:466–71.
28. Caroff SN, Hurford I, Lybrand J, Campbell EC. Movement disorders induced by antipsychotic drugs: implications of the CATIE schizophrenia trial. Neurol Clin. 2011;29(1):127–viii. https://doi.org/10.1016/j.ncl.2010.10.002.
29. Wenzel-Seifert K, Wittmann M, Haen E. QTc prolongation by psychotropic drugs and the risk of torsade de pointes. Dtsch Arztebl Int. 2011;108(41):687–93. https://doi.org/10.3238/arztebl.2011.0687.
30. Gadde KM, Parker CB, Maner LG, Wagner HR 2nd, Logue EJ, Drezner MK, et al. Bupropion for weight loss: an investigation of efficacy and tolerability in overweight and obese women. Obes Res. 2001;9:544–51.
31. Jacob S, Spinler SA. Hyponatremia associated with selective serotonin-reuptake inhibitors in older adults. Ann Pharmacother. 2006;40:1618–22.
32. Leth-Møller KB, Hansen AH, Torstensson M, Andersen SE, Ødum L, Gislasson G, et al. Antidepressants and the risk of hyponatremia: a Danish register-based population study. BMJ Open. 2016;6(5):e011200. https://doi.org/10.1136/bmjopen-2016-011200.
33. Sayyah M, Eslami K, AlaiShehni S, Kouti L. Cognitive function before and during treatment with selective serotonin reuptake inhibitors in patients with depression or obsessive-compulsive disorder. Psychiatry J. 2016;2016:5480391. https://doi.org/10.1155/2016/5480391.
34. Hill SK, Bishop JR, Palumbo D, Sweeney JA. Effect of second-generation antipsychotics on cognition: current issues and future challenges. Expert Rev Neurother. 2010;10(1):43–57. https://doi.org/10.1586/ern.09.143.
35. Newcomer JW. Second-generation (atypical) antipsychotics and metabolic effects: a comprehensive literature review. CNS Drugs. 2005;19(Suppl 1):1–93.
36. Creed F. How do SSRIs help patients with irritable bowel syndrome? Gut. 2006;55(8):1065–7. https://doi.org/10.1136/gut.2005.086348.
37. Parveen S, Javed MA. Stevens Johnson syndrome associated with lamotrigine. Pak J Med Sci. 2013;29(6):1450–2.
38. Herstowska M, Komorowska O, Cubała WJ, Jakuszkowiak-Wojten K, Gałuszko-Węgielnik M, Landowski J. Severe skin complications in patients treated with antidepressants: a literature review. Adv Dermatol Allergol/Postępy Dermatologii I Alergologii. 2014;31(2):92–7. https://doi.org/10.5114/pdia.2014.40930.
39. Wilson E, Lader M. A review of the management of antidepressant discontinuation symptoms. Ther Adv Psychopharmacol. 2015;5(6):357–68. https://doi.org/10.1177/2045125315612334.
40. Howland RH. Potential adverse effects of discontinuing psychotropic drugs. Part 3: antipsychotic, dopaminergic, and mood-stabilizing drugs. J Psychocsoc Nurs Ment Health Serv. 2010;48(8):11–4.
41. Howland RH. Potential adverse effects of discontinuing psychotropic drugs. Part 2: antidepressant drugs. J Psychocsoc Nurs Ment Health Serv. 2010;48(7):9–12.
42. Vitale SG, Laganà AS, Muscatello MR, La Rosa VL, Currò V, Pandolfo G, Zoccali RA, Bruno A. Psychopharmacotherapy in pregnancy and breastfeeding. Obstet Gynecol Surv. 2016;71(12):721–33. https://doi.org/10.1097/OGX.0000000000000369.
43. Diav-Citrin O, Shechtman S, Ornoy S, et al. Safety of haloperidol and penfluridol in pregnancy: a multicenter, prospective, controlled study. J Clin Psychiatry. 2005;66:317–22.
44. Reis M, Källén B. Maternal use of antipsychotics in early pregnancy and delivery outcome. J Clin Psychopharmacol. 2008;28:279–88.
45. Einarson A, Boskovich R. Use and safety of antipsychotic drugs during pregnancy. J Psychiatr Pract. 2009;15:183–92.

46. Coughlin CG, Blackwell KA, Bartley C, et al. Obstetric and neonatal outcomes after antipsychotic medication exposure in pregnancy. Obstet Gynecol. 2015;125:1224–35.
47. Kulkarni J, Worsley R, Gilbert H, et al. A prospective cohort study of antipsychotic medications in pregnancy: the first 147 pregnancies and 100 one year old babies. PLoS One. 2014;9:e94788.
48. Ban L, Gibson JE, West J, et al. Maternal depression, antidepressant prescriptions, and congenital anomaly risk in offspring: a population-based cohort study. BJOG. 2014;121:1471–81.
49. Ward RK, Zamorski MA. Benefits and risks of psychiatric medications during pregnancy. Am Fam Physician. 2002;66:629–36.
50. Enato E, Moretti M, Koren G. The fetal safety of benzodiazepines: an updated meta-analysis. J Obstet Gynaecol Can. 2011;33:46–8.
51. Telles-Correia D, Barbosa A, Cortez-Pinto H, Campos C, Rocha NBF, Machado S. Psychotropic drugs and liver disease: a critical review of pharmacokinetics and liver toxicity. World J Gastrointest Pharmacol Ther. 2017;8(1):26–38. https://doi.org/10.4292/wjgpt.v8.i1.26.
52. Reddy DS, Reddy MS. Serum lithium levels: ideal time for sample collection! Are we doing it right? Indian J Psychol Med. 2014;36(3):346–7. https://doi.org/10.4103/0253-7176.135399.
53. Chohan PS, Mittal R, Javed A. Antipsychotic medication and QT prolongation. Pak J Med Sci. 2015;31(5):1269–71. https://doi.org/10.12669/pjms.315.8998.

Chapter 3
Special Considerations for the Elderly

George T. Grossberg

Prescribing psychotropic medication for 85-year-olds is more challenging than in younger adults. Due to age-related changes in hepatic metabolism and renal excretion, older adults may require ½ to 1/3 the dose of medications that younger adults may need to see therapeutic benefits [1]. Older adults are also more likely to be on several prescriptions and over-the-counter medications – hence, the risk of drug-drug interactions is greater [2]. Lastly, older adults are more sensitive to common side effects of medications, even at low doses. The American Society of Consultant Pharmacists has adopted the saying that "any symptom in an elderly patient should be considered a drug side-effect until proven otherwise" [3]. They are particularly sensitive to sedating and cognitive-impairing side effects of commonly prescribed agents [1]. It is important for clinicians to be familiar with the Beers Criteria or Beers List of so-called good drugs and bad drugs in the elderly [4].

Basic Principles of Geriatric Psycho-pharmacotherapy

Document Target Symptoms

At the outset, it is important for clinicians to document the reason/reasons for prescribing medications – for what condition or target symptoms is the medication being prescribed? Have non-pharmacological or behavioral/environmental alternatives been considered? The latter is especially important before exposing dementia patients with neuropsychiatric symptoms such as agitation to neuroleptics. These agents in this population are associated with an increased risk of serious side effects

G. T. Grossberg, MD (✉)
Division of Geriatric Psychiatry, Department of Psychiatry & Behavioral Neuroscience,
St. Louis University School of Medicine, St. Louis, MO, USA
e-mail: george.grossberg@health.slu.edu

© Springer International Publishing AG, part of Springer Nature 2018
G. T. Grossberg, L. J. Kinsella (eds.), *Clinical Psychopharmacology for Neurologists*, https://doi.org/10.1007/978-3-319-74604-3_3

Table 3.1 Target symptoms for pharmacotherapy in the elderly

Pain
Lowered mood/depression
Cognitive impairment such as in Alzheimer's disease (AD)
Behavioral symptoms in AD
Agitation/aggressivity
Psychosis
Anxiety
Insomnia

and even mortality [5]. Because of these risks, Congress has passed legislation to mandate the Centers for Medicare and Medicaid Services (CMS) to implement ways to reduce the use of antipsychotic medications among dementia patients in nursing homes by 15% a year [6]. A variety of target symptoms are commonly identified in older adults, for which psychopharmacologic intervention may be considered. Some of these are listed in Table 3.1. It is important to consider the underlying cause(s) for neuropsychiatric symptoms before initiating pharmacotherapy. An example follows.

Case Study

Mrs. Z, an 85-year-old widow with moderate AD, is brought to the clinician by her daughter, with whom she lives, for recent onset agitation, yelling, especially during hands-on care (dressing, grooming, etc.). During the office visit, while the clinician and the daughter are helping the patient up to the exam table, she strikes out and yells. The clinician notes a tender, swollen knee. Anti-inflammatory medication resulted in amelioration of symptoms of agitation.

Ensure Close Collaboration Among Various Prescribers

According to the US FDA, older adults (greater than 65 years of age) represent 13.7% of the US population but consume nearly 40% of all prescribed and over-the-counter (OTC) remedies. On average, individuals over the age of 80 fill 18 prescriptions per year, and up to 25% of drug use in older adults is considered inappropriate or unnecessary, and nearly 40% of all annual drug reactions reported involve an older adult [7].

Older adults often have multiple medical comorbidities for which they may be seeing multiple healthcare providers. It is important for the prescribing clinician to be aware of *all* prescribed and (OTC) remedies their older patients may be exposed to and their dosages and indications.

Start One Medication at a Time

It is a dictum in geriatric prescribing to not start more than one new medication at a time. Since older patients are more vulnerable to side effects, if one starts two medications concurrently, it is hard to know which medication is causing the side effect. Geriatricians also disdain fixed combination medications for the same reason. We prefer being able to adjust the dose of each component of a combination medication, individually.

Start Low and Go Slow, But Go

Another dictum in geriatric pharmacotherapy is to start with the lowest dose possible and to titrate gradually. Often, the clinician may want to break the lowest-dose tablet in half and start with that. Until recently, the FDA did not require geriatric studies for new drug approval – consequently, the lowest dose manufactured was too high of a starting dose for 85-year-olds. At present, the FDA does require geriatric dosing data for newly approved compounds, but very few "truly geriatric" patients (those 80 + years of age) are included in the published trials.

As clinicians become more aware of the sensitivity of older adults to even modest doses of psychopharmacologic agents, they often underdose geriatric patients and obtain poor results. Though "start low and go slow" is the mantra, "but go" tells us to make sure to gradually build patients up to therapeutic levels and then give the drugs time to "kick-in." Unfortunately, for most psychotropic agents used in the elderly, e.g., antipsychotics, anxiolytics, sedative-hypnotics, newer antidepressants, cognitive enhancers, reliable serum levels to guide dosing are not available [8].

Dosing is guided by experience with the agent and geriatric clinical literature. Meaningful serum levels are available with some of the older antidepressants and with some of the mood stabilizers and anticonvulsants.

Hepatic and Renal Considerations

As part of "normal" aging, even without hepatic or renal disease, hepatic microsomal activity and renal excretion (often secondary to decreased renal blood flow) may decrease – necessitating "micro doses" of psychotropic medications. Since the vast majority of psychotropic medications are metabolized by the CYP-450 microsomal enzymes in the liver, and excreted by the kidneys, periodic monitoring, especially of renal functions, is recommended. Chronic kidney disease (CKD) is quite common in 85-year-olds and may necessitate periodic reevaluation of psychotropic dosing.

Knowledge of Available Formulations

The selection of the most appropriate psychotropic medications in a geriatric patient may often hinge on available formulations. As an example, patients with dementia may have difficulty swallowing pills. For them, a liquid or transdermal preparation may be more appropriate. As well, an older patient presenting acutely to the emergency room with severe psychosis and agitation may need a neuroleptic which is available in an IM form but which can be converted to a PO form if longer-term administration is recommended. Some psychotropic medications which come in capsules can be sprinkled in applesauce or pudding to facilitate adherence in patients who do not take pills or capsules well. Examples would include divalproex "sprinkles" and memantine XR. Some medications can also be crushed and administered in food to improve adherence. However, it is important to consult with a pharmacist to know which drugs are not to be crushed or to consult *Davis's Drug Guide* – Do Not Crush [9]. Examples of medications which should not be crushed include extended release, slow release, enteric-coated, and sublingual preparations.

Knowledge of Drug-Drug Interactions

Clinicians want to select a psychotropic agent with the lowest risk of drug-drug interactions, especially in the vulnerable older adult population. For example, the commonly prescribed antidepressant trazodone may produce hypotension in an older adult already on antihypertensives, as would the antipsychotic quetiapine. In a patient on modest doses of a tricyclic antidepressant such as amitriptyline, introduction of a potent CYP-450 2D6 blocker such as fluoxetine may dramatically elevate levels of the tricyclic, producing toxicity and even sudden death (due to cardiac standstill). Lastly, drugs known to induce hepatic enzymes – such as carbamazepine and phenytoin – can dramatically reduce blood levels of psychotropics metabolized by the liver such as the neuroleptics.

Assess Role of Gender, Lifestyle, Racial/Ethnic Differences in Drug Metabolism and Tolerance

A variety of factors can impact drug metabolism and tolerance. For example, olanzapine is cleared more rapidly by smokers [10]. Also, African-Americans require lower doses of lithium and often metabolize drugs more slowly, in general [11]. The FDA reissued an alert relative to an increased risk of Stevens-Johnson syndrome with carbamazepine in Asian-Americans. It is also known that some older adults are genetically poor metabolizers of drugs metabolized by the 2D6 hepatic microsomes, including tramadol, codeine, amitriptyline, fluoxetine, or paroxetine [11]. These patients may have seriously high serum levels of those drugs, even with modest doses.

Monitoring for Drug Response, Toxicity, and Interactions

It is important for clinicians to closely monitor geriatric patients who have been recently started on psychotropic medications. The use of a quantifiable assessment instrument which can be administered before, during, and after drug therapy is initiated may be useful. For example, administering the Geriatric Depression Scale [12] or the SLU-AMSAD [13] may enable the clinician to quantify improvement of depression with pharmacotherapy. Using a scale such as the SLUMS [14] or the MoCA [15] to quantify cognitive functions may be useful when prescribing cholinesterase inhibitors and/or memantine. Patient and family input relative to response is also vital.

The clinician should strive to minimize adverse reactions from psychotropic medications. Table 3.2 lists some of the most commonly implicated medications relative to propensity to produce adverse reactions in the elderly [3, 12].

The neuropsychiatric events which are most commonly seen as a consequence of drug toxicity in the elderly include oversedation, confusion, hallucinations, and delirium [3]. In dementia patients, especially in the more advanced stages,

Table 3.2 Medications most commonly implicated in producing adverse reactions in the elderly

Anticholinergics
Benzodiazepines
Antipsychotics
Opioids
Anticonvulsants
Warfarin – newer anticoagulants
Insulin
Digoxin
ACE inhibitors

Data from references [3, 11]

neuropsychiatric side effects of prescribed medications are often undetected and may present with accelerated cognitive decline and/or agitation and behavioral disturbances. These symptoms may result in additional antipsychotic medications being prescribed for the behavioral symptoms, e.g., antipsychotics for agitation. This can lead to even more drug toxicity, side effects, and functional deterioration.

Minimizing drug-drug interactions is particularly critical in older patients. The risk of drug-drug interactions is higher in older adults since they are often on multiple medications. Drug-drug interactions are often mediated by the CYP-450 system. An example would be an older patient on phenytoin who is prescribed quetiapine for psychosis. Since phenytoin is a potent inducer of CYP-450, 3A4, and quetiapine is a 3A4 substrate, quetiapine clearance can be increased up to five times, resulting in lack of efficacy of quetiapine. One can often substitute a safer alternate drug, one which has a low risk of drug-drug interactions. An example in the case cited would be to substitute levetiracetam for phenytoin. Electronic health record systems often warn clinicians about potential drug-drug interactions.

Avoid Introducing a Drug to Treat the Side Effects of Another Drug

Appropriate selection of psycho-pharmacotherapy will often prevent the need to use other medications to control drug-induced side effects. An example follows in the case study.

Case Study

Mr. G, an 85-year-old man, presents with major depression with psychotic features. The clinician starts sertraline 25 mg OD to be increased to 50 mg, daily in 1 week. Next, the clinician introduces risperidone 1 mg at bedtime to be increased to 2 mg at bedtime in 1 week. Mr. G develops extrapyramidal side effects (EPS) from the risperidone – stiffness and bradykinesia. The clinician starts benztropine 1 mg BID. After 2 days, Mr. G is brought to the emergency room with a full-blown delirium.

The above scenario could have been prevented if the clinician used microdoses of risperidone – e.g., 0.25 mg at bedtime to start and gradually increased to 0.5 mg at bedtime – or by using a drug such as aripiprazole in lieu of risperidone. Aripiprazole has a lower risk of producing Parkinsonian side effects than risperidone. The elderly are particularly sensitive to drugs which can produce EPS.

Table 3.3 Strategies to reduce medications in the elderly

Discontinue drugs which are ineffective or only marginally effective
Discontinue unnecessary medications
Consider non-pharmacological alternatives, when feasible
Discontinue medications which may have been effective in the past but may not provide continued benefits
Discontinue medications which are being used at subtherapeutic doses or on a trial basis, but are not working
Discontinue or reduce the dose of medications if the patient's health deteriorates such as with increasing dementia, frailty, or decline in renal or hepatic functions
Discontinue any and all medications which are not necessary to maintain life or comfort care in patients in the terminal stages of dementia

Adapted from Desai and Grossberg [11] with permission

Reducing Medication Burden

As noted previously, older adults consume three times their percentage in the population of prescribed and over-the-counter remedies [7]. Reducing medication burden in the elderly is an important goal. Table 3.3 lists strategies that may be useful in reducing medications in the elderly.

Periodic Drug Tapering and Discontinuation if Symptoms Are Well-Controlled

It is not unusual for medications, once started, to be continued for many years. As an example, one may encounter an older patient who has been on anticonvulsants for many years, and neither the patient or the family can even remember the last time the patient has had a seizure or for patients to be on subtherapeutic doses of medications for years without a clinician asking if the patient still needs to be on that medication.

Antipsychotic tapering and discontinuation, if possible, is particularly important in the elderly, especially in those with dementia. Antipsychotics continue to play a useful role in managing severe behavioral disturbances and psychosis in dementia patients [16]. However, in dementia patients who have had a good response to antipsychotics, dose reduction and discontinuation should not occur for 12 months, secondary to increased risk of relapse and hospitalization [17].

Although periodic drug tapering/discontinuation is generally recommended in the elderly, it is not always desirable. Examples would be discontinuing antidepressants in a patient with a history of recurrent depression. Discontinuing a mood stabilizer in a bipolar patient who has a previous history of relapse when this was attempted or obviously, abrupt discontinuation of benzodiazepines, narcotic analgesics or other psychotropic agents with severe discontinuation syndromes. Withdrawal and discontinuation syndromes tend to be particularly dangerous in frail elders and should be avoided.

Patient and Family Education

It is important to educate the older patient and her/his family about what side effects to look for with prescribed medications. The authors recommend sharing information about common side effects with patients and families but asking them to call if they experience what they believe are side effects of newly prescribed medications. To not automatically discontinue medications, call the clinician, who may advise that what the patient is experiencing is not a drug-related side effect. An example from the author's practice: 2 weeks after an Alzheimer's patient was started on a cholinesterase inhibitor, her family called the clinician, concerned that the new medication was causing confusion. Then the clinician asked if the patient was having any other symptoms; the family reported urinary frequency. Treatment of the patient's urinary tract infection resulted in clearing of her confusion.

It is also important to educate patients and families about having realistic expectations relative to pharmacotherapeutic interventions. They also need to know that many interventions take time to work, even once therapeutic doses are reached. Relative to expectations, the example of the anti-dementia agents is most apparent. Patients with Alzheimer's disease and their carers need to know that the cholinesterase inhibitors and/or memantine cannot halt disease progression or reverse existing symptoms. They may be able to stabilize symptoms in some patients and improve their quality of functioning. They are not a cure. Similarly, antidepressants, antipsychotics, and mood stabilizers can dramatically help bipolar patients, but they cannot *cure* bipolar affective disorders.

Patients and families also need to be told that many psychopharmacologic interventions take time to work or to have therapeutic effects, especially in the elderly, who often require more time to respond to psychiatric medications. Perhaps the best example is the need to counsel depressed elders being treated with antidepressants to be patient, since it may take 6–8 weeks and even up to 12 weeks for agents such as the SSRIs to have optimal effects [1]. Table 3.4 lists some common psychotropic medications used in the elderly and the amount of time required for them to show clinical benefits.

Table 3.4 Time to optimal response of psychoactive agents in the elderly

Agent	Time to optimal response
Antipsychotics	7–10 days (calming effect, minutes to hours)
Antidepressants	6–8 weeks (up to 12 weeks)
Benzodiazepines	Minutes to hours
Mood stabilizers	Days to weeks

Medication Cost/Reimbursement

Many older adults are living on limited incomes; consequently, affordability of prescribed medications always needs to be considered. The clinician needs to be aware of the fact that the lack of affordability of medication is a major reason for nonadherence [18]. The clinician needs to be aware of the cost of medications and should not prescribe medications for the elderly which are not affordable. If an older adult has to choose between putting food on the table and paying for expensive medication, food will win out.

It is also important to keep in mind that just because a medication is "generic" does not mean that it is not expensive. As an example, an older patient with severe OCD was told by the clinician that he may benefit from a trial of fluvoxamine, which would be inexpensive since it is "generic." When the patient found out that "generic" fluvoxamine would cost him $370.00 a month, he never filled the prescription.

Conclusion

Psycho-pharmacotherapy in the elderly is an art. But adhering to the basic principles cited in this chapter can make it safe, effective, rewarding, and even lifesaving.

References

1. Desai AK. Use of psychopharmacologic agents in the elderly. Clin Geriatr Med. 2003;19:697–719.
2. Desai AK, Grossberg GT. Herbals and botanicals in geriatric psychiatry. Am J Geriatr Psychiatr. 2003;11:498–506.
3. Gurwitz JH, Field TS, Avorn J, et al. Incidence and preventability of adverse drug events in nursing homes. Am J Med. 2005;118:251–8.
4. Steinman MA, Beizer JL, DuBeau CE, et al. How to use the AGS 2015 beers criteria – a guide for patients, clinicians, health systems, and payors. J Am Geriatr Soc. 2015;63(12):e1–7.
5. Schneider LS, Dagermen KS, Insel P. Risk of death with atypical antipsychotic drug treatment for dementia: meta-analysis of randomized, placebo-controlled trials. J Am Med Assoc. 2005;294:1934–43.
6. Mollot, RJ Butler D. Federal requirements and regulatory provisions relevant to dementia care and the use of antipsychotic drugs. Long-Term Care Community Coalition. 2012;1–21.
7. Task Force on Aging Research: Medications and Errors. https://www.ascp.com/sites/default/files/file_Task_Force_2009_Final--3.pdf (2009). Accessed Jan 2017.
8. Miller JJ. Serum levels of psychiatric drugs. Psychiatr Times. 2014;19:49.
9. Davis FA. DrugGuide.com. Accessed Jan 2017.
10. Bigos KL, Pollock BG, Coley KC, et al. Sex, race, and smoking impact olanzapine exposure. J Clin Pharmacol. 2008;48:157–65.

11. Desai AK, Grossberg GT. Psychiatric consultation in long-term care. Baltimore: Johns Hopkins University Press; 2010. p. 302.
12. Yesavage JA, Brink TL, Rose TL, et al. Development and validation of a geriatric depression screening scale: a preliminary report. J Psychiatr Res. 1983;17(1):37–49.
13. Chakkamparambil B, Chibnall JT, Graypel EA, et al. Development of a brief validated geriatric depression screening tool: the SLU "AM SAD". Am J Geriatr Psychiatr. 2015;23(8):780–3.
14. Tariq SH, Tumosa N, Chibnall JT, et al. The St. Louis University Mental Status (SLUMS) examination for detecting mild cognitive impairment and dementia is more sensitive than the Mini-Mental Status Examination (MMSE): a pilot study. Am J Geriatr Psychiatr. 2006;14:900–10.
15. Nasreddine ZS, Phillips NA, Bedirian V, et al. The Montreal Cognitive Assessment, MoCA: a brief tool for mild cognitive impairment. J Am Geriatr Soc. 2005;53(4):695–9.
16. Jennings L, Grossberg GT. Antipsychotics continue to have a place in the management of difficult behavior problems in patients with dementia. J Am Med Dir Assoc. 2013;14:447–9.
17. Devanand DP, Mintzer J, Schultz SK, et al. Relapse risk after discontinuation of risperidone in Alzheimer's disease. N Engl J Med. 2012;367(16):1497–507.
18. Musich S, Yan C, Yeh CS. Pharmaceutical cost-saving strategies and their association with medication adherence in a medicare supplement. J Gen Intern Med. 2015;30(8):1208–14.

Chapter 4
Antidepressants

Leigh Jennings

Depressive disorders are commonly comorbid with neurological illness and often underdiagnosed [1, 2]. Depression in neurology patients is associated with worse quality of life [3–5] and increased disability, pain, and somatic symptoms [6]. Conversely, remission of depression can improve outcomes [7]. Depression is also a risk factor for poor treatment adherence [8]. Treating depression is integral to the care of the neurology patient. For the purpose of this chapter, the terms "depression" and "clinical depression" will be used to refer to DSM-5 depressive disorders, including major depressive disorder and persistent depressive disorder.

Identifying Depression

Case Vignette: Part 1

Mrs. D. is a 48-year-old female with history of epilepsy and left temporal lobectomy 7 years ago who takes lacosamide 200 mg bid and aspirin 81 mg at home. Mrs. D. moved from a different state 3 months ago to help care for her grandson, and she needs to establish care with a new neurologist. She has been stable on the lacosamide with her last seizure 4 years ago. She has no other medical history or complaints. During the interview, the neurologist congratulates Mrs. D. on her new grandchild and asks how her move has been. She becomes slightly tearful and states that the move has been good but hard. She is enjoying her grandson but misses her friends and family back home.

L. Jennings, MD (✉)
Department of Psychiatry, Methodist Healthcare Systems, San Antonio, TX, USA

© Springer International Publishing AG, part of Springer Nature 2018   45
G. T. Grossberg, L. J. Kinsella (eds.), *Clinical Psychopharmacology for Neurologists*, https://doi.org/10.1007/978-3-319-74604-3_4

Depression Screening

Consider screening all patients for depression at their initial visit and regularly thereafter. One evidence-based approach is to ask two questions: (1) "During the past month, have you been bothered by feeling down, depressed, or hopeless?" (2) "During the past month, have you often been bothered by little interest or pleasure in doing things?" [9, 10] One or more "yes" responses are a positive screen. Self-report screening tools for depression may also be used. For adults, these include the Patient Health Questionnaire 2 (PHQ-2) [11] and Patient Health Questionnaire 9 (PHQ-9) [12] and the World Health Organization Well-Being Index (WHO-5) [13]. For older adults who retain cognitive function, consider the Geriatric Depression Scale (GDS-30 and GDS-15) [14] or the five-item SLU AMSAD [15].

In the vignette, the neurologist decides to assess for depression after the patient appears tearful when asked about a recent life event. Likewise, suspect depression may be present when the patient's symptoms, side effects, or disabilities exceed what is expected [16] or when the patient is having difficulty coping with the illness or adhering to treatment [17].

It is not uncommon for patients to minimize emotional distress, especially in the presence of loved ones. Interviewing the patient alone can sometimes be useful, as can asking family members what they have noticed. Although some patients may not relate to feeling sad or depressed, they will admit to feeling "bummed out," "stressed," or "not caring."

Subsyndromal Depression and Persistent Depressive Disorder

Case Vignette: Part 2

The neurologist is concerned about the possibility of depression in Mrs. D. and decides to assess her further. Mrs. D. reports feeling lonely and a little down for the past month. She has been visiting different churches each weekend, which she enjoys, but she has not found one she likes yet. She is feeling more tired than usual but thinks this is because she is not accustomed to caring for an infant. She is also having trouble falling asleep more than usual, but she notes no change in her appetite or concentration. She denies thoughts of death or suicide. Her son and his wife – with whom she lives – are supportive, she says, but they are busy, and she doesn't want to bother them with her problems. She is hopeful that things will improve soon. Mrs. D. has no history of depression, no other medical history, and she does not drink alcohol or use drugs.

The neurologist acknowledges that this is a big transition for Mrs. D. and that even positive life changes can be stressful. The neurologist asks Mrs. D. if there is anything she might do to reduce stress and increase support. Mrs. D. feels reticent to ask her son for help with the childcare, but she does agree to begin walking daily. She also agrees to reach out to friends back home and accepts a referral to see a counselor, so she has more support.

Subsyndromal Depression

Not all feelings of depression indicate a major depressive episode. It is normal to feel sad after a disappointment or loss or when meaningful activities or relationships are in flux. In the vignette, Mrs. D. is not clinically depressed, but she does have multiple risk factors for depression including a chronic medical illness, female gender, a role transition, a new household, a new city, and limited psychosocial support. The neurologist's role in this situation is to encourage healthy coping, offer resources, and ensure that Mrs. D. has close follow-up. Although referral to counseling for subclinical depressive symptoms is certainly not required, it makes sense for Mrs. D.'s situation. There is some data supporting the effectiveness of psychological interventions to prevent major depression in patients with subsyndromal symptoms like Mrs. D. [18].

Persistent Depressive Disorder (Dysthymia)

Had Mrs. D.'s depressive symptoms been occurring daily for 2 years or more, she might meet criteria for persistent depressive disorder (PDD), previously known as dysthymia. Diagnosis of PDD requires a depressed mood plus two or more of the following: (1) over- or under-eating, (2) insomnia or hypersomnia, (3) low energy or fatigue, (4) poor self-esteem, (5) decreased concentration or difficulty in making decisions, and (6) feelings of hopelessness. In the vignette, Mrs. D.'s unwillingness to "bother" her son could be interpreted as poor self-esteem. Symptoms must be present almost all day, almost every day, for at least 2 years, without interruption for more than 2 months [19]. Persistent depressive disorder is treated with antidepressants, alone or in combination with psychotherapy [20, 21].

Major Depressive Disorder

Case Vignette: Part 3

Mrs. D. misses her 1-month follow-up appointment and returns 3 months later. Now she is feeling even more fatigued. Her son has noticed and thinks it might be her epilepsy medication. Mrs. D.'s dose of lacosamide has not changed for many years, however. She has also been feeling increasingly sad and lonely for the past 6 weeks. Although Mrs. D. continues to care for her grandson, she is no longer enjoying herself. She wakes up before 5 a.m. every morning and lays in bed wondering if she made a mistake in moving. She has lost 10 lb without trying and has given up on finding a church. She is watching sermons on TV for hours each day instead. She has no social outlets beyond her son and his wife, whom she continues to describe as supportive. She did not see a counselor after her last visit, saying that her son convinced her it wasn't necessary.

Mrs. D. has never felt depressed like this in the past. She denies thoughts of suicide, and there is no evidence of psychosis. Mrs. D. has not had any seizures, but she has missed a few doses of lacosamide, which is unusual for her. She is not taking any new medications, and she continues to drink alcohol only rarely. Basic labs, including CBC, CMP, TSH, and UA, ordered at the previous visit are normal.

Diagnosing Major Depressive Disorder

Mrs. D. now meets criteria for major depressive disorder (see Diagnostic and Statistical Manual 5th edition) [22]. She is feeling increasingly sad and reports decreased pleasure and interest. She is experiencing poor sleep – specifically, early morning awakening, a classic symptom of depression. Mrs. D. is also ruminating about the past, which is also common in depression. She is doubting her ability to make decisions, and her social activity and relationships are significantly decreased compared to her previous level of function.

Mrs. D. has given up on finding a church community, as if she has concluded the endeavor is hopeless. Patients with depression frequently interpret seemingly neutral events in a negative way, for example, "I will never fit in here." Of particular concern, Mrs. D. has missed several doses of antiepileptic medication, possibly because she is feeling more tired and less motivated.

It is important to note here that Mrs. D.'s relationship with her son may not be as supportive as she suggests. Loved ones who neglect, criticize, or discount a patient can contribute negatively to a person's mood and life experience. Finally, it is not unusual for patients to attribute depressive symptoms to medication side effects or medical illness.

Assessing Depression Severity

After a diagnosis of a major depressive episode is made, consider its severity, which will guide treatment decisions. The American Psychiatric Association (APA) recommends that the patient's level of functional impairment determines whether depression is mild, moderate, or severe [23]. In neurology patients, it is important to consider whether depression is affecting the neurological condition, including treatment adherence (Table 4.1). The clinician may also take into account length of the depressive episode and factors such as past psychiatric history, family history, and social history, when determining depression severity.

Mrs. D. is experiencing mild to moderate impairment. Since she is also missing doses of her antiepileptic medication, the neurologist categorizes her episode as moderate in severity.

Table 4.1 Questions to assess depression severity and guide treatment

Which symptoms are most problematic?
Are there recent stresses or losses?
Are symptoms bothersome or impacting function? If so, to what extent?
Is neurological illness contributing to depression? If so, to what extent?
Is the patient adhering to neurological treatment?
Is there a personal or family history of depression? If so:
How severe? Is there a history of hospitalization, suicidal ideation, or suicide attempt?
What treatments, if any, have been effective in the past?

For patients with mild depression, the APA recommends treatment with antidepressants or psychotherapy. Regular exercise might also be considered for motivated patients, with close follow-up [23]. The NICE guidelines from the UK are more conservative for mild depression and suggest low-intensity psychosocial interventions, such as group exercise, as first-line treatments. NICE does support antidepressants for mild depressive episodes when (1) depression is complicating the care of a medical condition, (2) there is a history of moderate to severe depression, (3) symptoms have lasted 2 years or more (as in dysthymia), and (4) depression has not responded to other interventions [24].

Patients with moderate depression, like Mrs. D., should receive antidepressants or psychotherapy [23]. Patients with severe depression should generally receive medication. Antidepressants are especially effective for severe and possibly moderate depressive episodes, with less demonstrated benefit for patients with mild depression [25–27].

Completing the Assessment

Clinical Vignette: Part 3

The neurologist explains to Mrs. D. that treating depression is an important part of managing epilepsy. Since Mrs. D. had difficulty attending psychotherapy appointments in the past, she and the neurologist decide to try antidepressant medication. Mrs. D. says she is willing to see a psychiatrist, but her son doesn't believe in psychiatry, and she relies on him for transportation.

The neurologist is now considering treating Mrs. D.'s depression and decides to ask Mrs. D. a few more questions. Mrs. D. confirms she has no psychiatric history: she has never seen a psychiatrist or been diagnosed with depression or bipolar disorder. She has never considered or attempted suicide. She is unaware of any family history of these conditions, although her father was an alcoholic before she was born and always had a temper. She denies any history of significant mood elevation.

Table 4.2 Predictors of complicated treatment

History of sustained mood elevation or bipolar disorder
Family history of suicide or bipolar disorder
Active substance use disorder
Personality disorder or any patient who elicits a strong emotional response
More than one psychiatric disorder
History of severe or treatment-resistant depression
Suicidal ideation
Psychotic symptoms

Adapted from Kanner [28], with permission

There is no history of problematic use of alcohol or recreational drugs. The symptom that is bothering Mrs. D. most is fatigue.

The neurologist concludes that Mrs. D.'s depression is likely to be uncomplicated to treat and decides to start an antidepressant while continuing to encourage Mrs. D. to see a psychiatrist.

Although an antidepressant will not change Mrs. D.'s isolation, it might help her to consider options and take action on her behalf.

Discussion

Before starting an antidepressant, look for indications that depression will be complicated to treat (Table 4.2) [28]. It is essential to screen for a history of mood elevation, as major depressive episodes can occur in bipolar disorder. Patients with bipolar disorder who inadvertently receive antidepressants may experience a rapidly improving mood or feel anxious or agitated. To screen for a history of mood elevation, the clinician can ask, "have you ever experienced periods of time when you felt like you were on top of the world, and during that time you had plenty of energy, like the Energizer Bunny, and you didn't need to sleep as much?" If the answer is yes, inquire how long these episodes last and whether there was uncharacteristically risky or impulsive behavior. Mood elevation must be a significant departure from normal and persist for days or weeks to be suggestive of bipolar disorder.

If there is a safety concern such as active suicidal or homicidal ideation, or if the patient's function is markedly impaired, consider referring the patient to an emergency room for possible inpatient admission. Risk factors for suicide include previous suicide attempt, male gender, family history of psychiatric illness, substance abuse, hopelessness, more severe depression (e.g., with psychotic features), and access to lethal means (especially firearms) [29]. For more information on assessing suicide risk, the APA has published a practice guideline that is available on its website [30].

Prescribing an Antidepressant

Case Vignette: Part 4

The neurologist prescribes escitalopram 10 mg daily and asks Mrs. D. to call the office in 1 week and report how she is doing and to follow-up in person in 2–4 weeks. Mrs. D. is informed about the common side effects of escitalopram and educated that recovery from depression happens gradually, although she may start feeling better within a week or two [31]. The neurologist also warns about the possibility of feeling restless, very happy, or suicidal after starting the medication and instructs Mrs. D. what to do if these occur.

Selecting an Antidepressant

Antidepressants are considered to be equally efficacious; therefore, most clinicians choose an antidepressant by matching its side effect and safety profile with the patient's history and preferences. A patient with fatigue may benefit from an antidepressant reputed to be energizing, such as bupropion or venlafaxine, whereas a patient with poor sleep and appetite be a good candidate for mirtazapine. If an antidepressant was successful in treating a previous depressive episode, it is likely to be effective again [32]. Likewise, if a medication has been helpful for a close family member, consider starting there.

Some patients will have concerns about side effects. If the patient is wanting to avoid sexual dysfunction, consider bupropion, unless there is significant anxiety, in which case try mirtazapine. If the patient wants to avoid both sexual dysfunction and weight gain, consider duloxetine, unless there is hepatic dysfunction, in which case consider escitalopram – and so on.

Table 4.3 provides a comprehensive summary of how various comorbidities, symptoms, risks, and patient concerns may direct antidepressant choice.

The eight antidepressants described below are likely to be the most useful to neurologists. All are relatively well-tolerated, unlikely to cause drug-drug interactions, and affordable. Three (escitalopram, citalopram, sertraline) are SSRIs, two (venlafaxine, duloxetine) are SNRIs, and two (bupropion, mirtazapine) have unique mechanisms of action, creating specific advantages and liabilities. Starting and therapeutic doses for each agent are listed in Table 4.4.

Antidepressants for Neurologists

Escitalopram and citalopram are SSRIs that have less potential for pharmacokinetic interactions than other newer antidepressants and are commonly used in patients with medical comorbidities [33]. Escitalopram may cause mild 2D6 inhibition, but

Table 4.3 Choosing an antidepressant

Symptoms, side effects, comorbidities, concerns	Antidepressants to consider and to avoid
ADHD, comorbid	Bupropion [145]
Adherence concerns	See discontinuation syndrome
Anxiety disorder	Any SSRI or SNRI [146]
	Start at 1/2 the starting dose, and then increase after 1 week
Poor appetite	Mirtazapine [52]
Cardiac history (includes post-MI, CAD, CHF, LVH, hx arrhythmia, and congenital long QTc)	Sertraline [39] > mirtazapine [147]
	Bupropion is safe post-MI [148] but smoking cessation efficacy unclear [149]
	Avoid citalopram and possibly escitalopram due to QTc prolongation [35, 38]
	TCAs contraindicated [150]
Cost[a]	Less than $10: escitalopram, citalopram, fluoxetine, paroxetine, amitriptyline, nortriptyline
	$10–$20: sertraline, mirtazapine, venlafaxine XR
	$20–$30: duloxetine, bupropion XL
Diarrhea	Avoid sertraline [151]
Discontinuation syndrome [91]	Avoid paroxetine, venlafaxine (shorter-acting)
	Consider fluoxetine (longer-acting)
Energy or motivation low	Consider bupropion, venlafaxine, and fluoxetine
Gastrointestinal bleeding	See NSAIDs
Headache (chronic) [152]	Amitriptyline > venlafaxine
Hepatic impairment [153]	Consider escitalopram and citalopram (least risk of hepatotoxicity); avoid duloxetine, bupropion, and amitriptyline (greatest risk)
Hypertension	Monitor blood pressure with SNRIs, bupropion
Hyponatremia [86]	Consider mirtazapine; monitor serum sodium regularly
Nausea	Consider mirtazapine [154] and bupropion [155]
NSAIDs [80]	Consider adding PPI to SSRIs and SNRIs, esp. if there are risk factors for GI bleed [81]
Overdose risk	Avoid TCAs [156]
Pain	Duloxetine [45][b] > amitriptyline [53] > venlafaxine [41]
Pregnancy	Consider psychotherapy; avoid paroxetine [157] (Category D); refer to psychiatry
Seizure risk	Bupropion [95], TCAs contraindicated
Sexual dysfunction	Consider bupropion [158], mirtazapine [159], and duloxetine [160], possibly vortioxetine [161] and vilazodone [162]
Smoking cessation	Bupropion[b] [47]
Weight gain [74]	Bupropion > fluoxetine; avoid mirtazapine and paroxetine

[a]Cost is for uninsured patient, according to GoodRx.com at time of press
[b]FDA approval for this indication

Table 4.4 Therapeutic daily dosing of commonly prescribed antidepressants

Antidepressant	Starting dose	Therapeutic range	Maximum dose
Escitalopram	10 mg (5 mg)	10–20 mg	20 mg (10 mg)
Citalopram	20 mg (10 mg)	20–40 mg	40 mg (20 mg)
Sertraline	50 mg (25 mg)	50–150 mg	200 mg (100 mg)
Venlafaxine ER	37.5 mg	75–225 mg	225 mg (150 mg)
Desvenlafaxine	50 mg	50–100 mg	100 mg
Duloxetine	20–30 mg	60–120 mg	120 mg
Levomilnacipran [163]	20 mg	40–120 mg	120 mg
Mirtazapine	15 mg (7.5 mg)	30–45 mg	45 mg
Bupropion XL	150 mg	150–450 mg	450 mg
Vortioxetine	10 mg (5 mg)	10–20 mg	20 mg
Vilazodone [164]	10 mg	20–40 mg	40 mg
Amitriptyline	25 mg	150–300 mg	300 mg
Nortriptyline	50 mg (25 mg)	50–150 mg[a]	150 mg

Adapted from Schatzberg and Debattista [33] and Taylor et al. [55], with permission
Doses in parentheses are for older adults
[a]Titrate to plasma level of 50–150 ng/mL. Efficacy is reduced outside of this range

the clinical significance of this is questionable [34]. Escitalopram also causes mild QTc prolongation (4.5 ms at 10 mg/day and 6.6 ms at 20 mg/day), causing some experts to exercise caution with at-risk patients, as below [35, 36]. The maximum recommended dose of escitalopram for older adults and patients with hepatic dysfunction is 10 mg/day [34].

Citalopram is a racemic mixture of two enantiomers, one of which is escitalopram. In 2011, the FDA published a warning about its dose-dependent risk of QTc prolongation (8.5 ms at 20 mg/day and 12.6 ms at 40 mg/day) [37]. Citalopram should therefore be avoided in patients with recent myocardial infarction, uncompensated heart failure, bradycardia, hypokalemia, hypomagnesemia, and in combination with other drugs known to prolong QTc [38]. The maximum recommended dose of citalopram is 20 mg/day in older adults and 40 mg/day in adults [37].

Sertraline was used in clinical trials for treating depression after myocardial infarction and is considered to be safe and effective in this population [39]. Unlike many antidepressants, sertraline has a linear dose-response curve, with increasing response up to 200 mg per day. Sertraline is also a mild 2D6 inhibitor and may increase TCA levels slightly [40]. Sertraline is FDA-approved for major depression, posttraumatic stress disorder, premenstrual dysphoric disorder, and several anxiety disorders [40].

Venlafaxine is an SNRI that is most conveniently prescribed in its once-daily, extended-release formulation. Venlafaxine is FDA-approved for several anxiety disorders in addition to depression and is sometimes used off-label for neuropathic pain [41], vasomotor symptoms of menopause [42], and migraine prophylaxis [43]. Venlafaxine has few drug-drug interactions and may cause or exacerbate hypertension [44]. Monitor blood pressure after initiating venlafaxine and other SNRIs.

Duloxetine is an SNRI that is FDA-approved for major depression, generalized anxiety disorder, fibromyalgia, diabetic neuropathy, and chronic musculoskeletal pain. Duloxetine can cause hepatic toxicity and therefore should not be prescribed in patients with hepatic insufficiency or who are heavy drinkers [45]. Duloxetine is a moderately potent 2D6 inhibitor and can increase TCA levels two- to threefold [46].

Bupropion is FDA-approved for smoking cessation [47] in addition to major depression. Unlike other antidepressants, bupropion may not be effective for anxiety disorders. Bupropion is a moderate 2D6 inhibitor and can increase blood levels when combined with other antidepressants, including TCAs [48]. Bupropion is contraindicated in patients with epilepsy [49].

Mirtazapine has prominent sedative effects and is associated with increased appetite and weight gain [50]. Cigarette smoking, phenytoin, and carbamazepine can induce mirtazapine's metabolism [51], and CYP3A4 inhibitors such as ketoconazole can increase blood levels [52]. Because bupropion and mirtazapine do not inhibit the reuptake of serotonin, they do not cause many of the side effects commonly associated with SSRIs and SNRIs.

Amitriptyline is a first-generation, tricyclic antidepressant commonly used off-label at low doses for pain syndromes, including neuropathy [53] and migraine headaches [54]. Antidepressant doses are higher and range from 150 to 300 mg/day. Blood levels associated with antidepressant response range from 100 to 250 ng/ml. Amitriptyline is started at 25 mg and increased by 25 mg every few days until its therapeutic dose of 150 mg is reached. Like other tricyclic antidepressants, amitriptyline can cause fatal cardiac arrhythmias in overdose. Its use should be avoided in suicidal patients. All tricyclic antidepressants are 2D6 substrates and may become toxic or even fatal if combined with a CYP2D6 inhibitor. Blood levels are drawn 8–12 h after the patient's last dose and should be monitored closely [33]. Polypharmacy should be avoided. Amitriptyline and other tricyclic antidepressants also cause adverse effects related to their antihistaminic, anticholinergic, and alpha-1 blocking actions that may limit their utility, especially for older adults [33].

Evaluating and Adjusting Treatment

Case Vignette: Part 5

Mrs. D. calls the office in 1 week and says she is feeling nauseated when she takes the escitalopram. She is advised to take the medication with food. She returns after 4 weeks and reports she is feeling a little better. She still feels profoundly sad, overwhelmed, and helpless at times, but the depression is lessening its grip. Mrs. D. is still watching sermons online and not attending church. One positive development is that Mrs. D. has been able to convince her son and his wife to hire a babysitter one or two afternoons a week.

Evaluating Treatment Response

To assess a patient's response to depression treatment, ask about the target symptoms identified in the initial assessment, the patient's level of functioning, and status of neurological illness. Depression scales, discussed at the end of this chapter, may be helpful to track improvement. Patients should be seen regularly and encouraged to call if any unusual symptoms emerge.

Continuing or Increasing the Antidepressant

The most common reason for antidepressant treatment failure is giving an insufficient dose for an inadequate period of time. An adequate trial of an antidepressant requires 4–6 weeks of daily use at a therapeutic dose [56]. If the patient's symptoms are partially improved after this time period, increase the dose or continue to monitor. Patients should be reevaluated approximately every 4 weeks and medications adjusted until depression symptoms are completely in remission. Mrs. D. has been taking escitalopram for 4 weeks and is having a partial response. Her neurologist could continue the current dose but decides to increase to 20 mg.

A partial response at the maximum tolerated dose should prompt the clinician to (1) change antidepressants, (2) add psychotherapy, or (3) refer to psychiatry. (Antidepressant augmentation is a fourth option but beyond the scope of this chapter.)

Changing Antidepressants, if Not Effective

If depression is not improved after an adequate time period, ensure the patient is taking the medication regularly before documenting a failed trial in the chart. A second antidepressant is chosen in a similar manner as the first. Most antidepressants can be safely cross-tapered, with dose adjustments every 3–7 days as tolerated. Certain antidepressants require more caution when switching: TCA doses should be reduced by half before a new antidepressant is added at its starting dose, and the TCA tapered. Because of fluoxetine's long half-life and 2D6 inhibition, consider stopping it for 1 week before starting a new antidepressant [55].

Goals and Duration of Treatment

Case Vignette: Part 6

Mrs. D. returns after 4 more weeks. She is feeling much improved. Her energy is returning, and she is only waking up early approximately twice per week. She is enjoying caring for her grandson again, and she has found a church she likes. She reports her son has seen the difference in his mother and is grateful for the depression treatment. The neurologist acknowledges Mrs. D. for her persistence with treatment and continues her current dose of escitalopram.

Treat Residual Symptoms Fully

Mrs. D. is feeling better, but she is still experiencing mild depressive symptoms in the form of sleep disturbance. Patients who experience residual symptoms after a depressive episode are more likely to experience a recurrence of depression in the next year (74% versus 26%) [57]. Residual symptoms are also associated with a greater lifetime burden of illness, including impairment in work and relationships [57]. Depressive symptoms should therefore be treated proactively until completely resolved. Since Mrs. D. has been taking the antidepressant only 8 weeks and improving steadily, continuing the present dose is appropriate. If residual symptoms do not improve, the neurologist could add psychotherapy or refer to psychiatry.

Duration of Treatment

Patients commonly want to know how long they will need to take antidepressants. Antidepressants should be continued at the same dose for 6–9 months following full symptom remission [58], to prevent return of depression when the risk is highest [59]. After this time period, patients with a single lifetime episode of depression can start to slowly taper the antidepressant. Ideally, this should not occur during a major life transition or other stressful time.

Patients with a greater risk of relapse and recurrence may benefit from longer-term maintenance pharmacotherapy. These patients include individuals with a chronic medical illness, two or more episodes of depression in a few years, three or more lifetime episodes, and/or residual symptoms [23]. Psychotherapy can also be useful for preventing depression recurrence when an antidepressant is stopped or when added to an antidepressant during maintenance [60]. Psychotherapy also effectively prevents relapse when continued after acute phase treatment with pharmacotherapy [61].

Psychotherapy

Evidence-based psychotherapies for depression include cognitive behavioral therapy (CBT), interpersonal therapy (IPT), problem-solving therapy (PST), and mindfulness-based cognitive therapy (MBCT). Cognitive behavioral therapy (CBT) is a structured therapy that helps patients examine and challenge faulty thinking while incorporating skills such as diaphragmatic breathing and activity scheduling. Interpersonal therapy (IPT) focuses on resolving relationship and role conflicts that may be contributing to depression. Problem-solving therapy (PST) teaches patients how to solve psychosocial difficulties and helps them to regain a sense of control over life's challenges.

Ideally, the clinician is familiar with several skilled psychotherapists to whom patients can be referred.

For depression of mild to moderate severity, psychotherapy is as effective as antidepressants [62]. For depression that is severe or recurrent, combining psychotherapy with medication is superior to psychotherapy alone [63].

Adverse Effects

Case Vignette: Part 7

Mrs. D. follows up in 2 months and her depression is in full remission. At her 4-month follow-up appointment, Mrs. D. says that she would like to begin dating. She has heard that antidepressants can cause problems with sexual function, however, and wants to know if she needs to stop the medication. The neurologist explains that some individuals taking antidepressants experience sexual difficulties; however if she does, there are various options to regain her sexual function.

Common Adverse Effects

Like all medications, antidepressants can cause adverse effects [64]. Common side effects of antidepressants initially include nausea, feeling activated, and sedation. These issues are typically self-limiting and can usually be addressed by taking the medication with food or at a different time of the day [65]. If side effects are intolerable, reduce the dose by half and attempt to increase in another week.

Sexual dysfunction, including difficulties with desire, arousal, and orgasm, occurs in 30–60% of patients taking antidepressants [66]. Many patients will not spontaneously report sexual dysfunction, so it is important to ask [67]. Sexual dysfunction tends to occur early and persist. Various strategies exist to address antidepressant-related sexual dysfunction, including decreasing the dose of medication, changing antidepressants, exercising before sex, and scheduling regular sexual activity and brief drug holidays [68]. Adding bupropion at doses of 300 mg/day can improve antidepressant-related sexual dysfunction for both genders [69], and phosphodiesterase inhibitors have been shown to be helpful for men [70] and possibly for women [71].

If changing the antidepressant or antidepressant dose, monitor the patient's mood carefully. The antidepressants least likely to cause sexual dysfunction, according to one meta-analysis [72], include bupropion, mirtazapine, escitalopram, and duloxetine (in the order of increasing dysfunction).

Weight gain tends to build gradually over time when it occurs in patients taking antidepressants [73]. Mirtazapine and paroxetine cause the most weight gain and bupropion, the least [74].

Treatment-emergent *hypertension* is a possible side effect when starting SNRIs, especially venlafaxine [75]. Monitor blood pressure regularly, and consider changing antidepressants or treating hypertension if blood pressure rises.

Serious Adverse Effects

The clinician should remain vigilant for less common but potentially serious adverse reactions. *Akathisia* can be distressing and even dangerous when accompanied by suicidal ideation [76]. Suicidal thoughts and behaviors may newly emerge, especially in patients under 25 years of age [77]. Rapidly improving mood and energy are concerning for an evolving *manic episode*. Eye pain or vision changes may indicate *acute angle-closure glaucoma*, an ophthalmic emergency. Risk factors for acute angle closure include advanced age, female gender, farsightedness, Asian or Eskimo ethnicity, family history of closed-angle glaucoma, and narrow anterior chambers [78]. If any of these symptoms occur, stop the antidepressant, and consider referral to an emergency room.

Other Adverse Effects

Although the absolute risks are low, SSRIs and SNRIs are associated with an increased risk of *upper gastrointestinal bleeding*, especially in combination with NSAIDs [79], aspirin, or antiplatelet agents [80]. The use of a proton-pump inhibitor (PPI) may offset this risk [81]. Serotonergic antidepressants are also associated with an elevated risk of *perioperative bleeding* [82]. Switching to mirtazapine or bupropion may reduce bleeding risk [82]. Discontinuation of antidepressants 2 weeks before surgery is not routinely recommended but may be considered in situations where the risk of bleeding is high and depression is stable [82].

The risk of *serotonin syndrome* is greatest when combining a monoamine oxidase inhibitor (MAOI) with other serotonergic medications; consequently these should never be prescribed together [83].

In practice, most non-MAOI antidepressants can be combined safely with other serotonergic medications, including tramadol and triptans. To be cautious, warn patients taking two or more serotonergic agents about the possibility of serotonin syndrome. Although the FDA has specifically warned about combining triptans with antidepressants [84], the American Headache Society has critiqued this advisory as relying upon case reports of serotonin syndrome that did not meet diagnostic criteria [85]. *Hyponatremia* is another possible side effect of serotonergic antidepressants, with the risk increasing for older adults and in patients taking diuretics or who are volume depleted [86].

Discontinuation Syndrome

Stopping an antidepressant after several weeks of regular use may cause a discontinuation, or withdrawal, syndrome. Although not dangerous, discontinuation symptoms can be uncomfortable and potentially disruptive to a patient's life. Common discontinuation symptoms are summarized by the acronym FINISH and include flu-like symptoms (e.g., fatigue and myalgias), insomnia, nausea, imbalance (e.g., dizziness), sensory disturbances (e.g., paresthesias), and hyperarousal [87]. Rebound depression and suicidality have also been reported [88].

Patients should be informed about the possibility of discontinuation symptoms and advised not to stop medications abruptly. When completing therapy, clinicians should taper the medication over several months while monitoring mood closely [89]. For patients who are very uncomfortable during discontinuation, one or more daily doses of fluoxetine 20 mg (which has a long half-life and self-tapers) may help ease symptoms [90]. Shorter-acting antidepressants such as paroxetine and venlafaxine are the most likely to cause a discontinuation syndrome [91].

Neurological Illnesses

Epilepsy

The International League Against Epilepsy (ILAE) recommends screening patients with epilepsy for depression at every visit and treating depression promptly when identified [92]. This proactive approach reflects an elevated risk of suicide compared to the general population [93]. Epilepsy patients with the greatest suicide risk include those with psychiatric comorbidity and those diagnosed with epilepsy in the past 6 months [94]. The highest rates of depression occur in patients with treatment-resistant epilepsy, in whom depression is a more significant predictor of quality of life than seizure control [3].

Second-generation antidepressants are generally safe in patients with epilepsy [95], with the exception of bupropion. Although only immediate-release bupropion has been associated with increased seizures, all formulations of bupropion are contraindicated in patients with epilepsy [96].

Antidepressants may cause clinically significant interactions with antiepileptic drugs (AEDs). For example, fluoxetine and fluvoxamine can increase levels of phenytoin and valproic acid [97], and phenytoin and carbamazepine decrease levels of mirtazapine [98, 99], vilazodone [100], and TCAs [33]. Carbamazepine induces bupropion metabolism [101]. Checking serum levels of antiepileptic medications can help neurologists ensure that AEDs remain therapeutic. Drug-drug interactions are explored further in Chap. 11.

Recommended screening tools for persons with epilepsy include the Neurologic Depressive Disorder Inventory in Epilepsy (NDDI-E) [102] and the PHQ-2 [92].

Parkinson's Disease

Comorbid depression in Parkinson's disease is associated with increased disability [103], less quality of life [104], earlier treatment of motor dysfunction [105], and increased mortality [106]. Antidepressants are commonly used to treat depression in Parkinson's disease, although evidence supporting their efficacy is mixed [17, 107]. Some experts believe that bupropion may be useful, because of its pro-dopamine effects [108]. Pramipexole may be useful for depression in patients with persistent motor symptoms [109]. Finally, CBT appears to be a promising treatment for depression in Parkinson's disease [110]. The WHO-5 [111], PHQ-2 [112], PHQ-9, Beck Depression Inventory (BDI-II), GDS-30, and GDS-15 are all validated as screening tools, when used with Parkinson's-specific cutoff points [113].

Stroke

Approximately one-third of patients will exhibit some depressive symptoms 1 year after a stroke [114], and between 14% and 24% of patients will meet criteria for major depressive disorder within 5 years following a cerebrovascular event [115]. Some experts [115] believe that frontal, left-sided strokes are more likely to cause depression in the acute phase, despite recent meta-analyses that have found no association [116, 117].

Poststroke depression is correlated with worse functional outcomes [116], greater cognitive impairment [118], and increased mortality [119]. Remission of depression is associated with improved function [7] and cognition [120]. A 2008 Cochrane review found that antidepressants are efficacious in treating poststroke depression [121]. Brief psychosocial therapies may also be helpful to improve depressive symptoms [122] and coping [123]. Both antidepressants and psychosocial therapies show promise for depression prevention [124]. In stroke patients, the PHQ-9 is more sensitive for depression screening than the PHQ-2 [125].

Multiple Sclerosis

Depression in patients with multiple sclerosis is associated with increased fatigue [126], worse cognition [127], decreased quality of life [4], and reduced adherence to treatment [128]. Patients with multiple sclerosis have an increased risk for suicide, especially young males in the first 5 years following diagnosis [129]. CBT has been well-studied in patients with multiple sclerosis and has been shown to be effective, as have other talk therapies [130]. Only a few trials have studied antidepressant efficacy (with mixed results), although anecdotal data supports their use [131]. A consensus group from the National Multiple Sclerosis Society recommends combining medication and psychotherapy [132].

Two "yes" answers on the two-question clinical screen (described in "Depression Screening," above) have a sensitivity of 99% for depression [10]. The Hospital Anxiety and Depression Scale (HADS) [133] and the Beck Fast Screen [134] have also been validated for screening patients with multiple sclerosis.

Scales for Evaluating Treatment Response

Depression outcome scales provide a summary score based upon symptom frequency and can be used to track treatment response. Validated outcome scales include the nine-item Patient Health Questionnaire (PHQ-9) [135], the Clinically Useful Depression Outcome Scale (CUDOS) [136], and the World Health Organization Well-Being Index (WHO-5) [13]. Other validated self-report measures include the Beck Depression Inventory (BDI-II) [137] and Hospital Anxiety and Depression Scale (HADS) [138], but these scales require a fee, making them less practical for clinical use.

Of note, outcome scales should not be used to determine whether depression is mild, moderate, or severe. These categories differ widely by instrument, have not been empirically validated, and may overstate depression severity [139].

Antidepressant Overview

Selective serotonin reuptake inhibitors (SSRIs) include fluoxetine (Prozac), paroxetine (Paxil), sertraline (Zoloft), citalopram (Celexa), escitalopram (Lexapro), and fluvoxamine (Luvox). Fluoxetine and paroxetine are moderate CYP2D6 inhibitors. Fluvoxamine is a strong CYP2D6 inhibitor most commonly used for obsessive-compulsive disorder.

Serotonin norepinephrine reuptake inhibitors (SNRIs) include venlafaxine (Effexor), duloxetine (Cymbalta), desvenlafaxine (Pristiq), milnacipran (Savella), and levomilnacipran (Fetzima). Milnacipran is FDA-approved for fibromyalgia only. Its L-enantiomer, levomilnacipran, was FDA-approved for depression in 2013. Desvenlafaxine is the first metabolite of venlafaxine and is not metabolized by the CYP450 system.

Novel antidepressants include bupropion (Wellbutrin, Zyban, Contrave) and mirtazapine (Remeron). Bupropion enhances norepinephrine and dopamine transmission, although its exact mechanism of action is unknown [49]. Bupropion is FDA-approved for depression and smoking cessation and was recently approved for weight loss in combination with low-dose naltrexone [140]. Mirtazapine indirectly enhances serotonin (especially 5-HT1) and norepinephrine transmission by blocking central alpha-2 adrenergic and postsynaptic 5-HT2 and 5-HT3 receptors [50].

Serotonin "plus" antidepressants include vortioxetine (Trintellix) and vilazodone (Viibryd). More recently on the market, these antidepressants combine serotonin reuptake inhibition with specific receptor actions. The relative advantages and liabilities of these agents will emerge with more clinical experience.

Tricyclic antidepressants (TCAs) are first-generation antidepressants that inhibit the reuptake of norepinephrine primarily and serotonin secondarily. TCAs also have antagonist activity at histamine, muscarinic, and alpha-1 receptors and can cause related adverse effects. TCAs can cause lethal arrhythmias in overdose and should not be used in patients with cardiac conduction abnormalities. TCAs are metabolized by CYP2D6, and blood levels can become toxic and even lethal when administered with 2D6 inhibitors such as fluoxetine and paroxetine. TCAs include amitriptyline (Elavil) and nortriptyline (Pamelor). Nortriptyline is not as anticholinergic as amitriptyline and is often better tolerated [33].

Monoamine oxidase inhibitors (MAOIs) are first-generation antidepressants used for treatment-resistant depression. MAOIs can cause a life-threatening serotonin syndrome or hypertensive crisis when combined with serotonergic agents or foods containing tyramine, respectively. Antidepressant MAOIs include phenelzine, isocarboxazid, and tranylcypromine. Selegiline (Emsam) is a transdermal patch that requires fewer dietary restrictions than other MAOIs. Non-antidepressant MAOIs include methylene blue [141] and linezolid [142]. MAOIs should not be combined with antidepressants. Oral selegiline at doses therapeutic for Parkinson's disease (10 mg/day or less) is selective for the MAO-B receptor, making it less dangerous than its less selective counterparts. However, serotonin syndrome can occur rarely [143], and the FDA recommends against combining oral selegiline with serotonergic antidepressants [144].

Clinical Pearls

- Depression can negatively affect quality of life and function in patients with neurological disorders. Resolution of depression may reverse these effects.
- A clinical interview is required to diagnose depression. Always consider how recent stressors, medical illness, medications, and substances may be contributing.

- Patients with mild to moderate depression can be treated with psychotherapy or antidepressants. Patients with severe depression should be prescribed antidepressants, with or without psychotherapy.
- Depression severity is determined based upon the patient's degree of impairment.
- An antidepressant may be chosen based upon a desired side-effect profile.
- Escitalopram and sertraline are relatively well-tolerated SSRIs with few drug-drug interactions.
- Venlafaxine, duloxetine, bupropion, mirtazapine, and amitriptyline are non-SSRI antidepressants with unique advantages and liabilities.
- Antidepressants with the least incidence of sexual dysfunction include bupropion, mirtazapine, escitalopram, and duloxetine (in the order from less to more dysfunction).

References

1. Fink P, Hansen MS, Sondergaard L, Frydenberg M. Mental illness in new neurological patients. J Neurol Neurosurg Psychiatry. 2003;74:817–9.
2. Thielscher C, Thielscher S, Kostev K. The risk of developing depression when suffering from neurological diseases. Ger Med Sci. 2013;11:Doc02.
3. Luoni C, Bisulli F, Canevini MP, De Sarro G, Fattore C, Galimberti CA, et al. Determinants of health-related quality of life in pharmacoresistant epilepsy: results from a large multicenter study of consecutively enrolled patients using validated quantitative assessments. Epilepsia. 2011;52(12):2181–91.
4. Fernández-Jiménez E, Arnett P. Impact of neurological impairment, depression, cognitive function and coping on quality of life of people with multiple sclerosis: a relative importance analysis. Mult Scler. 2015;21(11):1468–72.
5. Schrag A. Quality of life and depression in Parkinson's disease. J Neurol Sci. 2006;248(1–2):151–7.
6. Carson AJ, Ringbauer B, Mackenzie L, Warlow C, Sharpe M. Neurological disease, emotional disorder, and disability: they are related: a study of 300 consecutive new referrals to a neurology outpatient department. J Neurol Neurosurg Psychiatry. 2000;68:202–6.
7. Chemerinski E, Robinson RG, Arndt S, Kosier JT. The effect of remission of poststroke depression on activities of daily living in a double-blind randomized treatment study. J Nerv Ment Dis. 2001;189:421–5.
8. DiMatteo RM, Lepper HS, Croghan TW. Depression is a risk factor for noncompliance with medical treatment: meta-analysis of the effects of anxiety and depression on patient adherence. Arch Intern Med. 2000;160:2101–7.
9. Whooley MA, Avins AL, Miranda J, Browner WS. Case-finding instruments for depression. Two questions are as good as many. J Gen Intern Med. 1997;12:439–45.
10. Mohr DC, Hart SL, Julian L, et al. Screening for depression among patients with multiple sclerosis: two questions may be enough. Mult Scler. 2007;13:215–9.
11. Manea L, Gilbody S, Hewitt C, North A, Plummer F, Richardon R, et al. Identifying depression with the PHQ-2: a diagnostic meta-analysis. J Affect Disord. 2016;203:382–95. The sensitivity of the PHQ-2 using a cutoff of 2 in primary care is 0.91
12. Mitchell AJ, Yadagarfar M, Gill J, Stubbs B. Case finding and screening clinical utility of the Patient Health Questionnaire (PHQ-2 and PHQ-9) for depression in primary care: a diagnostic meta-analysis of 40 studies. B J Psychiatry Open. 2016;2:127–38.

13. Topp CW, Ostergaard SD, Songergaard S, Bech P. The WHO-5 well-being index: a systematic review of the literature. Psychother Psychosom. 2015;84:167–76.
14. Wancata J, Alexandrowicz R, Marquart B, Weiss M, Frederich F. The criterion validity of the geriatric depression scale: a systematic review. Acta Psychiatr Scand. 2006;114:398–410. The sensitivity of the GDS-30 is 0.753 and the specificity is 0.770. The sensitivity of the GDS-15 is 0.805 and the specificity is 0.750
15. Chakkamparambil B, Chibnall JT, Graypel EA, Manepalli JN, Bhutto A, Grossberg GT. Development of a brief validated geriatric screening tool: the SLU "AM SAD". Am J Ger Psych. 2015;23(8):780–3. The sensitivity of the AM SAD in this study is 0.75 and the specificity is 0.62
16. Fragoso YD, Adoni T, Anacleto A, da Gama D, Goncalves MVM, Palma da Cunha Matta P, et al. Recommendations on diagnosis and treatment of depression and anxiety in patients with multiple sclerosis. Pract Neurol. 2014;0:1–6. *Recommended reading
17. Marsh L. Depression and Parkinson's disease: current knowledge. Curr Neurol Neurosci Rep. 2013;13(12):409. *Recommended reading
18. Cuijpers P, Smit F, van Straten A. Psychological treatments of subthreshold depression: a meta-analytic review. Acta Psychiatr Scand. 2007;115(6):434–41.
19. American Psychiatric Association. Diagnostic and statistical manual of mental disorders. 5th ed. Arlington: American Psychiatric Association; 2013. p. 168–71.
20. Kriston L, von Wolff A, Westphal A, Hölzel LP, Härter M. Efficacy and acceptability of acute treatments for persistent depressive disorder. Depress Anxiety. 2014;31:621–30.
21. Jobst A, Brakemeier EL, Buchheim A, Caspar F, Cuijpers P, Ebmeier KP, et al. European psychiatric association guidance on psychotherapy in chronic depression across Europe. Eur Psychiatry. 2016;33:18–36.
22. American Psychiatric Association. Diagnostic and statistical manual of mental disorders. 5th ed. Arlington: American Psychiatric Association; 2013. p. 160–8.
23. American Psychiatric Association. Practice guideline for the treatment of patients with major depressive disorder. 3rd ed. Arlington: American Psychiatric Association; 2010.
24. National Institute for Health and Care Excellence (NICE). Depression in adults with a chronic physical health problem: recognition and management. London: NICE; 2009.
25. Fournier JC, RJ DR, Hollon SD, Dimidjian S, Amsterdam JD, Sheldon RC, et al. Antidepressant drug effects and depression severity: a patient-level meta-analysis. JAMA. 2010;303:47–53. The effect size for mild depression was 0.11 and for moderate depression, 0.17
26. Kirsch I, Deacon BJ, Huedo-Medina TB, Scoboria A, Moore TJ, Johnson BT. Initial severity and antidepressant benefits: a meta-analysis of data submitted to the Food and Drug Administration. PLoS Med. 2008;5(2):e45.
27. Vöhringer PA, Ghaemi SN. Solving the antidepressant efficacy question: effect sizes in major depressive disorder. Clin Ther. 2011;33(12):B49–61.
28. Kanner AM. Management of psychiatric and neurological comorbidities in epilepsy. Nat Rev Neurol. 2016;12:106–16.
29. Hawton K, Casanas I, Comabella C, Haw C, Saunders K. Risk factors for suicide in individuals with depression: a systematic review. J Affect Disord. 2013;147(1):17–28.
30. American Psychiatric Association. Guideline III. Assessment of suicide risk. In: Practice guidelines for the psychiatric evaluation of adults, 3rd ed. Arlington: American Psychiatric Association; 2015. http://psychiatryonline.org/doi/pdf/10.1176/appi.books.9780890426760.
31. Lam RW. Onset, time course and trajectories of improvement with antidepressants. Eur Neuropsychopharmacol. 2012;22(Suppl 3):S492–8.
32. Sacchetti E, Conte G, Guarneri L. Are SSRI antidepressants a clinically homogenous class of compounds? Lancet. 1994;344(8915):126–7.
33. Schatzberg A, Debattista C. Manual of clinical psychopharmacology. 8th ed. Arlington: American Psychiatric Publishing; 2015.
34. Lexapro ®(escitalopram oxalate). [package insert from internet]. Irvine: Allergan USA., 2016. [revised Jan 2017; cited 20 Mar 2017]. Available from: http://www.accessdata.fda.gov/drugsatfda_docs/label/2017/021323s047lbl.pdf.

35. Sheeler RD, Ackerman MJ, Richelson E, Nelson TK, Staab JP, Tangalos EG, et al. Considerations on safety concerns about citalopram prescribing. Mayo Clin Proc. 2012;87(11):1042–5.
36. Medicines and Healthcare Products Regulatory Agency (MHRA). Citalopram and escitalopram: QT interval prolongation—new maximum daily dose restrictions (including in elderly patients), contraindications, and warnings. Drug Saf Updat. 2011;5:A1.
37. US Food and Drug Administration. FDA drug safety communication: revised recommendations for Celexa (citalopram hydrobromide) related to a potential for abnormal heart rhythms with high doses. March 8, 2012. Accessed on 1 Jan 2017: http://www.fda.gov/Drugs/DrugSafety/ucm297391.htm.
38. Celexa® (citalopram hydrobromide). [package insert from internet]. St. Louis: Forest Laboratories., July 8, 2014. Accessed on 1 Jan 2017: http://www.accessdata.fda.gov/drugsatfda_docs/label/2014/020822Orig1s046lbl.pdf.
39. Shapiro PA, Lesperance F, Frasure-Smith N, O'Connor CM, Baker B, Jiang JW, et al. An open-label preliminary trial of sertraline for treatment of major depression after acute myocardial infarction (the SADHAT trial). Sertraline Anti-Depressant Heart Attack trial. Am Heart J. 1999;137:1100–6.
40. Zoloft® (sertraline hydrochloride). [package insert from internet]. New York: Pfizer, 2016. [revised Oct 2016; cited 23 Dec 2016]. Available from: http://labeling.pfizer.com/ShowLabeling.aspx?id=517.
41. Aiyer R, Barkin RL, Bhatia A. Treatment of neuropathic pain with venlafaxine: a systematic review. Pain Med. 2016;00:1–14.
42. Joffe H, Guthrie KA, LaCroix AZ, Reed SD, Ensrud KE, Manson JE. Randomized controlled trial of low-dose estradiol and the SNRI venlafaxine for vasomotor symptoms. JAMA Intern Med. 2014;174(7):1058–66.
43. Ozyalcin SN, Talu GK, Kiziltan E, Yucel B, Ertas M, Disci R. The efficacy and safety of venlafaxine in the prophylaxis of migraine. Headache. 2005;45:144–52.
44. Effexor®(venlafaxine hydrochloride tablets). [package insert from internet]. Philadelphia: Wyeth Pharmaceuticals; 2015. [revised Feb 2015; cited 1 Jan 2017.] Available at: http://www.accessdata.fda.gov/drugsatfda_docs/label/2016/020699s106lbl.pdf.
45. Cymbalta® (duloxetine hydrochloride oral capsule, delayed release pellets). [package insert from internet]. Indianapolis: Eli Lilly; 2008. [revised 13 June 2008; cited 1 Jan 2017]. Available at: http://www.accessdata.fda.gov/drugsatfda_docs/label/2008/022148lbl.pdf.
46. Patroneva A, Connolly SM, Fatato P, Pederson R, Jiang Q, Guico-Pabia C, et al. An assessment of drug-drug interactions: the effect of desvenlafaxine and duloxetine on the pharmacokinetics of the CYP2D6 probe desipramine in healthy subjects. Drug Metab Dis. 2008;36:2484–91.
47. Zyban® (bupropion hydrochloride sustained-release tablets). [package insert on the internet]. Research Triangle Park: GlaxoSmithKline; 2016. [revised June 2016; cited 1 Jan 2017]. Available from: http://www.accessdata.fda.gov/drugsatfda_docs/label/2016/020711s044lbl.pdf.
48. Jefferson JW, Pradko JF, Muir KT. Bupropion for major depressive disorder: pharmacokinetic and formulations considerations. Clin Ther. 2005;27:1685–95.
49. Wellbutrin XL® (bupropion hydrochloride extended release tablets). [package insert from internet]. Research Triangle Park: GlaxoSmithKline; 2016. [revised April 2016; cited 12 March 2017]. Available from: http://www.accessdata.fda.gov/drugsatfda_docs/label/2016/018644s050,020358s057lbl.pdf.
50. Croom KF, Perry CM, Plosker GL. Mirtazapine: a review of its use in major depression and other psychiatric disorders. CNS Drugs. 2009;23:427–52.
51. Lind AB, Reis M, Bengtsson F, Johnzier-Perey M, Powell Golay K, Ahlner J, et al. Steady-state concentrations of mirtazapine, N-desmethylmirtazapine, 8-hydroxymirtazapine and their enantiomers in relation to cytochrome P450 2D6 genotype, age and smoking behaviour. Clin Pharmacokinet. 2009;48:63–70.

52. Remeron® (mirtazapine oral tablet). [package insert from internet]. Whitehouse Station: Merck & Co.; 2016. [revised July 2016; cited 12 March 2017]. Available at: http://www.accessdata.fda.gov/drugsatfda_docs/label/2016/020415s030lbl.pdf.
53. Moore RA, Derry S, Aldington D, Cole P, Wiffen PJ. Amitriptyline for neuropathic pain in adults. Cochrane Database Syst Rev. 2015;7:CD008242.
54. Keskinbora K, Aydinli I. A double-blind randomized controlled trial of topiramate and amitriptyline either alone or in combination for the prevention of migraine. Clin Neurol Neurosurg. 2008;110:979–84.
55. Taylor D, Paton C, Kapur S, editors. The Maudsley prescribing guidelines in psychiatry. 12th ed. West Sussex: Wiley; 2015.
56. Sackeim HA, Roose SP, Burt T. Length of antidepressant trials in late-life depression. J Clin Psychopharmacol. 2005;25(4 Supplement 1):S34–7.
57. Judd LL, Schettler PJ, Rush AJ, Coryell WH, Fiedorowicz JG, Solomon DA. A new empirical definition of major depressive episode recovery and its positive impact on future course of illness. J Clin Psychiatry. 2016;77(8):1065–73.
58. Crismon ML, Trivedi M, Pigott TA, Rush AJ, Hirschfeld RM, Kahn DA, et al. The Texas medication algorithm project. Report of the Texas consensus conference panel on medication treatment of major depressive disorder. J Clin Psychiatry. 1999;60:142–56.
59. McGrath PJ, Stewart JW, Petkova E, Quitkin FM, Amsterdam JD, Fawcett J, et al. Predictors of relapse during fluoxetine continuation or maintenance treatment of major depression. J Clin Psychiatry. 2000;61:518–24.
60. Guidi J, Tomba E, Fava GA. The sequential integration of psychotherapy and pharmacotherapy in the treatment of major depressive disorder: a meta-analysis of the sequential model and a critical review of the literature. Am J Psychiatry. 2016;173:128–37.
61. Beshai S, Dobson KS, Bockting CLH, Quigley L. Relapse and recurrent prevention in depression: current research and future prospects. Clin Psychol Rev. 2011;31:1349–60.
62. Qaseem A, Barry M, Kansagara D. Nonpharmacologic versus pharmacologic treatment of adult patients with major depressive disorder: a clinical practice guideline from the American College of Physicians. Ann Intern Med. 2016;164:350–9.
63. Thase ME, Greenhouse JB, Frank E, Reynolds CF, Pilkonis PA, Hurley K, et al. Treatment of major depression with psychotherapy or psychotherapy-pharmacotherapy combinations. Arch Gen Psychiatry. 1997;54:1009–15.
64. Carvalho AF, Sharma MS, Brunoni AR, Vieta E, Fava GA. The safety, tolerability, and risks associated with the use of newer generation antidepressant drugs: a critical review of the literature. Psychother Psychosom. 2016;85:270–88. *Excellent review with free full text available at https://www.karger.com/Article/FullText/447034
65. Beasley CM Jr, Sayler ME, Weiss AM, Potvin JH. Fluoxetine: activating and sedating effects at multiple fixed doses. J Clin Psychopharmacol. 1992;12(5):328–33.
66. Gregorian RS, Golden KA, Bahce A, Goodman C, Kwong WJ, Khan ZM. Antidepressant-induced sexual dysfunction. Ann Pharmacother. 2002;36(10):1577–89.
67. Kikuchi T, Uchida H, Suzuki T, Watanabe K, Kashima H. Patients' attitudes toward side effects of antidepressants: an internet survey. Eur Arch Psychiatry Clin Neurosi. 2011;261:103–9.
68. Clayton AH, Alkis AR, Parikh NB, Votta JB. Sexual dysfunction due to psychotropic medications. Psych Clin North Am. 2016;39(3):427–63. *Helpful overview including physiology and nonpharmacologic approaches
69. Taylor MJ, Rudkin L, Bullemor-Day P, Lubin J, Chukwujekwu C, Hawton K. Strategies for managing sexual dysfunction induced by antidepressant medication. Cochrane Database Syst Rev. 2013;31(5):CD003382.
70. Fava M, Nurnberg HG, Seidman SN, Holloway W, Nicholas S, Tseng L, et al. Efficacy and safety of sildenafil in men with serotonergic antidepressant-associated erectile dysfunction: results from a randomized, double-blind, placebo-controlled trial. J Clin Psychiatry. 2006;67(2):240–6.
71. Nurnberg HG, Hensley PL, Heiman JR, et al. Sildenafil treatment of women with antidepressant-associated sexual dysfunction: a randomized controlled trial. JAMA. 2008;300(4):395–404.

72. Serretti A, Chiesa A. Treatment-emergent sexual dysfunction related to antidepressants: a meta-analysis. J Clin Psychopharmacol. 2009;29(3):259–66.
73. Blumenthal SR, Castro VM, Clements CC, Rosenfield HR, Murphy SN, Fava M, et al. An electronic health records study of long-term weight gain following antidepressant use. JAMA Psychiat. 2014;71(8):889–96.
74. Fava M. Weight gain and antidepressants. J Clin Psychiatry. 2000;61(suppl 1):37–41.
75. Thase ME. Effects of venlafaxine on blood pressure: a meta-analysis of original data from 3744 depressed patients. J Clin Psychiatry. 1998;59(10):502–8.
76. Hawthorne JM, Caley C. Extrapyramidal reactions associated with serotonergic antidepressants. Ann Pharmacoth. 2015;49(10):1136–52.
77. US Food and Drug Administration. FDA proposes new warning about suicidal thinking, behavior, in young adults who take antidepressant medications. [news release] Silver Spring: US Food and Drug Administration, 2007. Accessed 1 Feb 2017 at: http://www.fda.gov/NewsEvents/Newsroom/PressAnnouncements/2007/ucm108905.htm.
78. Ah-kee EY, Egong E, Shafi A, Lim LT, Li Yim JF. A review of drug-induced acute angle closure glaucoma for non-ophthalmologists. Qatar Med J. 2015;6:1–8.
79. Anglin R, Yuan Y, Moayyedi P, Tse F, Armstrong D, Leontiadis GI. Serotonin reuptake inhibitors with concurrent nonsteroidal anti-inflammatory use: a systemic review and meta-analysis. Am J Gastroenterol. 2014;109:811–9. For SSRI use alone, NNH = 3,177 for low-risk patients, NNH = 881 for high-risk patients. For SSRIs and NSAIDs together, NNH = 645 for low-risk patients, NNH = 179 for high-risk patients.
80. Jiang H, Chen H, Hu X, Yu Z, Yang W, Deng M, et al. Use of selective serotonin reuptake inhibitors and risk of upper gastrointestinal bleeding: a systematic review and meta-analysis. Clin Gastroenterol Hepatol. 2015;13:42–50.
81. Targownik LE, Bolton JM, Metge CJ, Leung S, Sareen J. Selective serotonin reuptake inhibitors are associated with a modest increase in the risk of upper gastrointestinal bleeding. Am J Gastroenterol. 2009;104(6):1475–82. https://doi.org/10.1038/ajg.2009.128.
82. Jeong B, Kim S, Kim S, Kim J, Shin I, Yoon J. Use of serotonergic antidepressants in patients undergoing surgery. Psychosomatics. 2014;55:213–20.
83. Buckley N, Dawson AH, Isbister GK. Serotonin syndrome. BMJ. 2014;348:g1626.
84. FDA Alert. Combined use of 5-hydroxytryptamine receptor agonists (triptans), selective serotonin reuptake inhibitors (SSRIs) or selective serotonin-norepinephrine reuptake inhibitors (SNRIs) may result in life-threatening serotonin syndrome. 2006. [cited 29 Jan 2017]. Available from: http://www.fda.gov/Drugs/DrugSafety/PostmarketDrugSafetyInformationforPatientsandProviders/DrugSafetyInformationforHeathcareProfessionals/ucm085845.htm.
85. Evans WR, Tepper SJ, Shapiro RE, Sun-Edelstein C, Tietjen GE. The FDA alert on serotonin syndrome with use of triptans combined with selective serotonin reuptake inhibitors and selective norepinephrine reuptake inhibitors: American Headache Society position paper. Headache. 2010;50:1089–99.
86. De Picker L, Van Den Eede F, Dumont G, Moorkens G, Sabbe BG. Antidepressants and the risk of hyponatremia: a class-by-class review of literature. Psychosomatics. 2014;55(6):536–47.
87. Berber MJ. FINISH: remembering the discontinuation syndrome. Flu-like symptoms, insomnia, nausea, imbalance, sensory disturbances, and hyperarousal (anxiety/agitation). J Clin Psychiatry. 1998;59:255.
88. Tint A, Haddad PM, Anderson IM. The effect of rate of antidepressant tapering on the incidence of discontinuation symptoms: a randomised study. J Psychopharmacol. 2008;22(3):330–2.
89. Ninan PT, Musgnung J, Messig M, Buckley G, Guico-Pabia CJ, Ramey TS. Incidence and timing of taper/posttherapy-emergent adverse events following discontinuation of desvenlafaxine 50 mg/d in patients with major depressive disorder. Prim Care Companion CNS DIsord. 2015;17(1): https://doi.org/10.4088/PCC.14m01715.
90. Schatzberg AF, Blier P, Delgado PL, Fava M, Had-dad PM, Shelton RC. Antidepressant discontinuation syndrome: consensus panel recommendations for clinical management and additional research. J Clin Psychiatry. 2006;67(suppl 4):27–30. [G]

91. Warner CH, Bobo W, Warner C, Reid S, Rachal J. Antidepressant discontinuation syndrome. Am Fam Physician. 2006;74:449–56. 457

92. Kerr MP, Mensah S, Besag F, de Toffol B, Ettinger A, Kanemoto K, et al. International consensus clinical practice statements for the treatment of neuropsychiatric conditions associated with epilepsy. Epilepsia. 2011;52(11):2133–8.

93. Jones JE, Hermann BP, Barry JJ, Gilliam FG, Kanner AM, Meador KJ. Rates and risk factors for suicide, suicidal ideation, and suicide attempts in chronic epilepsy. Epilepsy Behav. 2003;4:S31–8.

94. Christensen J, Vestergaard M, Mortensen PB, Sidenius P, Agerbo E. Epilepsy and the risk of suicide: a population-based case control study. Lancet Neurol. 2007;6:693–8.

95. Alper KR, Schwartz KA, Kols RL, Khan A. Seizure incidence in psychopharmacological clinical trials: an analysis of Food and Drug Administration (FDA) summary basis of approval reports. Biol Psychiatry. 2007;62:345–54.

96. Wellbutrin® (bupropion hydrochloride oral tablet). [package insert from internet]. Research Triangle Park: GlaxoSmithKline; 2016. [revised April 2016; cited 1 Jan 2017]. Available at: http://www.accessdata.fda.gov/drugsatfda_docs/label/2016/018644s050,020358s057lbl.pdf.

97. Spina E, Pisani F, de Leon J. Clinically significant pharmacokinetic drug interactions of antiepileptic drugs with new antidepressants and new antipsychotics. Pharmacol Res. 2016;106:72–86.

98. Spaans E, van den Heuvel MW, Schnabel PG, Peeters P, Chin-Kon-Sung U, Colbers E, et al. Concomitant use of mirtazapine and phenytoin: a drug-drug interactions study in healthy male subjects. Eur J Chn Pharmacol. 2002;58:423–9.

99. Sitsen J, Maris F, Timmer C. Drug-drug interaction studies with mirtazapine and carbamazepine in healthy male subjects. Eur J Drug Metab Pharmacokinet. 2001;26:109–21.

100. Boinpally R, Gad N, Gupta S, Periclou A. Influence of CYP3A4 induction/inhibition on the pharmacokinetics of vilazodone. Clin Ther. 2014;36(11):1638–49.

101. Ketter TA, Jenkins JB, Schroeder DH, Pazzaglia PJ, Marangell LB, George MS, et al. Carbamazepine but not valproate induces bupropion metabolism. J Clin Psychopharmacol. 1995;15:327–33.

102. Gilliam FG, Barry JJ, Hermann BP, Meador KJ, Vahle V, Kanner AM. Rapid detection of major depression in epilepsy: a multicentre study. Lancet Neurol. 2006;5:399–405.

103. Pontone GM, Bakker CC, Chen S, Mari Z, Marsh L, Rabins P, et al. The longitudinal impact of depression on disability in Parkinson disease. Int J Geriatr Psychiatry. 2016;31:458–65.

104. Menza M, Dobkin RD, Marin H, Mark MH, Gara M, Buyske S, et al. The impact of treatment of depression on quality of life, disability and relapse in patients with Parkinson's disease. Move Disord. 2009;24:1325–32.

105. Ravina B, Camicioli R, Como PG, Marsh L, Jankovic J, Weintraub D, et al. The impact of depressive symptoms in early Parkinson disease. Neurology. 2007;69:342–7.

106. Hughes TA, Ross HF, Mindham RH, Spokes EG. Mortality in Parkinson's disease and its association with dementia and depression. Acta Neurol Scand. 2004;110:118–23.

107. Connolly BS, Lang AE. Pharmacological treatment of Parkinson disease: a review. JAMA. 2014;311(16):1670–83.

108. Dyduch A, Załuska M. Depression in Parkinson's disease: the effectiveness and risk of pharmacotherapy. Clin Rev Psychogeriatr. 2015;15:147–53.

109. Barone P, Poewe W, Albrecht S, Debieuvre C, Massey D, Rascol O, et al. Pramipexole for the treatment of depressive symptoms in patients with Parkinson's disease: a randomised, double-blind, placebo-controlled trial. Lancet Neurol. 2010;9(6):573–80.

110. Armento ME, Stanley MA, Marsh L, Kunik ME, York MK, Bush AL, et al. Cognitive behavioral therapy (CBT) for depression and anxiety in Parkinson's disease: a clinical review. J Park Dis. 2012;2:135–51.

111. Schneider CB, Pilhatsch M, Rifati M, Jost WH, Wodarz F, Ebersbach G, et al. Utility of the WHO-Five Well-being Index as a screening tool for depression in Parkinson's disease. Mov Disord. 2010;25:777–83.

112. Chagas MHN, Crippa JAS, Loureiro SR, Hallak JEC, de Meneses-Gaya C, Machado-de-Sousa JP, et al. Validity of the PHQ-2 for the screening of major depression in Parkinson's disease: two questions and one important answer. Aging Ment Health. 2011;7:838–43.

113. Williams JR, Hirsch ES, Anderson K, Bush AL, Goldstein SR, Grill S, et al. A comparison of nine scales to detect depression in Parkinson disease: which scale to use? Neurology. 2012;78:998–1006.

114. Hackett ML, Pickles K. Part I: frequency of depression after stroke: an updated systematic review and meta-analysis of observational studies. Int J Stroke. 2014;9:1017–25.

115. Robinson RG, Jorge RE. Post-stroke depression: a review. Am J Psychiatry. 2016;173:221–31.

116. Kutlubaev MA, Hackett ML. Part II: predictors of depression after stroke and impact of depression on stroke outcome: an updated systematic review of observational studies. Int J Stroke. 2014;9:1026–36.

117. Wei N, Yong W, Li X, et al. Post-stroke depression and lesion location: a systematic review. J Neurol. 2015;262:81–90.

118. Robinson RG, Bolla-Wilson K, Kaplan E, Lipsey JR, Price TR. Depression influences intellectual impairment in stroke patients. Br J Psychiatry. 1986;148:541–7.

119. Bartoli F, Lillia N, Lax A, Crocamo C, Mantero V, Carrà G, et al. Depression after stroke and risk of mortality: a systematic review and meta-analysis. Stroke Res Treat. 2013;862978.

120. Kimura M, Robinson RG, Kosier JT. Treatment of cognitive impairment after poststroke depression: a double-blind treatment trial. Stroke. 2000;31:1482–6.

121. Hackett ML, Anderson CS, House A, Xia J. Interventions for treating depression after stroke. Cochrane Database Syst Rev. 2008; (4):CD003437.

122. Mitchell PH, Veith RC, Becker KJ, Buzaitis A, Cain KC, Fruin M, et al. Brief psychosocial-behavioral intervention with antidepressant reduces poststroke depression significantly more than usual care with antidepressant: living well with stroke: randomized, controlled trial. Stroke. 2009;40:3073–8.

123. Visser MM, Heijenbrok-Kal MH, Van't Spijker A, Lannoo E, JJV B, et al. Problem-solving therapy during outpatient stroke rehabilitation improves coping and health-related quality of life. Stroke. 2016;47:135–42.

124. Towfighi A, Obviagele B, El Husseini N, Hackett ML, Jorge RE, Kissela BM, et al. Poststroke depression: a scientific statement for healthcare professionals from the American Heart Association/American Stroke Association. Stroke. 2017;48:e30–43.

125. Meader N, Moe-Byrne T, Llewellyn A, Mitchell AJ. Screening for post- stroke major depression: a meta-analysis of diagnostic validity studies. J Neurol Neurosurg Psychiatry. 2014;85:198–206.

126. Brown RF, Valpiani EM, Tennant CC, Dunn SM, Sharrock M, Hodgkinson S, et al. Longitudinal assessment of anxiety, depression, and fatigue in people with multiple sclerosis. Psychol Psychother. 2009;82(Part 1):41–56.

127. Arnett PA, Higginson CI, Voss WD, Wright B, Bender WI, Wurst JM, et al. Depressed mood in multiple sclerosis: relationship to capacity-demanding memory and attentional functioning. Neuropsychology. 1999;13:434–46.

128. Tarrants M, Oleen-Burkey M, Castelli-Haley J, et al. The impact of comorbid depression on adherence to therapy for multiple sclerosis. Mult Scler Int. 2011;2011:271321.

129. Stenager EN, Stenager E, Koch-Henrikson N, Brønnum-Hansen H, Hyllested K, Jensen K, et al. Suicide and multiple sclerosis: an epidemiological investigation. J Neurol Neurosurg Psychiatry. 1992;55:542–5.

130. Fiest KM, Walker JR, Bernstein CN, Graff LA, Zarychanski R, Abou-Setta AM, et al. Systematic review and meta-analysis of interventions for depression and anxiety in persons with multiple sclerosis. Mult Scler Relat Disord. 2016;5:12–26.

131. Feinstein A. Multiple sclerosis and depression. Mult Scler J. 2011;17(11):1276–81.

132. Goldman Consensus Group. The Goldman consensus statement on depression in multiple sclerosis. Mult Scler. 2005;11:328–37.

133. Honarmand K, Feinstein A. Validation of the hospital anxiety and depression scale for use with multiple sclerosis patients. Mult Scler. 2009;15:1518–24.

134. Benedict RH, Fishman I, McClellan MM, Bakshi R, Weinstock-Guttman B. Validity of the Beck Depression Inventory-Fast Screen in multiple sclerosis. Mult Scler. 2003;9:393–6.
135. Lowe B, Unutzer J, Callahan CM, Perkins AJ, Kroenke K. Monitoring depression treatment outcomes with the Patient Health Questionnaire-9. Med Care. 2004;42:1194–201.
136. Zimmerman M, Chelminski I, McGlinchey JB, Posternak MA. A clinically useful depression outcome scale. Compr Psychiatry. 2008;49:131–40.
137. Beck AT, Steer RA, Ball R, Ranieri W. Comparison of Beck Depression Inventories -IA and -II in psychiatric outpatients. J Pers Assess. 1996;67(3):588–97.
138. Bjelland I, Dahl AA, Haug TT, Neckelmann D. The validity of the Hospital Anxiety and Depression scale: an updated literature review. J Psychosom Res. 2002;52:69–77.
139. Zimmerman M, Martinez JH, Friedman M, Boerescu DA, Attiullah N, Toba C. How can we use depression severity to guide treatment selection when measures of depression categorize patients differently? J Clin Psychiatry. 2012;73(10):1287–91.
140. Contrave® (bupropion hydrochloride; naltrexone hydrochloride; extended release oral tablet). [package insert from internet] La Jolla: Orexigen Therapeutics; 2014. [cited 9 March 2017]. Available at: http://www.accessdata.fda.gov/drugsatfda_docs/label/2014/200063s000lbl.pdf.
141. Ramsay RR, Dunford C, Gillman PK. Methylene blue and serotonin toxicity: inhibition of monoamine oxidase A (MAO A) confirms a theoretical prediction. Br J Pharmacol. 2007;152(6):946–51.
142. Lawrence KR, Adra M, Gillman PK. Serotonin toxicity associated with the use of linezolid: a review of postmarketing data. Clin Infect Dis. 2006;42:1578–83.
143. Richard IH, Kurlan R, Tanner C, Factor S, Hubble J, Suchowersky O, et al. Serotonin syndrome and the combined use of deprenyl and an antidepressant in Parkinson's disease. Parkinson study group. Neurology. 1997;48(4):1070–7.
144. Eldepryl® (selegeline hydrochloride oral tablet). [package insert from internet]. Tampa: Somerset Pharmaceuticals; 2008. [cited 12 March 2017]. Available at: https://www.access-data.fda.gov/drugsatfda_docs/label/2008/020647s006s007lbl.pdf.
145. Wilens TE, Haight BR, Horrigan JP, Hudziak JJ, Rosenthal NE, Connor DF, et al. Bupropion XL in adults with attention-deficit/hyperactivity disorder: a randomized, placebo-controlled study. Biol Psychiatry. 57(7):793–801.
146. American Psychiatric Association. Practice guideline for the treatment of patients with panic disorder, 2nd. American Psychiatric Association: Washington, DC, 2010. Accessed 1/18/17 at http://psychiatryonline.org/pb/assets/raw/sitewide/practice_guidelines/guidelines/panicdisorder.pdf.
147. Honig A, Kuyper AMG, Schene AH, van Melle JP, de Jonge P, Tulner DM, et al. Treatment of post-myocardial infarction depressive disorder: a randomized, placebo-controlled trial with mirtazapine. Psychosom Med. 2007;69:606–13.
148. Eisenberg MJ, Grandi SM, Gervais A, O'Loughlin J, Paradis G, Rinfret S, et al. Bupropion for smoking cessation in patients hospitalized with acute myocardial infarction: a randomized, placebo-controlled trial. J Am Coll Cardiol. 2013;61:524–32.
149. Grandi SM, Eisenberg MJ, Joseph L, O'Loughlin JO, Paradis G, Filion KB. Cessation treatment adherence and smoking abstinence in patients after acute myocardial infarction. Am Heart J. 2016;173:35–40.
150. Thanacoody HK, Thomas SH. Tricyclic antidepressant poisoning: cardiovascular toxicity. Toxicol Rev. 2005;24:205–14.
151. Cipriani A, La Ferla T, Furukawa TA, Signoretti A, Nakagawa A, Churchill R, et al. Sertraline versus other antidepressive agents for depression. Cochrane Database Syst Rev. 2010;(4):CD006117.
152. Smitherman TA, Walters AB, Maizels M, Penzien DB. The use of antidepressants for headache prophylaxis. CNS Neurosci Ther. 2011;5:462–9.
153. Voican CS, Corruble E, Naveau S, Perlemuter G. Antidepressant-induced liver injury: a review for clinicians. Am J Psychiatry. 2014;171:404–15.
154. Watanabe N, Omori IM, Nakagawa A, Cipriani A, Barbui C, Churchill R, et al. Mirtazapine versus other antidepressive agents for depression. Cochrane Database Syst Rev. 2011; CD006528.

155. Nieuwstraten CE, Dolovich LR. Bupropion versus selective serotonin-reuptake inhibitors for treatment of depression. Ann Pharmacother. 2001;35(12):1608–13.
156. Kerr GW, McGuffie AC, Wilkie S. Tricyclic antidepressant overdose: a review. Emerg Med J. 2001;18(4):236–41.
157. Marks DM, Park MH, Ham BJ, Han C, Patkar AA, Masand PS, et al. Paroxetine: safety and tolerability issues. Expert Opin Drug Saf. 2008;7(6):783–94.
158. Patel K, Allen S, Haque M, Angelescu I, Baumeister D, Tracy DK. Bupropion: a systematic review and meta-analysis of effectiveness as an antidepressant. Ther Adv Psychopharmacol. 2016;6(2):99–144.
159. Gartlehner G, Gaynes B, Hansen RA, Thieda P, DeVeaugh-Geiss A, Krebs EE, et al. Comparative benefits and harms of second-generation antidepressants: background paper for the American college of physicians. Ann Int Med. 2008;149(10):734–50.
160. Clayton A, Kornstein S, Prakash A, Mallinckrodt C, Wohlreich M. Changes in sexual functioning associated with duloxetine, escitalopram, and placebo in the treatment of patients with major depressive disorder. J Sex Med. 2007;4:917–29.
161. Jacobsen PL, Mahableshwarkar AR, Palo WA, Chen Y, Dragheim M, Clayton AH. Treatment-emergent sexual dysfunction in randomized trials of vortioxetine for major depressive disorder or generalized anxiety disorder: a pooled analysis. CNS Spect. 2016;21(5):367–78.
162. Clayton AH, Kennedy SH, Edwards JB, Gallipoli S, Reed CR. The effect of vilazodone on sexual function during the treatment of major depressive disorder. J Sex Med. 2013;10(10):2465–76.
163. Fetzima® (levomilnacipran extended-release oral capsule). [package insert from internet]. Irvine: Allergan USA; 2016. [cited 19 Nov 2017]. Available at: https://www.accessdata.fda.gov/drugsatfda_docs/label/2017/204168s004lbl.pdf.
164. Viibryd® (vilazodone hydrochloride oral tablet). [package insert from internet]. Irvine: Allergan USA; 2017. [cited 19 Nov 2017]. Available at: https://www.accessdata.fda.gov/drugsatfda_docs/label/2017/022567s020lbl.pdf.

Chapter 5
Anxiolytics

David A. Beck and Christine L. Beck

Anxiety will frequently be encountered in the clinical setting as the prevalence in the general population is approximately 2% [1], while in the elderly, the prevalence range is between 10% and 20% [2]. This makes anxiety disorders more common in the elderly than either dementia or major depressive disorder [2]. In the healthcare setting, there is an even greater presence of anxiety disorders. Anxiety disorders are associated with an increased risk of depression, the perception of worse physical or mental health compared to peers, an increased use of healthcare resources as well as a greater number of comorbidities. These contribute to a lower quality of life [3]. Other studies of the general population found decreased role functioning at work and in family, in addition to decreased quality of life for people with generalized anxiety disorder (GAD) [4]. Finally, there may be physiological effects as late-life GAD is associated with increased risk of stroke and other cardiovascular diseases [5, 6].

The relationship between anxiety and dementia is complex. For some patients, it should be noted anxiety may be a harbinger of dementia, partially because of patients being aware of their difficulties [7]. Anxiety increases the risk of progression of mild cognitive impairment (MCI) to Alzheimer's disease [8]. There are other anxiety disorders; however, the focus here will be on GAD and panic disorder. As can be seen from Table 5.1, rates of anxiety are high in many neurological conditions. Thus, there is a paramount need to understand the available treatment options. As the following case history demonstrates, anxiety is often seen in the setting of another illness, making management even more difficult.

D. A. Beck, MD (✉)
Departments of Psychiatry and Behavioral Neuroscience and Internal Medicine,
Saint Louis University School of Medicine, St. Louis, Missouri, USA
e-mail: david.beck@health.slu.edu

C. L. Beck, RN, BSN, FNP Candidate 2019
Maryville University, St. Louis, MO, USA

© Springer International Publishing AG, part of Springer Nature 2018
G. T. Grossberg, L. J. Kinsella (eds.), *Clinical Psychopharmacology for Neurologists*, https://doi.org/10.1007/978-3-319-74604-3_5

Table 5.1 Rates of anxiety in neurological conditions

Neurological condition	Rates of anxiety	References
Seizure disorders	Panic disorder: 5.7–70%	[9]
	GAD: 9.1–39%	
Multiple sclerosis	Pooled mean prevalence of anxiety: 22.1%	[10]
Migraine headaches	GAD: 21.9%	[11]
Strokes	10-year prevalence of anxiety: 32–38%	[12]
Parkinson's disease	Anxiety in early, drug naïve Parkinson's patients: 15.8%	[13]
Major neurocognitive disorder, Alzheimer's type	Pooled prevalence of anxiety: 39%	[14]
Major neurocognitive disorder, vascular type	Anxiety: 28%	[15]

Case Study

The patient is a 67-year-old married, Caucasian, man, retired physician. He had severe Parkinson's disease requiring placement of a deep brain stimulator. He had an anxiety attack at the time of placement of the deep brain stimulator, which he described as psychological torture. At his first clinic visit, he described feeling antsy, on edge, and tense which worsened as the day went on. He also had a persistent low-level anxiety. Distraction would help. He reported feeling anxious about a quarter of the time. He was worried about falling and had fallen two times in the week prior to the appointment. Crowds bothered him as he worried about a need to stop quickly. He had sleep apnea but was compliant with CPAP and described his sleep as fine. He reported to having power naps in the afternoon though stated it did not help his energy. Appetite was not changed, but he was much less active and therefore had gained a lot of weight. He reported no symptoms of depression. He did report violent dreams which he acted on. He denied feeling restless. His muscles would become tense with activity. Alcohol use was one to two drinks per week, and there was no history of substance misuse.

Significant medications were carbidopa-levodopa 25–250 1½ tablets at 6 am and 1 tablet QID and pramipexole 1.5 mg TID. Clonazepam 0.5 mg BID as needed was added at the first clinic visit.

He was involved in an intensive occupational therapy program to prevent falls so felt he did not have time to participate in psychotherapy. Instead, he was encouraged to engage in exercise, yoga, and massage.

At a 1 month follow-up, he had taken only one dose of clonazepam and felt better within 20–30 min. He was pleased with his status, and no changes were made. Two months later, he had used only 4.5 tablets of the clonazepam, all used in the afternoon or evening. He also admitted to taking ½ tablet with alcohol and becoming very confused. He reported feeling restless several times per day. However, he requested no medication changes.

Case Points

Anxiety symptoms occur in 5–60% of Parkinson's patients [16]. Most frequently seen are GAD, panic disorder, and social phobia [17, 18]. Interestingly, an anxiety disorder may occur long before the motor symptoms of Parkinson's are evident [19]. Additionally, anxiety disorders can easily lead to social withdrawal.

Patients frequently present with features of both GAD and panic disorder and rarely fulfill the complete *Diagnostic and Statistical Manual of Mental Disorders 5th Edition* (DSM-5) [20] criteria for either diagnosis.

Although clonazepam is often not a first-line agent, it did produce an adequate response for the patient. With such intermittent and mild symptoms, it did not make sense to place the patient on a scheduled medication that could lead to increased falls and other side effects.

Evaluation

While there are evidence psychotherapies, especially cognitive behavioral therapy (CBT) or medications can be used to treat anxiety disorders, this chapter focuses only on medication management. Some patients with GAD do not respond well to medications for reasons which will be discussed later. In a 2011 review, 25–40% of patients did not respond to existing medications in clinical trials [21].

The first step begins with evaluation. The evaluation starts with the patient interview. It is necessary to determine if the patient has panic disorder symptoms or GAD symptoms. The key feature of panic disorder is the abrupt onset of fear with at least four co-occurring symptoms. The essence of GAD is persistent worry with at least three symptoms over a period of 6 months. Risk of suicide can be increased in anxiety patients, so suicidality should be assessed.

For GAD, the symptoms must cause significant distress or impairment in role functioning. For both GAD and panic disorder, the symptoms should not be due to any medications, illegal drugs, or underlying medical illnesses. Additionally, neither of these should be better explained by the presence of another mental disorder.

It is important to question the patient or family about a multitude of other physical conditions which can lead to anxiety. Neurological patients, especially those with communication difficulties, may appear anxious due to restlessness from elimination difficulties such as constipation or incontinence. Those with aphasia may be angry or anxious due to frustration of inability to make themselves be understood. Pain can make patients hypermobile and thus appear anxious.

A careful review of medications is imperative. Several classes of medications can provoke an anxiety condition or unmask an underlying anxiety disorder (Table 5.2). If possible, gradually taper and discontinue any medications which may be contributing to the anxiety symptoms.

Table 5.2 Medications associated with anxiety symptoms

Medication class	Examples	Anxiety prevalence	Comments	Major metabolic pathways
Neurologic				
	Carbidopa-levodopa	Anxiety 2–8%		
	Ropinirole	Anxiety 2–6% in advanced Parkinson's when used with levodopa		CYP1A2
	Pramipexole	Not listed as significant	May worsen restless leg syndrome in 10–12%; akathisia 2–3%	
	Phenobarbital		Agitation and anxiety present but frequency not defined	CYP2C9
	Phenytoin	Not defined		CYP2C19 CYP2C9
	Levetiracetam		>10% behavioral problems which includes anxiety, restlessness, and irritability	
	Rivastigmine	Transdermal: agitation 1–4%	Oral: restlessness 1–3%; nonlinear pharmacokinetics at doses >3 mg BID	
		Oral: anxiety 1–5%		
	Memantine	XR formulation: anxiety 4%		
Psychiatric				
	Bupropion	Anxiety 3–8%	Agitation 2–32%	CYP2B6
	Haloperidol		Frequency not defined	CYP3A4
	Aripiprazole	Anxiety 17%	Akathisia 2–25%; agitation 19%	CYP2D6 CYP3A4
Stimulants				
	Methylphenidate	Anxiety 8%	Irritability 6–11%; restlessness 3%	
	Modafinil	Anxiety 5%; dose related	Nervousness 7%; agitation 1%; hyperkinesia 1%	CYP3A4
	Caffeine		Agitation and restlessness, appears serum concentration related	CYP1A2
Sedative				
	Alprazolam		Irritability 33%; akathisia 2%	CYP3A4

(continued)

Table 5.2 (continued)

Medication class	Examples	Anxiety prevalence	Comments	Major metabolic pathways
Cardiovascular				
	Digitalis	Frequency not defined		CYP3A4
	Amiodarone		Tremor up to 40%	CYP3A4 CYP2C8
	Clonidine		Irritability 5–9%; nervousness 1–3%	
Endocrine				
	Levothyroxine	Frequency not defined	Nervousness, irritability frequency not defined	
	Testosterone	Frequency not defined	Irritability 2%; aggression 1%	
	Conjugated estrogen	Anxiety 6%		CYP1A2 CYP3A4
	Tamoxifen	Anxiety 6%	Insomnia 9%	CYP2D6 CYP2C9 CYP3A4
Respiratory				
	Albuterol	Anxiety <3%	Nervousness 4–15%	
	Theophylline	Frequency not defined		CYP1A2
	Diphenhydramine		Frequency of excitement, nervousness, restlessness not defined	CYP2D6
	Pseudoephedrine		Frequency of CNS stimulation, excitability, nervousness not defined	
Analgesics				
	Celecoxib	Anxiety <2%		CYP2C9
	Tramadol	Anxiety up to 5%	CNS stimulation 7–14%; agitation and restless up to 5%	CYP2D6 CYP3A4
	Oxycodone	Anxiety 1–5%	Irritability 1–5%	CYP3A4
Antispasmodics				
	Baclofen	Anxiety <1%	Agitation and tremor up to 1%	
	Cyclobenzaprine	Anxiety <1%	Irritability 1–3%	CYP1A2 CYP2D6 CYP3A4
	Oxybutynin		Restlessness and irritability not defined	
Gastrointestinal				
	Metoclopramide	Not significant	Restless in approximately 10% and rare akathisia	

Data from online.lexi.com accessed 12/20/16 and 2/14/17

As can be seen from the above table, many medications produce anxiety or symptoms that can easily be mistaken for anxiety. Akathisia is easily mistaken for anxiety with its sense of inner restlessness; however, it does not have the psychological features of anxiety, such as fear and worry. Irritability is also a symptom that is easy to mistake for anxiety. With it though, you will see an angry affect versus a fearful affect. Major metabolic pathways were included to emphasize the importance of being aware that anxiety may arise when a medication is added to an already complex medication regimen. An unexpected medication may produce anxiety by inhibiting the metabolism of one of the above agents and raising their blood level. Particular attention should be paid to medications for Parkinson's disease; due to their dopaminergic effects, they can be quite activating and cause patients to be anxious. Levetiracetam can produce anxiety symptoms as well.

Obtain lab work to ensure an undetected medical condition is not evoking the anxiety. Labs such as CBC, electrolyte levels, thyroid-stimulating hormone level, and blood glucose levels are all needed for a complete evaluation. Anemia can lead to anxiety symptoms, especially if hemoglobin is less than 10. Thyrotoxicosis is a classical condition leading to anxiety. In addition, anyone with hypoxia may be anxious, and the hypoxia may be the result of respiratory insufficiency from the underlying neurological condition. Adjust treatment plans to treat any newly discovered underlying illness.

The use of an anxiety scale to document baseline severity and treatment response is also recommended. It is best to find a scale that is not cumbersome to work with and applies to the patient's condition.

Anxiety Assessment Instruments

There are numerous anxiety scales with the clinical setting determining which scale is used. Each scale has its own unique focus and advantages/disadvantages. The challenge of most scales is its use in patients with physical illnesses, like the Parkinson's patient of the case study. In fact, anxiety scales have been criticized as not being particularly useful in Parkinson's disease [22]. The GAD committee for DSM-5 recommended using the generalized anxiety disorder 7 (GAD-7) as a screening tool [23]. Finally, although these scales are trying to measure anxiety, it is difficult to differentiate between anxiety and depression. This is only a brief overview of commonly used scales.

GAD-7

The GAD-7 is a valid tool to test for anxiety in both clinical and research settings [24]. In the GAD-7 individuals rate how often they experienced a symptom during the previous 2 weeks. The response ranges from "not at all" (0), "several days" (1), "more than half the days" (2), and "nearly every day" (3). A score of 10 gives acceptable sensitivity and specificity for GAD. GAD-7 was developed for ease of testing [24].

The Hospital Anxiety and Depression Scale (HADS)

The Hospital Anxiety and Depression Scale (HADS) is also composed of seven items. The focus of the HADS is for outpatients age 16–65 years old. Questions are directed at how individuals feel at the current moment, based on a four-point scale for each answer. Total scores range from 0 to 21. Less than 7 is normal, 8–10 is mild anxiety, 11–14 is moderate anxiety, and 12–21 is severe anxiety. A score of greater than 9 is considered positive for significant anxiety. This can either be a self-administered test or given by an interviewer. The HADS has been shown to have high reliability, validity, and sensitivity. The advantage is the brevity and ease of testing. The major disadvantage is the decrease in validity in the elderly population [25].

Zung Self-Rating Anxiety Scale

The Zung Self-Rating Anxiety Scale was originally developed by WK Zung. This is a self-administered test composed of 20 questions. Each question is on a four-point scale. Individuals answer each question with an answer ranging from a little of the time to most of the time with corresponding numerical scores from 1 to 4. Scores below 45 indicate norm, 45–59 is minimal to moderate anxiety, 60–74 is moderate to severe anxiety, and greater than 75 is extreme anxiety. The advantage of the Zung is the fact it is a self-administrated test, therefore, decreasing the bias of administration [26].

State-Trait Anxiety Inventory (STAI)

The State-Trait Anxiety Inventory (STAI) is another self-reported test. There are versions for both children and adults. There are two subscales; one scale evaluates the individual in their current state (S-anxiety), while the trait anxiety (T-anxiety) takes into account the general state one feels. Unlike the previous tests, the STAI is a much longer test made up of 40 items, 20 items of S-anxiety and 20 items of T-anxiety. S-anxiety items are scored for feelings at the current moment from "not at all" (1) to "very much" (4). The T-anxiety scores for the frequency of feelings scored from "almost never" (1) to "almost always" (4). A higher score suggests a greater degree of anxiety. A score of 39–40 indicates significant anxiety in the S-anxiety scale. The STAI has poor validity at differentiating between anxiety and depression; this is one of the greatest disadvantages to this test. The STAI has been well researched and has been used extensively in generalized anxiety disorder [25].

Beck Anxiety Inventory (BAI)

The Beck Anxiety Inventory (BAI) is also a self-reported scale. Similar to previous scales, individuals rate symptoms on a four-point scale from "not at all" (0) to "severely" (3). The individual answers a total of 21 items as they have experienced in the previous week. Scores are from 0 to 63. Less than 9 is clinically not significant, 10–18 indicates mild to moderate anxiety, 19–29 indicates moderate to severe anxiety, and 30 and above are indicative of severe anxiety. Due to the focus on somatic symptoms, the BAI is effective with older adults. A possible drawback of using this scale is the fact it is copyright protected [25].

Geriatric Anxiety Inventory

The Geriatric Anxiety Inventory is a 20-item self-report scale, and responses are simply yes or no. One point is scored for each positive response. A cutoff point of 10/11 produces acceptable specificity and sensitivity for GAD. The advantage of this scale is less response options make it more user friendly [27]. The Geriatric Anxiety Inventory has been validated in Parkinson's patients [28].

Medication Management

General Guidelines

Anxiety patients require much education and support to provide for a successful medication trial. Patients with anxiety disorders are sensitive to medications and are vigilant of bodily sensations, which they tend to label as side effects. The patient should be warned that one side effect at the beginning of treatment, especially SSRIs, is a short-term increase of anxiety. Due to this, the provider might want to consider adding a benzodiazepine for a short period. One additional benefit of using BZDs is improvement in sleep. Extensive education on side effects is one key to success of medication management. Patients need to be forewarned by the provider of the common side effects as there is a tendency of these patients to develop any side effect listed on the pharmacy information sheets. Assuring the patient of your availability and willingness to work with them through the side effects may improve medication adherence.

For patients who do not respond to medication therapy, the clinician should first consider nonadherence to treatment. Again, it cannot be overemphasized that anxiety patients are very sensitive to the side effects of medications and they are very sensitive to bodily sensations which they frequently attribute to medication side effects. Commonly, they will have adjusted their medication dosage downward in between appointments. Additional considerations for nonresponse include substance abuse, underlying undiagnosed medical condition, personality disorder, inadequate dose, or simply having chosen the wrong medication.

Medication options for the treatment of anxiety include selective serotonin reuptake inhibitors (SSRIs), serotonin/norepinephrine reuptake inhibitors (SNRIs), buspirone, and benzodiazepines. Agents are chosen based primarily on patient factors. Considerations include success of past treatments for the patient, response of family members, and history of substance abuse. Because of addictive potential, benzodiazepines should be avoided in those with any history of substance abuse, especially alcohol. The most recent treatment guidelines for GAD indicate SSRIs and SNRIs may have similar efficacy [29].

An additional factor to heavily weigh is the patient's age. With medication management in the elderly, there are two key points. The first is to gradually decrease medications with anxiety-causing properties. The second is the adage of "start low and go slow." In the geriatric population, the beginning dose should be ¼ to ½ the dose of an adult. Additionally, as the dose is being increased, the increments should remain ¼ to ½ of a dose increase for a healthy, younger adult.

It is best to see patients every 1–2 weeks when starting medications such as the SSRIs or SNRIs. Doses should be increased at each visit if the patient is tolerating adequately. The goal would be to reach the target dose in about 4 weeks. Of note, patients will frequently need higher doses of medication to treat anxiety than what would be used for depression. If a patient has no response after about 2 weeks at a good therapeutic dose, the practitioner should consider changing to an alternate agent. If there is only a partial response at about 2 weeks, then consider adding a medication to augment the original agent. Although the focus here is on medication interventions, psychotherapy can be a very useful augmentation strategy or primary treatment, especially if the patient is exquisitely sensitive to medications. If the patient does not respond to the above in about 6 weeks, then consider a referral to a psychiatrist (APA guidelines). A major problem is that up to half of the patients do not have an adequate response to medications [30]. Therefore, these techniques may need to be frequently invoked. Figure 5.1 presents the approach to GAD. Figure 5.2 presents the approach to panic disorder.

It is recommended that medications be continued for at least a year to provide an opportunity to achieve remission [23]. Medications for anxiety should always be tapered to prevent withdrawal symptoms or recurrence, unless there is a compelling medical reason to not taper. When considering a taper of medications, take into account the severity of the patient's presenting symptoms, how long they have been stable, current stressors, and their wishes regarding a taper. When a decision is made to taper therapy, it should be done slowly over 3–4 months (APA guidelines).

Selective Serotonin Reuptake Inhibitors

Some of the most common medicines used to manage anxiety disorders are the serotonin reuptake inhibitors (SSRIs). In general, the SSRIs are well tolerated; however, there is moderate risk of gastrointestinal side effects, which are primarily decreased appetite and nausea at the start of treatment. It needs to be noted that SSRIs may cause GI/other bleeding [31]. Insomnia can be a major symptom of

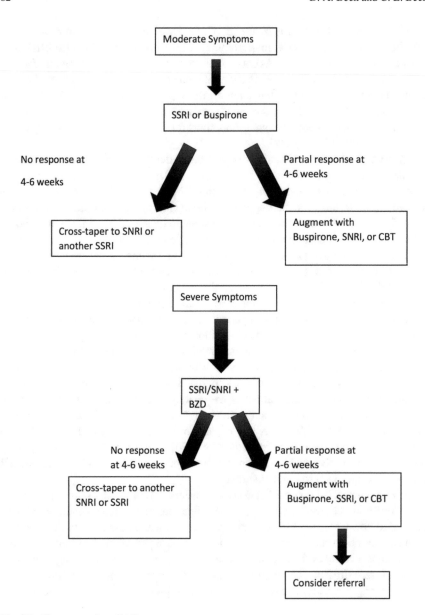

Fig. 5.1 The approach to GAD

GAD. In fact, one study showed that treating the insomnia specifically with hypno-sis improved the response [32].

A meta-analysis looking at panic disorder found citalopram, sertraline, parox-etine, fluoxetine, and venlafaxine effective for panic symptoms: citalopram the least effective, venlafaxine the most effective, and the other three being of intermediate effectiveness. For anxiety symptoms in general, the rank order of effectiveness was

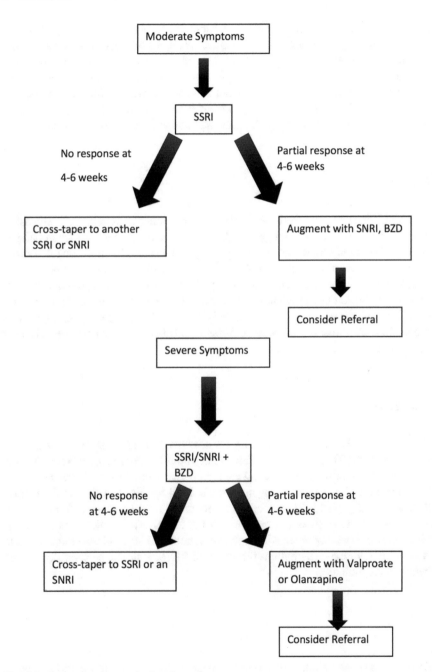

Fig. 5.2 The approach to panic disorder

paroxetine, fluoxetine, fluvoxamine, citalopram, venlafaxine, and mirtazapine. Based on having newer options, monoamine oxidase inhibitors (MAOIs) and tricyclic antidepressants (TCAs) should not be used as first-line therapy, and their use should be limited, so they will not be discussed further here. Fluoxetine may be more effective than other SSRIs in patients with a shorter duration of illness. The effectiveness of paroxetine and venlafaxine may increase over time [33]. The specifics of individual agents will now be discussed and are summarized in Table 5.3.

Fluoxetine

Fluoxetine dose range is from 10 to 80 mg daily. It tends to be relatively well tolerated and has a half-life in a range of 7 days, which may be an advantage in patients who are marginally adherent. It has significant CYP2D6 inhibition such that drug-drug interactions may be problematic. A feature relatively unique to fluoxetine is long term; it can be associated with an apathy syndrome. This syndrome may be particularly difficult to assess in neurological patients, some of whom tend to suffer from lack of motivation from the underlying neurological condition. There is a preparation of fluoxetine for weekly dosage, so this may be even more helpful if medication adherence is an issue.

Paroxetine

Paroxetine can be particularly helpful for selected patients. Like fluoxetine, it has significant CYP2D6 inhibition, so it may have multiple drug-drug interactions. It is associated with more sedation and weight gain than other SSRIs. There are no data to indicate that doses over 20 mg are more helpful for GAD. Although the recommended starting dose is 10 mg, clinically it can be useful to start at 5 mg or even 2.5 mg to ease side effect burden. Since it has sedative properties, it is best to be given after the evening meal. Although paroxetine's half-life is in the range of 24 h, it has more withdrawal symptoms than other SSRIs, so it should be carefully tapered before discontinuation.

Sertraline

Sertraline has been studied in multiple anxiety disorders and has a wide range of FDA indications for anxiety disorders. It is administered in the morning. Drug-drug interactions seem to be less than with some of the other SSRIs. A notable side effect of sertraline is diarrhea upon initiation of treatment. This information needs to be conveyed by the prescriber. Although guidelines are to start at 25 mg daily, frequently, older patients tolerate sertraline better if started at 12.5 mg daily.

Table 5.3 Medications for anxiety disorders

Class	Medication	FDA indication	Dose range	Positives	Negatives
SSRIs					
	Fluoxetine	Yes panic disorder; no GAD	10–60 mg daily; may increase by 10 mg/week	Long half-life so better for minimally compliant patients	Multiple drug-drug interactions
	Paroxetine	GAD and panic disorder	10–60 mg daily; increase dosage weekly	May be more effective than other meds	Drug-drug interactions
	Fluvoxamine	Obsessive Compulsive Disorder, Social Phobia	25–200 mg daily; increase by 25 mg weekly		Drug-drug interactions; wide dose range
	Sertraline	Yes panic disorder; no GAD	25–200 mg daily; may increase by 25 mg weekly	Fewer drug-drug interactions than other SSRIs	Wide dose range
	Citalopram	Not labeled for any anxiety disorders but used off-label	10–40 mg daily; increase by 10 mg weekly	Few drug- drug interactions; relatively less GI upset	Questionable QT prolongation at doses >20 mg
	Escitalopram	Yes GAD; no panic disorder	10–20 mg daily; start at 10 mg and increase to 20 mg in 1 week	Narrow dose range; few drug-drug interactions; minimal GI upset	Possible QT prolongation
SNRIs					
	Venlafaxine	GAD and panic disorder but only ER formulation	ER 37.5–225 mg daily; may increase by 37.5 mg or 75 mg weekly	Can use in Parkinson's disease; few drug-drug interactions	May increase diastolic blood pressure
	Duloxetine	GAD only	60–120 mg daily; increase by 30 mg weekly	Multiple indications	Drug-drug interactions
Other antidepressants					
	Mirtazapine	None	15–45 mg at bedtime; increase by 15 mg every 1–2 weeks	No abuse potential; helps sleep; may quickly alleviate insomnia	Not indicated; sedation; weight gain
	Vilazodone	None	10–40 mg daily; increase by 10 mg weekly	Narrow dose range	Cost
	Vortioxetine	None	10–20 mg daily	No dose adjustment needed for geriatric or renal patients	Cost

(continued)

Table 5.3 (continued)

Class	Medication	FDA indication	Dose range	Positives	Negatives
Benzodiazepines					
	Clonazepam	Panic disorder	0.25–4 mg BID maximum dosage; increase by 0.25 mg q 3 days	Multiple uses	Long half-life; may accumulate
	Lorazepam	Anxiety disorders	1 mg BID to TID maximum dosage 10 mg/day	Multiple uses	Wide dose range
	Alprazolam	GAD and panic disorder	0.25–0.5 mg TID to maximum of 4 mg/day; may increase 0.25–0.5 mg every 4 days	Quickly effective	Short half-life, so patients may withdraw before next dose
			Panic: 5–6 mg/day-10 mg/day		
Antihistamine					
	Hydroxyzine	Anxiety	50–100 mg QID	May be used as needed; nonaddictive; older drug so inexpensive	Increase confusion; paradoxical reactions
Non-benzodiazepine anxiolytic					
	Buspirone	GAD	7.5–30 mg BID; increase every 3 days by 2.5 mg	Low side effect profile; No abuse potential	Effects may be delayed; wide dose range
Anticonvulsants					
	Gabapentin	None	300 mg daily to maximum 3600 mg daily; increase as tolerated	No hepatic metabolism	Needs adjustment for renal impairment
	Pregabalin	None (GAD in Europe)	75 mg BID to maximum 300 mg BID; increase weekly	No hepatic metabolism	Abuse potential
Antipsychotics					
	Quetiapine XR	None	50–300 mg at bedtime; increase by 50 mg every 3 days	Wide range of use	Weight gain; black box warning; QT prolongation

Data from online.lexi.com accessed 12/20/16 and 2/14/17

Citalopram

Citalopram tends to be very well tolerated with few drug-drug interactions. It, however, should be avoided in those with certain cardiac disorders and has been associated with QT prolongation and sudden death. Dosages of citalopram and escitalopram have been capped for those 60 and older. These recommendations have been somewhat controversial [34]. Although the recommended starting dose is 10 mg daily, there tends to be better tolerance when starting at 5 mg daily.

Escitalopram

Escitalopram is chemically closely related to citalopram. Although it does not have FDA approval for panic disorder, the American Psychiatric Association (APA) guidelines include the use of citalopram and escitalopram for panic disorder (APA guidelines).

Fluvoxamine

Fluvoxamine is included in the APA guidelines for treatment of panic disorder. This medication can be sedating, so it is best to give it after the evening meal. Clinically it is less familiar to most practitioners as it is not indicated for depression.

Serotonin/Norepinephrine Reuptake Inhibitors

In the Parkinson's patient, a serotonin/norepinephrine reuptake inhibitor (SNRI) may be a preferred agent as the SSRIs have the potential to decrease dopamine transmission in the brain. The most commonly used SNRI is venlafaxine. Duloxetine will also be discussed.

Venlafaxine

Venlafaxine was the first SNRI to be FDA approved. It has a reputation of more quickly alleviating anxiety than the SSRIs. It is relatively well tolerated. It like the SSRIs can produce significant GI side effects. It does have the potential to raise diastolic blood pressure, especially at higher doses. There is some evidence that venlafaxine may help with diabetic neuropathic pain [35], so it may be a good choice in those with anxiety and neuropathic pain. It has two formulations, immediate release (IR) and extended release (ER). Extended release tends to be better tolerated with less GI upset. A major problem with venlafaxine IR is the short half-life such that patients may go into withdrawal with increased anxiety and flu-like symptoms prior to the next dose. Even though the ER is generic, some insurances will require a prior authorization. Only the ER formulation has been studied and approved for use in anxiety disorders.

Duloxetine

Duloxetine is an additional SNRI and has an indication for GAD. It has a wide range of indications including depression, neuropathic pain, musculoskeletal pain, and fibromyalgia. It may be a particularly attractive medication for patients with any of those disorders. Unlike venlafaxine, it has no or minimal effect on blood pressure. About one-third of the patients given duloxetine experience sedation. It may be best to start by giving a dose after the evening meal. GI upset can occur so it should be given after meals; however, it may produce less GI side effects than venlafaxine. The major problem with duloxetine is profound inhibition of CYP2D6. This inhibition can lead to drug-drug interactions, thus should not be given with SSRIs. Like venlafaxine, duloxetine has efficacy in diabetic neuropathy [35]. This is a medication that might best be started at 30 mg in the evening. Additionally, it should be used with caution in patients with renal insufficiency. Two newer SNRIs are desvenlafaxine and levomilnacipran although neither has an indication for use in anxiety disorders.

Other Antidepressants

Mirtazapine

Mirtazapine is not formally indicated for any anxiety disorders. However, a relatively recent review found evidence for its effectiveness in panic disorder [36]. Clinically the authors have seen improvements in GAD as well. It may be particularly useful for anxiety-associated insomnia. Anxiety patients will commonly complain of GI upset. Mirtazapine could be a good choice for those patients, as it is associated with less GI upset than SSRIs or SNRIs. Some patients may respond to doses as low as 7.5 mg at bedtime. Theoretically, patients should have less sedation as the dose is increased; however, that is not always seen. Unfortunately, it tends to produce weight gain making it not a good choice for those with diabetes or other metabolic disorders.

Vilazodone

Vilazodone is an SSRI in addition to a 5-HT1A receptor agonist, approved for major depression. Doses of 20–40 mg daily have been shown to be effective for the anxiety symptoms of GAD but not the associated disability. The most frequent side effects were GI related, nausea, and diarrhea [37]. It has extensive liver metabolism and a long half-life. It does not have an indication for anxiety disorders. With its relatively tight dose range and ability to be titrated weekly, it can quickly reach a maximum therapeutic dose. Vilazodone should be taken after eating to both decrease its GI side effects and improve its absorption. It also has less sexual dysfunction compared to either the SSRIs or SNRIs.

Vortioxetine

A meta-analysis of vortioxetine in the treatment of GAD concluded its effects were inconsistent. Only four studies were included. It did separate from placebo in those with more severe anxiety. So, this would be an alternative medication; however, the evidence for it is weak [38]. In a head-to-head trial with duloxetine and placebo, duloxetine separated from placebo, and there was only a weak signal for efficacy of vortioxetine 10 mg daily. Vortioxetine, however, was well tolerated [3]. It has a long half-life and is metabolized by the liver. This medication also has a very narrow dose range and can quickly be titrated so can reach maximum dosage within 2 weeks. In CYP2D6 poor metabolizers, its maximum dose is 10 mg per day. In clinical practice, the dosage can be started at 5 mg per day. It should not be used in those with severe hepatic impairment.

Benzodiazepines (BZDs)

Benzodiazepines are a class which can quickly alleviate anxiety symptoms, whether it is GAD, non-specific anxiety, or panic disorder. Caution must be observed in the use of these medications because of the increased potential for abuse. They are remarkably similar, with main difference being onset of action and half-life. Additionally, BZDs have fewer GI side effects than SSRIs or SNRIs; in fact, at times they are used to treat nausea. One major concern with BZDs is their side effects of dizziness, unsteadiness which can increase falls, as well as cognitive impairment in older adults.

Diazepam

Historically, one of the most frequently prescribed BZDs is diazepam. This drug has a long half-life and active metabolites which may lead to accumulation, which may be especially pronounced in the elderly and can lead to confusion. It is subject to extensive liver metabolism. With the presence of active metabolites and extensive liver metabolism, diazepam is used much more frequently than should be the case. It does have a quick onset of action and is associated with significant abuse potential. It has many other uses such as in seizure disorders, as a muscle relaxant, and for some sleep disorders. Thus, it may be a good choice in those settings. It is listed in the APA guidelines as useful in panic disorder. Patients may respond to doses lower than listed in Table 5.3. Patients may in fact do well with just one or two doses per day.

Oxazepam

An often-overlooked benzodiazepine is oxazepam as it is an older medication. It does seem to have less abuse potential, which may be due to slower absorption. Although GI upset is not common with BZDs, oxazepam seems to have even less than others. It does have a short half-life with minimal if any liver metabolism, hence ideal for those with hepatic impairment. With its slow onset of action, it may be useful in patients who are overly concerned about dizziness or unsteadiness. Due to its short half-life, it is best given three to four times per day with dosing based on the severity of the anxiety.

Clonazepam

Clinically clonazepam is used for both anxiety and some seizure disorders. Additionally, it is used for restless leg syndrome, rapid eye movement (REM) sleep behavior disorder and other sleep disorders, muscle spasms, mood stabilization, and tremor as off-label uses. It has a long half-life and may accumulate in older patients. It seems to have moderate abuse potential. It is extensively metabolized by the liver. In clinical settings, it can be dosed daily to BID with the last dose given at bedtime.

Lorazepam

This medication is also commonly used for anxiety disorders and is among one of the best known antianxiety agents. Its advantage is an intermediate half-life and minimal hepatic metabolism. Due to its intermediate half-life, some patients may benefit from once-daily dosing given at bedtime. Most often it is prescribed every 8 h. It can be used in seizure disorders and in chemotherapy-induced nausea and vomiting.

Alprazolam

Alprazolam is a short-acting BZD with a moderate to high abuse potential. It is widely used with indications for both GAD and panic disorder; with the advantage, it quickly quells symptoms. Disadvantages would be the need for multiple doses through the day, usually every 6–8 h. Occasional patients may metabolize this medication very quickly and need four to six doses per day. Those patients may have increased anxiety before the next scheduled dose due to withdrawal effects. Another disadvantage of alprazolam is a relatively wide dose range so it may take a long time to titrate to clinical effectiveness. Finally, it can be difficult to taper and stop this medication. To avoid withdrawal, it may need to be tapered very slowly.

Antihistamines

Hydroxyzine

Hydroxyzine is one of the oldest antianxiety medications. Its effectiveness is comparable to benzodiazepines and buspirone [29]. It has a syrup formulation, so it can be given in doses as low as 10 mg or even less. These ultra-low doses would be useful in a debilitated patient. Additionally, hydroxyzine may help with nausea. One of the disadvantages is it can lower the seizure threshold so it would need to be used with caution in those with a seizure disorder. As it is antihistaminic/anticholinergic, it should be used with caution in the elderly as it may produce or increase confusion.

Non-benzodiazepine Anxiolytic

Buspirone

Buspirone is in a class by itself. It is indicated for GAD. It has a very benign side effect profile and does not create the GI side effects which are prevalent with the SSRIs and SNRIs. It also has minimal, if any, drug-drug interactions. It can be useful as an augmenting agent for depression. With the significant overlap between anxiety and depression, this may be a useful feature. However, it is not indicated and should not be used in panic disorder or on an as needed basis. Another drawback is it may need dosage adjustment in patients with renal or hepatic disorders. There are two significant problems with buspirone. The first is a wide dose range; on occasions, patients may respond to doses as low as 5 mg daily and then not do as well at higher doses. The lower doses may be tried in those who are debilitated or in the elderly. However, most patients require high doses, and in fact, many require the maximum dose of 30 mg BID. Therefore, dose titration can be a major issue. The second problem with buspirone is the time to response is delayed with onset of action taking 2 weeks or more. The time to response is typically longer than SSRIs or SNRIs.

Anticonvulsants

Gabapentin

Gabapentin is not formally indicated for any anxiety disorders but is included in the APA guidelines. It does have an indication as an adjunctive agent for partial onset seizures, so is a medication neurologists are familiar with. It also has an indication for postherpetic neuralgia. For those who are frail, the dose can be started as low as 100 mg at bedtime. It is relatively well tolerated, and there are no common drug-drug interactions, so it may be an option for those who are very ill. Dosages do need to be adjusted for renal impairment but not hepatic impairment. Of note, its bio-availability may decrease at higher daily doses.

Pregabalin

Pregabalin is structurally similar to gabapentin. In Europe, it has received approval for GAD in addition to neuropathic pain. However, in the US, the FDA has only approved it for fibromyalgia, and it does not have a formal indication for anxiety. The British guidelines indicate pregabalin has efficacy in both acute and chronic GAD [39]. Pregabalin is also generally well tolerated [40]. It has a short half-life and no hepatic metabolism with few drug-drug interactions. It is usually given two to three times per day. It does need to be dose adjusted for renal insufficiency. This would be another medication which may be considered as a third or fourth line agent.

Antipsychotics

Quetiapine

For those who do not respond to other treatments, quetiapine may be considered, as it has some short-term efficacy [41]. There are studies showing quetiapine XR used off-label is effective for GAD [42]. Required dosage is lower for anxiety disorders than in other psychiatric disorders. It is used in an array of psychiatric disorders. There are several difficulties for this medication including sedation and weight gain. One must be aware of its potential to produce orthostatic hypotension, especially early in treatment. It also has a reputation of worsening Parkinson's symptoms in patients though probably less so than other antipsychotics. It is also associated with

QT prolongation. At this point, there is little evidence for the effectiveness of other second-generation antipsychotics in the treatment of GAD [43].

Miscellaneous

In terms of refractory panic disorder, there is good evidence for the augmentation effect of cognitive behavioral therapy (CBT). There is some support for the use of olanzapine as a single agent. Pindolol, divalproex sodium, aripiprazole, and olanzapine may be effective as augmenting agents [44]. However, based on the metabolic side effect burden associated with the second-generation antipsychotics, they should be considered only in refractory cases of anxiety or panic disorder [29]. An additional caveat is the black box warning concerning increased mortality relative to the use of all antipsychotics, even in low doses, in dementia patients. Consequently, antipsychotic use for anxiety should be avoided for this population.

Clinical Pearls

1. Rule out substance abuse, medication side effects, and medical illnesses which could be contributing to anxiety symptoms.
2. For mild to moderate anxiety, use an SSRI with few side effects such as escitalopram, citalopram, or sertraline.
3. For severe anxiety, use an SSRI or venlafaxine with a benzodiazepine.
4. For extreme anxiety, use a BZD to provide the patient with quick relief of symptoms.
5. For those with substance abuse issues, avoid the use of BZDs, and try to manage with an SSRI or SNRI.
6. BZDs are the most effective for the acute management of anxiety. Most other medications have delayed effect due to dose titration and time to onset of action.
7. For patients who do not respond to any of the above agents, consider one of the atypical agents.
8. Beware of drug-drug interactions.
9. Buspirone has no role in the management of acute anxiety or panic disorder.

Conclusion

Anxiety will frequently be seen by clinicians. The presentation of an anxiety disorder will rarely be clear cut. Additionally, there can be multiple co-occurring physical illnesses, medications, or substance use, all of which can worsen the anxiety disorder. The clinician does have multiple medications in addition to psychotherapy to help the patient. These patients require education, support, and patience to manage their illness. However, successful treatment can markedly increase their quality of life.

References

1. Kessler RC, et al. Twelve-month and lifetime prevalence and lifetime morbid risk of anxiety and mood disorders in the United States. Int J Methods Psychiatr Res. 2012;21(3):169–84.
2. Cassidy K-L, Rector NA. The silent geriatric giant: anxiety disorders in late life. Geriatr Aging. 2008;11(3):150–6.
3. Mahableshwarkar AR, et al. A randomised, double-blind, placebo-controlled, duloxetine-referenced study of the efficacy and tolerability of vortioxetine in the acute treatment of adults with generalised anxiety disorder. Int J Clin Pract. 2014;68(1):49–59.
4. Hoffman DL, Dukes EM, Wittchen HU. Human and economic burden of generalized anxiety disorder. Depress Anxiety. 2008;25(1):72–90.
5. Lambiase MJ, Kubzansky LD, Thurston RC. Prospective study of anxiety and incident stroke. Stroke. 2014;45(2):438–43.
6. Tully PJ, Cosh SM, Baune BT. A review of the affects of worry and generalized anxiety disorder upon cardiovascular health and coronary heart disease. Psychol Health Med. 2013;18(6):627–44.
7. Wands K, et al. A questionnaire investigation of anxiety and depression in early dementia. J Am Geriatr Soc. 1990;38(5):535–8.
8. Rosenberg PB, et al. The association of neuropsychiatric symptoms in MCI with incident dementia and Alzheimer disease. Am J Geriatr Psychiatry. 2013;21(7):685–95.
9. Diprose W, Sundram F, Menkes DB. Psychiatric comorbidity in psychogenic nonepileptic seizures compared with epilepsy. Epilepsy Behav. 2016;56:123–30.
10. Boeschoten RE, et al. Prevalence of depression and anxiety in multiple sclerosis: a systematic review and meta-analysis. J Neurol Sci. 2017;372:331–41.
11. Seo JG, Park SP. Validation of the generalized anxiety disorder-7 (GAD-7) and GAD-2 in patients with migraine. J Headache Pain. 2015;16:97.
12. Ayerbe L, et al. Natural history, predictors and associated outcomes of anxiety up to 10 years after stroke: the South London Stroke Register. Age Ageing. 2014;43(4):542–7.
13. Isais-Millan S, et al. Prevalence of neuropsychiatric disorders in drug-naive subjects with Parkinson's disease (PD). Gac Med Mex. 2016;152(3):357–63.
14. Zhao QF, et al. The prevalence of neuropsychiatric symptoms in Alzheimer's disease: systematic review and meta-analysis. J Affect Disord. 2016;190:264–71.
15. Bandyopadhyay TK, et al. Neuropsychiatric profiles in patients with Alzheimer's disease and vascular dementia. Ann Indian Acad Neurol. 2014;17(3):325–30.
16. Prediger RD, et al. Anxiety in Parkinson's disease: a critical review of experimental and clinical studies. Neuropharmacology. 2012;62(1):115–24.
17. Schrag A, Jahanshahi M, Quinn N. What contributes to quality of life in patients with Parkinson's disease? J Neurol Neurosurg Psychiatry. 2000;69(3):308–12.
18. Dissanayaka NN, et al. Anxiety disorders in Parkinson's disease: prevalence and risk factors. Mov Disord. 2010;25(7):838–45.
19. Shiba M, et al. Anxiety disorders and depressive disorders preceding Parkinson's disease: a case-control study. Mov Disord. 2000;15(4):669–77.
20. American Psychiatric Association: Diagnostic and Statistical Manual of Mental Disorders, Fifth Edition. Arlington, VA, American Psychiatric Association, 2013.
21. Baldwin DS, Waldman S, Allgulander C. Evidence-based pharmacological treatment of generalized anxiety disorder. Int J Neuropsychopharmacol. 2011;14(5):697–710.

22. Leentjens AF, et al. Anxiety rating scales in Parkinson's disease: critique and recommendations. Mov Disord. 2008;23(14):2015–25.
23. Allgulander C. Generalized anxiety disorder: a review of recent findings. J Exp Clin Med. 2012;4(2):88–91.
24. Spitzer RL, et al. A brief measure for assessing generalized anxiety disorder: the GAD-7. Arch Intern Med. 2006;166(10):1092–7.
25. Julian LJ. Measures of anxiety: State-Trait Anxiety Inventory (STAI), Beck Anxiety Inventory (BAI), and Hospital Anxiety and Depression Scale-Anxiety (HADS-A). Arthritis Care Res. 2011;63(S11):S467–72.
26. Zung WW. A rating instrument for anxiety disorders. Psychosom J Consult Liaison Psychiatry. 1971;12:371–9.
27. Pachana NA, et al. Development and validation of the geriatric anxiety inventory. Int Psychogeriatr. 2007;19(1):103–14.
28. Matheson SF, et al. Validity and reliability of the geriatric anxiety inventory in Parkinson's disease. Australas J Ageing. 2012;31(1):13–6.
29. Katzman MA, et al. Canadian clinical practice guidelines for the management of anxiety, post-traumatic stress and obsessive-compulsive disorders. BMC Psychiatry. 2014;14(Suppl 1):S1.
30. Buoli M, et al. New approaches to the pharmacological management of generalized anxiety disorder. Expert Opin Pharmacother. 2013;14(2):175–84.
31. Jiang HY, et al. Use of selective serotonin reuptake inhibitors and risk of upper gastrointestinal bleeding: a systematic review and meta-analysis. Clin Gastroenterol Hepatol. 2015;13(1):42–50.e3.
32. Pollack M, et al. Eszopiclone coadministered with escitalopram in patients with insomnia and comorbid generalized anxiety disorder. Arch Gen Psychiatry. 2008;65(5):551–62.
33. Andrisano C, Chiesa A, Serretti A. Newer antidepressants and panic disorder: a meta-analysis. Int Clin Psychopharmacol. 2013;28(1):33–45.
34. Rector TS, et al. Outcomes of citalopram dosage risk mitigation in a veteran population. Am J Psychiatry. 2016;173(9):896–902.
35. Rudroju N, et al. Comparative efficacy and safety of six antidepressants and anticonvulsants in painful diabetic neuropathy: a network meta-analysis. Pain Physician. 2013;16(6):E705–14.
36. Rafael CF, et al. Current pharmacological interventions in panic disorder. CNS Neurol Disord Drug Targets. 2014;13(6):1057–65.
37. Gommoll C, et al. Vilazodone in patients with generalized anxiety disorder: a double-blind, randomized, placebo-controlled, flexible-dose study. Int Clin Psychopharmacol. 2015;30(6):297–306.
38. Pae CU, et al. Vortioxetine, a multimodal antidepressant for generalized anxiety disorder: a systematic review and meta-analysis. J Psychiatr Res. 2015;64:88–98.
39. Baldwin DS, et al. Evidence-based pharmacological treatment of anxiety disorders, post-traumatic stress disorder and obsessive-compulsive disorder: a revision of the 2005 guidelines from the British Association for Psychopharmacology. J Psychopharmacol. 2014;28(5):403–39.
40. Montgomery S, et al. Efficacy and safety of pregabalin in elderly people with generalised anxiety disorder. Br J Psychiatry. 2008;193(5):389.
41. Stein DJ, et al. Efficacy and tolerability of extended release quetiapine fumarate (quetiapine XR) monotherapy in patients with generalised anxiety disorder: an analysis of pooled data from three 8-week placebo-controlled studies. Hum Psychopharmacol. 2011;26(8):614–28.
42. Mezhebovsky I, et al. Double-blind, randomized study of extended release quetiapine fumarate (quetiapine XR) monotherapy in older patients with generalized anxiety disorder. Int J Geriatr Psychiatry. 2013;28(6):615–25.
43. Albert U, et al. Role and clinical implications of atypical antipsychotics in anxiety disorders, obsessive-compulsive disorder, trauma-related, and somatic symptom disorders: a systematized review. Int Clin Psychopharmacol. 2016;31(5):249–58.
44. Freire RC, et al. Treatment-resistant panic disorder: a systematic review. Expert Opin Pharmacother. 2016;17(2):159–68.

Chapter 6
Sedatives and Hypnotics

William Maurice Redden

Sleep-related problems, in particular insomnia, have been problematic for ages. The prevalence of sleep disorders is high on a global level, with rates of 56% in the USA, 31% in Western Europe, and 23% in Japan [1]. Insomnia may be characterized by its duration: acute (or transient) or chronic (occurs at least three times a week and lasts for at least 1 month). Some 30% of the population will report at least occasional episodes of sleep disruption, but only 10% of the population meets the specific diagnostic criteria for an insomnia disorder. Chronic insomnia is multifactorial and highly individualized, making it a challenging condition to treat. It is associated with an often significant decrease in quality of life and can interact with comorbid conditions to worsen overall health and increase morbidity [2].

Sedatives and hypnotics are two different classes of drugs that are often used together or interchangeably. However, they each have different meanings and are meant to produce a different effect. Sedatives are drugs or chemicals that produce a relaxing and calming effect. Hypnotic compounds have the desired effects of producing sleepiness by causing one to fall asleep and maintain sleep. There are medications that can cause either state or even both, thereby leading to the blurring of the terms, with the most commonly used being sedative-hypnotics. Barbiturates and benzodiazepines are the two major categories of sedative-hypnotics. There are other types of medications that have similar mechanisms of action that are used and will be discussed in this chapter as well.

Several sleep disorders, including insomnia, are highly prevalent among patients with neurologic diagnoses, such as Parkinson's disease, epilepsy, multiple sclerosis, and Alzheimer's disease [3]. Insomnia is a common comorbidity in epilepsy that can adversely impact seizure control and has negative associations with quality of life [4]. In addition, people with insomnia have higher incidences and risks of

W. M. Redden, MD (✉)
Department of Psychiatry and Behavioral Neuroscience, Saint Louis University
School of Medicine, St. Louis, MO, USA
e-mail: wredden@slu.edu

© Springer International Publishing AG, part of Springer Nature 2018   97
G. T. Grossberg, L. J. Kinsella (eds.), *Clinical Psychopharmacology for Neurologists*, https://doi.org/10.1007/978-3-319-74604-3_6

hospitalization for stroke compared with those with a normal sleep pattern [5]. Therefore, clinicians need to recognize that assessment and treatment of insomnia in complex patients may also lead to better management of their primary conditions. This chapter will explore the current treatment options available for insomnia as well as how to choose the most appropriate agent.

Normal Sleep Cycle

There are two states of sleep: non-rapid eye movement (NREM) sleep and rapid eye movement (REM) sleep. NREM sleep is divided into four stages, each representing a continuum of relative depth. Stages 3 and 4 are referred to as slow-wave sleep (SWS), which is most commonly believed to be the restorative part of sleep. This stage is then followed by REM sleep that consists of slow alpha activity and is the stage that is associated with dreaming [6]. The transition from wakefulness to sleep occurs when going into NREM sleep then transitioning to REM sleep. After a period of REM sleep, a brief arousal or awakening may occur before entry again into NREM sleep. Over the course of the night, four to six cycles of NREM to REM sleep typically occur, with each cycle lasting about 80–110 min [7]. Sleep disorders occur when this system is dysfunctional. Benzodiazepine use, especially on a short-term basis, changes both sleep architecture and sleep quality. These changes include increased stage 2 sleep, decrease in slow-wave sleep, and prolonged REM sleep latency [8].

Definition and Classification of Insomnia

Insomnia is a subjective or patient-reported complaint of problems with sleep: either falling asleep, staying asleep, or a combination of both. The *International Classification of Sleep Disorders*, Third Edition *(ICSD-3)* diagnostic criteria for insomnia specify (1) a complaint of difficulty initiating or maintaining sleep or waking up too early. Sleep is chronically non-restorative or of poor quality, (2) poor sleep despite adequate opportunity and circumstances for sleep and (3) at least one pathophysiological abnormality causing daytime impairment such as fatigue, difficulty with attention, and daytime sleepiness. The ICSD-3 delves further in classifying chronic insomnia as a condition where the criteria for insomnia are met plus a duration of 3 months and a frequency of at least three times per week [9].

It has been suggested that about 30% of the general population complains of sleep disruption, while approximately 10% have associated symptoms of daytime functional impairments consistent with the diagnosis of insomnia [10].

Brief History of Sedatives and Hypnotics

Barbiturates

Prior to the discovery of barbiturates, several agents were used for their sedative and hypnotic properties. These included alkaloids derived from opioids, chloral hydrate, and bromides [11]. At one point, barbiturates were the gold standard for treatment of insomnia as well as for the management of seizures [12]. It was not until the mid-1950s that the Narcotics Expert Committee at the World Health Organization stated that barbiturates were habit forming and could produce a drug addiction dangerous to public health. That announcement led to recommendations that included barbiturates only being dispensed by a prescription which included the number of refills as well as a record being kept of such prescriptions [13].

Benzodiazepines

The first benzodiazepine, chlordiazepoxide, was identified in 1955 [14]. Since then, benzodiazepines have been the agents used most commonly to treat anxiety and sleep disorders.

There are current concerns that these agents are being abused and overprescribed. Clinicians should also be focused on the potential for physical and psychological dependence as well as withdrawal/tolerance concerns [15].

Sedative and Hypnotics in Clinical Practice

We will discuss the treatment algorithms for using hypnotics and sedatives with the following case:

> *Ms. SH is a 51-year-old female who presents to your clinic with the chief complaint of feeling tired during the day. After further questioning, it is revealed that she has not been sleeping well at night. This has been a problem since her mid-30s, but now is causing more impairment in her daily functioning. She has noticed difficulty concentrating at work which has led to her making more errors that usual. When she gets home, she is often too exhausted to help with activities around the house.*

Before prescribing medications, a thorough evaluation should be done to rule out any secondary or comorbid causes of insomnia. Therefore, the practitioner should get a detailed history of the patient's sleep problem, followed by a complete physical exam including neurological assessment. Then any pertinent diagnostic labs (such as TSH, CMP, CBC) should be done. Also if there are any abnormal findings on neurological examination (such as abnormal movements or unilateral weakness), imaging should be done as well. Hilty et al. also recommend asking specific

Table 6.1 Sleep hygiene recommendations

Maintain a regular sleep-wake cycle (go to bed at the same time each night and wake at the same time each morning)
Avoid exercise within 3 h of bedtime
Avoid caffeine after lunch
Avoid nicotine at least 2 h before bedtime
Use the bed for only sleeping and sex; do not read or watch TV in bed
If not asleep within 15–30 min, get out of bed and walk around

questions that would include as follows: (1) Do you have problems falling asleep or staying asleep? (2) Do you frequently awaken and is that associated with anything, for example, pain? (3) Do you wake up tired or refreshed despite many hours of sleep [16]?

> *Ms. SH denies any other signs and symptoms of mood disorder or other conditions that may impact sleep. Upon more detailed questions relative to her sleep habits, it is determined that she has trouble falling asleep and is easily awoken in the middle of the night and has trouble getting back to sleep.*

Nonpharmacologic Treatment Options for Insomnia

The first treatment recommendation should be to encourage good sleep hygiene (Table 6.1), to increase daytime activity, and to search for any secondary or reversible causes such as depression, anxiety, gastroesophageal reflux, or thyroid disorders.

Cognitive Behavioral Therapy for Insomnia

Cognitive behavioral therapy for insomnia (CBT-I) is a nonpharmacological approach to treatment comprised of several strategies which include establishing a learned association between the bed and sleeping through stimulus control, restoring homeostatic regulation of sleep through sleep restriction, and altering anxious sleep-related thoughts through cognitive restructuring. It is conveyed over the course of four to eight sessions that occur weekly or every other week for 30–60 min each session. In general, CBT-I is at least as effective for treating insomnia when compared with sleep medications, and its effects may be more durable than medications [17]. The effective nature of CBT-I along with minimal side effects should make this treatment option highly attractive; however, factors such as cost, lack of available CBT practitioners, and potential problems with patient motivation and adherence may make the use of behavioral techniques difficult [18].

Ms. SH has stressed the importance to her of getting sleep and says she does not have the time to invest in therapy. She wants something that will work immediately. She has tried over-the-counter sleep products without success. There is no previous history of being on any prescribed medications for sleep. Upon further questioning she admits to drinking a glass of wine 3–4 times per week, but denies any other substance use and there is no history of abusing prescribed medications.

Medication Options

Currently, the benzodiazepines (BZD) and non-benzodiazepine receptor agonists (non-BzRA) are the main FDA-approved treatment choices for insomnia. Initially, these medications were meant for short-term or intermittent use; however, clinical experience has shown that these medications are often used for much longer periods or even chronically. The main treatment goals are (1) to improve sleep quality and quantity and (2) to improve insomnia-related daytime impairments [9].

Benzodiazepines (BDZ)

Benzodiazepines are FDA-approved for both the treatment of insomnia and anxiety (Table 6.2). At times, multiple benzodiazepines are used to treat both conditions. This can enhance the addictive potential as well as increase the tolerance for either medication [19]. There are currently five FDA-approved benzodiazepines for the treatment of insomnia (estazolam, flurazepam, quazepam, temazepam, and triazolam) [20].

Temazepam is the most common BDZ prescribed for insomnia [21]. It is absorbed more slowly and metabolized more quickly than other benzodiazepines, which leads to reduced awakenings during the night and increased sleep duration [22].

Estazolam significantly increases total sleep time and reduces time awake during sleep in a dose-dependent manner (0.25, 0.5, 1.0, and 2.0 mg) [23]. In long-term studies, estazolam 2.0 mg remained an effective hypnotic for at least 6 weeks of continuous nightly administration with no evidence of clinically significant tolerance [24]. Vogel et al. found estazolam 1 mg nightly appears to be a safe and

Table 6.2 Benzodiazepine receptor agonists

Drug (trade name)	Half-life	Dose range	Elderly
Estazolam (Prosom)	15–20 h	0.5–2 mg	1 mg
Flurazepam (Dalmane)	2.3 h (active metabolite 100 h)	15–30 mg	15 mg
Quazepam (Doral)	39–72 h	15 mg	7.5 mg
Temazepam (Restoril)	5–11 h	15–30 mg	7.5–15 mg
Triazolam (Halcion)	2–3 h	0.25–1 mg	0.125–0.5 mg

Data from Heel et al. [92], Cohn et al. [93], Pakes et al. [28], Pierce and Shu [24]

effective hypnotic for elderly patients with insomnia. Those patients had rebound insomnia the first night after discontinuation, but sleep parameters (wake time after sleep onset and total sleep time) returned to normal the following night. Also, there was no effect on daytime performance or anterograde memory [25]. Flurazepam has shown moderate improvement in sleep, in short-term use, but with higher risk of adverse effects of somnolence and hypokinesia (the following morning) when compared with estazolam [26]. Flurazepam significantly increased total sleep time while reducing the latency to stage 1 sleep, the number of awakenings in the night, and the amount of wakefulness after sleep onset as well as decreased REM sleep [27].

Triazolam is an older benzodiazepine with a short half-life, 2–3 h. In the past it has been used to treat acute or chronic insomnia, situational insomnia in hospitalized patients, and insomnia associated with other disease states [28]. Triazolam has been shown to decrease sleep latency and the number of nocturnal awakenings while increasing total sleep time in patients with insomnia [29]. In contrast, quazepam has a long half-life, 39–72 h due to two active metabolites. It is useful for inducing and maintaining sleep for acute and chronic insomnia with less incidence of rebound insomnia when discontinued [30].

Z-Drugs

With several pharmacologic treatment options available, trying to decide which agent to start can be challenging, as each may offer specific benefits versus their potential side effects (Table 6.3). Non-benzodiazepines receptor agonists (non-BzRA) offer a better safety profile, and most studies have shown them to be non-habit forming [31]. Zolpidem was the first of this class of medication to be developed and FDA-approved in 1992. The non-BzRA work at the GABA receptor site where they also have preferential subtype selectivity by binding to omega receptors [32].

The other agents in this class include zaleplon, zopiclone (not available in the United States), eszopiclone, and now the various formulations of zolpidem (immediate release vs extended release, sublingual and nasal).

Zolpidem decreases sleep latency and increases total sleep time and sleep efficiency without adversely affecting sleep architecture [33]. The optimal dose of zolpidem is 10 mg at bedtime and 5 mg for elderly patients. The hypnotic effects have been shown to be active at low doses, and there was a decrease in percent of time spent in rapid eye movement sleep at much higher doses (20 mg) [34]. While zolpidem has fewer side effects than the benzodiazepines, it may be associated with rebound insomnia, next-day residual effects, and complex sleep-related behaviors [35]. There has been growing concern relative to zolpidem causing daytime automatisms and sleep-related parasomnias. These behaviors involve confusion, amnesia, or somnambulism which has lead patients to "sleepwalk," "sleep eat," and even "sleep drive" [36, 37]. These events do not occur very often but clinicians should be aware of the risks.

Table 6.3 Non-benzodiazepine receptor agonists and other sedatives

Drug (trade name	Mechanism of action	Dose range	Special considerations
Eszopiclone (Lunesta)	Non-BzRA	2–3 mg	Unpleasant taste
Zaleplon (Sonata)	Non-BzRA	5–10 mg	Low risk of withdrawal symptoms and rebound insomnia
Zolpidem (Ambien)	Non-BzRA	5–10 mg	Comes in several forms including nasal spray, concern for sleep-related behaviors
		6.25–12.5 mg (CR)	
Ramelteon (Rozerem)	MT_1 and MT_2 agonist	8 mg	Short half-life, no abuse potential
Trazodone	$5HT_2$, $alpha_1$, H_1 antagonist	25–200 mg	Risk of orthostasis, dizziness, priapism
Mirtazapine (Remeron)	$5HT_{2-3}$, $alpha_{1-2}$, H_1, M_1, NE antagonist	7.5–30 mg	Risk of increased weight and appetite
Doxepin (Silenor)	H_1, $5HT_2$, $alpha_1$, M_1 antagonist	3–6 mg (capsules)	Risk of orthostatic hypotension, dry mouth, delirium
		10–100 mg (tablets)	
Suvorexant (Belsomra)	$Orexin_{1-2}$ antagonist	5–20 mg	Low risk of withdrawal symptoms and rebound insomnia, chance of abnormal dreams
Quetiapine (Seroquel)	$5HT_{1-2}$, D_{1-2}, $alpha_{1-2}$, H_1 antagonist	50–200 mg	Indicated for schizophrenia and bipolar disorder, increased risk of weight gain, dry mouth, EPS
Gabapentin (Neurontin)	Interacts at the GABA transporter, decreases glutamate	100–900 mg	Anticonvulsant, not effective as mood stabilizer, recent reports of abuse risk

Data from FDA prescribing information; Asnis et al. [69], Stahl [94]
MT melatonin receptor, *5HT* serotonin, *H* histamine, *M* muscarinic receptor, *NE* norepinephrine

Zopiclone is a non-BzRA that has been recognized as an effective and well-tolerated hypnotic agent. It has a relatively low risk of causing residual clinical effects (such as difficulty in waking or reduced morning alertness) as well as a decreased incidence of rebound insomnia [38].

Eszopiclone is the stereoisomer of zopiclone which is effective at reducing sleep onset time as well as improving overall sleep maintenance [39]. Within this same study, it was discovered there was little indication that eszopiclone was associated with withdrawal effects or rebound insomnia. There is also evidence that eszopiclone is beneficial in long-term use for chronic insomnia with enhanced quality of life, reduced work limitations, and reduced global insomnia severity [40]. The most commonly reported adverse effects include bitter taste, dizziness, and dry mouth, with low risk for tolerance [41]. If both options are available, eszopiclone is as efficacious as zopiclone in the treatment of insomnia, increasing total sleep time as well as sleep efficiency as evidenced by polysomnography [42].

Zaleplon has been shown to be efficacious in promoting sleep initiation, but less so in promoting sleep maintenance. Elie et al. demonstrated that zaleplon is an effective treatment option for patients with difficulty falling asleep by reducing sleep latency. They also validated the favorable safety profile of zaleplon as shown by the absence of rebound insomnia and withdrawal symptoms after treatment was stopped. Interestingly, they have also shown that zolpidem was associated with higher incidence of withdrawal symptoms and rebound insomnia than with placebo. These withdrawal symptoms consisted of depressed mood, muscle pain, a peculiar taste, loss of memory, and olfactory discrimination [43]. Zaleplon has a rapid onset of action and undergoes rapid elimination, which may explain its more favorable safety profile [44].

This class of medication has been shown to be effective up to 12 months with evidence in improvement in daytime functioning and with little risk of rebound insomnia after discontinuation [45–47]. Overall, prolonged use of non-BzRA has been shown to be well tolerated without evidence of tolerance [45].

Orexin Antagonist

Orexin neuropeptides are secreted from the lateral hypothalamus and are critical for maintaining normal wakefulness. When they are malfunctioning or destroyed, they can cause narcolepsy as they play a vital role in keeping people awake [48].

Suvorexant is the first dual receptor orexin antagonist that was FDA-approved in 2014. Dual orexin receptor antagonists block the activity of orexin 1 and 2 receptors to both reduce the threshold to the transition of sleep and attenuate orexin-mediated arousal [49]. Initially, the pharmaceutical company which developed suvorexant requested approval of doses between 20 and 40 mg. But after much debate and discussion, it was determined that this drug provides maximum benefit with low risk of tolerance/dependence at doses less than 20 mg per night [50].

Suvorexant is indicated for the treatment of insomnia characterized by difficulties with sleep onset and poor sleep maintenance. The recommended dose is 10 mg at bedtime which can provide up to 7 h of sleep. The maximum recommended dose is 20 mg per 24 h [51]. Suvorexant is generally safe and well tolerated for chronic use (longer than 3 months [52]).

Melatonin

Melatonin (5-methoxy-N-acetyltryptamine) is endogenously synthesized, secreted by the pineal gland and plays a key role in maintaining regular circadian rhythms [53]. In most studies exogenous melatonin reduced sleep onset latency to a greater extent in people with delayed sleep phase syndrome than in people with insomnia. Otherwise, melatonin was not effective in treating most primary sleep disorders with short-term use (4 weeks or less) [54].

Ramelteon is a melatonin receptor agonist that has high affinity for MT1 and MT2 receptors [55]. At doses of 4–32 mg, ramelteon had statistically significant reductions in latency to persistent sleep (LPS) and increases total sleep time (TST). Also, at these same doses, there were no next-day residual effects, as compared with placebo. The most commonly reported adverse events were headache, somnolence, and sore throat [56]. The FDA-recommended dose of ramelteon is 8 mg nightly. One concerning side effect to be mindful of is that ramelteon can affect road-tracking performance (the number of subjects who slid off the track), visual attention and/or psychomotor speed, subjective sleepiness, and equilibrium function with acute treatment [57].

Sedating Antidepressants

We have been using sedating antidepressants such as trazodone, amitriptyline, and doxepin to treat insomnia. However, there have been little if any double-blind, placebo-controlled studies to validate their use. Buscemi et al. conducted a meta-analysis on drugs used for the treatment of chronic insomnia. The analysis suggested that sedating antidepressants, particularly doxepin and trazadone, may have a role in the management of chronic insomnia [54].

Some reasons that clinicians prescribe antidepressants off-label for insomnia include (1) the benefit of using a single medication with sedating properties to manage both a psychiatric or medical disorder and concurrent insomnia, (2) using a medication with sedating properties to offset sleep difficulties caused by another medication, and (3) avoiding the use of hypnotics due to concerns about dependency and side effects [58].

Trazodone at doses of 25–50 mg has been shown to have modest effects on insomnia [59]. In a double-blind, placebo-controlled study using trazodone 50 mg prior to bedtime, Roth et al. demonstrated that compared to placebo, trazodone was associated with fewer nighttime awakenings, decreased minutes of stage 1 sleep, and fewer self-reports of difficulty sleeping. However high doses of trazodone (200–300 mg) may cause some concerning side effects including significant impairments of short-term memory, difficulty with verbal learning, and some trouble with equilibrium and orthostasis, in both the adult and geriatric populations [60].

Doxepin is a tricyclic antidepressant that at low doses selectively antagonizes histaminic receptors, which is believed to cause its sedative effects. In the first placebo-controlled, double-blind, polysomnographic study, low-dose doxepin (25–50 mg) was shown to improve sleep efficiency and increase total sleep over 4 weeks. There was an increase in stage 2 sleep without significantly affecting total REM sleep. Withdrawal and rebound symptoms were seen when doxepin was stopped abruptly. Therefore, it is recommended to slowly taper off this medication. In addition, some severe side effects of leukopenia, thrombocytopenia, and elevated liver enzymes were observed [61]. In three large, well-designed phase III trials in adult or elderly patients with chronic primary insomnia, oral, low-dose doxepin 3 or 6 mg capsules once daily improved wake time after sleep onset, total sleep time, and sleep efficiency to a significantly greater extent than placebo [62]. This led to the FDA approval of doxepin as Silenor. Being a tricyclic, anticholinergicity, cardiotoxicity, and overdose potential need to be kept in mind.

Mirtazapine is tetracyclic antidepressant that blocks the noradrenergic alpha2-auto- and heteroreceptors responsible for controlling noradrenaline and serotonin release. It also has a low affinity for serotonin (5-HT)1A receptors but potently blocks 5-HT2 and 5-HT3 receptors. The blockade of 5-HT2 and 5-HT3 receptors along with histamine-1 receptors prevents development of the side effects associated with nonselective 5-HT activation and may contribute to its calming and sleep-improving effects [63]. In patients without primary sleep disorders, mirtazapine has been shown to increase sleep efficiency by increasing slow-wave sleep time while decreasing stage 1 sleep time. In addition, there was no significant effect on rapid eye movement sleep variables [64]. Mirtazapine may also be effective in treating insomnia in patients who are also depressed. This medication improves sleep disturbance as well as counteracts the key biological symptoms of depression due to its unique pattern of neurotransmitter modulation [65]. In depressed patients, the acute effects of mirtazapine on improvement of sleep efficiency are evident, and these effects may persist with chronic use as well [66].

Esmirtazapine (Org 50081), which was in development for the treatment of insomnia, is the maleic acid salt of the S(+) enantiomer of mirtazapine. As esmirtazapine has a shorter half-life (10 h) than racemic mirtazapine, it is anticipated that esmirtazapine will have a smaller risk for residual sedative effects the next day. In a 6-week, double-blind, randomized, polysomnography (PSG) study, esmirtazapine was associated with consistent and sustained improvements in sleep in adults with primary insomnia. Overall, it was well tolerated, and there was minimal residual daytime effect [67]. However, its clinical development was stopped in 2010 for strategic reasons [68].

Other medications have been tried off-label due to their sedating properties. The primary agents include quetiapine and gabapentin. Thus far, there has been limited evidence for their efficacy in treating insomnia. However, it may be beneficial to use such medications off-label for insomnia when patients also have a comorbid medical condition for which the drug is FDA-approved, e.g., neuropathy with gabapentin [69]. Obviously, one needs to consider the risks of using sedating antipsychotics for insomnia, which include increased mortality in geriatric patients with dementia.

Major Side Effects and Concerns

Rebound Insomnia

When sedatives or hypnotics, especially those with short-half lives, are abruptly discontinued, some patients may experience insomnia worse than it was prior to treatment. This usually lasts one to two nights. To avoid this, it is recommended to taper down the medication dosage over a few nights.

Residual Effects

Another concern associated with the use of hypnotics is residual effects such as daytime sleepiness and impairment of psychomotor and cognitive functioning the morning following taking the medication.

It seems that compounds with longer half-lives greatly increase these risks, but those with shorter half-lives have also been associated [70].

Memory Loss

Morning sedation and difficulties with memory have always been concerns associated with benzodiazepines. They may be failure of memory consolidation rather than failure of retrieval, and those with shorter sleep latency may have better memory consolidation than those who stayed up more during the night [71].

Falls

Hypnotics and sedatives may significantly contribute to falls, since these drugs affect balance and can produce body sway even after a single dose. This effect is dose-dependent and made worse by addition of other psychoactive drugs or alcohol [72].

Chronic Use Issues and Concerns

Sedatives and hypnotics have the potential for misuse and abuse due to the euphoric feelings they can cause. Occasionally, patients may intentionally exaggerate their symptoms to get these medications. Presentations of intentional malingering may include resisting access to outside medical records; nonadherence with diagnostic or treatment recommendations; reemergence, or a worsening of symptoms when medication dose is due to be reduced; and when evidence from medical testing disputes information provided by the patient [73].

Treatment of Alcohol- and Substance-Dependent Patients

There are high prevalence rates (36–91%) of insomnia in alcohol-dependent patients [74]. Alcohol withdrawal-related insomnia is common among this patient population and is related to a lifetime co-occurring diagnosis of insomnia. There is a 50%

prevalence rate among individuals who meet lifetime criteria for both alcohol dependence and alcohol withdrawal insomnia [75].

When addressing treatment options in this complex patient population, one should make sure to (1) emphasize that abstinence is necessary and is reasonable, (2) target other modifiable causes including poor sleep hygiene, (3) include behavioral therapy as an appropriate treatment option, and (4) when selecting medications, try at all cost to avoid benzodiazepine receptor antagonists due to their addictive properties in this addiction-prone population [76].

Trazodone is an antidepressant that is often used off-label for treating insomnia. However, in patients with alcohol dependency, it has been shown that despite short-term benefits in sleep quality, trazodone may impede improvements in alcohol consumption and lead to increased drinking when stopped [77].

Use in the Elderly

As we age, our sleep cycle patterns change. It usually takes one longer to fall asleep and we also see more frequent awakenings during the night. Older adults often display a different circadian pattern, usually going to bed earlier and waking up earlier than their younger counterparts. Sleep architecture changes include spending an increased proportion of time in stages 1 and 2 sleep and a decreased proportion of time in stage 3 sleep and REM sleep (the deeper stages) [78].

Sleep disturbances, particularly among older persons, often may be secondary to coexisting diseases and are associated with an increasing number of respiratory symptoms and physical disabilities [79].

Long-term benzodiazepine use includes the risks of developing tolerance or dependence, rebound insomnia, residual daytime sedation, cognitive impairment, and motor incoordination/fall risk, which are magnified in the elderly. Therefore, it is recommended that benzodiazepines be used for short-term (usually <35 days) management of insomnia in the elderly [10].

However, recent studies have shown that elderly patients with persistent/chronic insomnia are also at greater risk for the development of new-onset depression [80]. In addition, the risk of falls and fractures is higher in the elderly when prescribed zolpidem, being almost twice as high as in those patients who are prescribed benzodiazepines [81, 82].

General Prescribing Recommendations

There are several factors that should be assessed before deciding which medication to prescribe for insomnia. Comorbid conditions can guide clinicians on what medications are appropriate or not. For example, in patients with severe pulmonary disease, CNS-sedating medications should be avoided if possible [69]. Or in patients with coexisting anxiety and insomnia who may already be on a benzodiazepine, adding a melatonin receptor agonist or an orexin antagonist might be beneficial.

When prescribing medications which may be misused or abused, trying to obtain records from previous providers and information from significant others is useful. Also, obtaining a detailed substance abuse history including sharing medications with a friend or family member or of legal issues stemming from drug use is vital [73].

Middle-age persons may be more susceptible to the effects of alcohol and sedative-hypnotic drug interactions by engaging in risky drinking behaviors (i.e., binge drinking) when compared to the older patient population. Despite the lower overall prevalence, older persons may be particularly susceptible to additive CNS-depressant effects due to physiologic changes in drug and alcohol metabolism. Therefore, clinicians should carefully consider patients' level and pattern of alcohol consumption before prescribing sedatives and/or hypnotics [83].

Drugs with shorter time to peak blood concentration (tmax) will probably have a more rapid onset of action and aid sleep onset, whereas those with longer half-lives (t1/2) can provide better sleep maintenance but have the potential for daytime hangover. Therefore, medication treatment should be focused on patient's symptom pattern and treatment goals (acute vs chronic). Starting with a short- to intermediate-acting BZA or non-BzRA followed by ramelteon is advised. If the initial agents are not successful, then try another medication in the same class. If that proves unsuccessful, then switch classes of medications. Clinicians should consider using sedating mediations such as antidepressants, antipsychotics, or anticonvulsants when treating comorbid conditions for which these drugs are appropriate [84] (Fig. 6.1). It is also recommended that all patients with insomnia be offered the option of CBT-I as an initial treatment [85].

After a, thorough discussion of benefits, risk and the option of short-term use versus long-term use, it was decided to start Ms. SH on a non-BzRA. It was agreed that this would be for short-term use during which period she would also practice healthy sleep habits. She was advised to avoid alcohol and other sedating medications with her non-BzRA.

Considerations of Use in Comorbid Neurological Conditions

In patients with Parkinson's disease, non-motor symptoms, including fatigue, depressed mood, and autonomic instability, are most closely and independently associated with reported insomnia [86]. Disrupted sleep, early morning awakenings, and non-restorative sleep are the most common insomnia symptoms in Parkinson's patients [87]. Therefore, at times, patients may be on two or more psychoactive mediations that may cause sedation. For example, a patient may be on levodopa/carbidopa therapy and/or an anticholinergic drug, but still complain of difficulty sleeping. In this instance using a short-acting BZA or non-BzRA could be beneficial and improve quality of life for the patient. As with the use of any controlled substance, the ongoing screening for aberrant behavior, monitoring of treatment compliance, documentation of medical necessity, and the adjustment of treatment to clinical changes are essential [88].

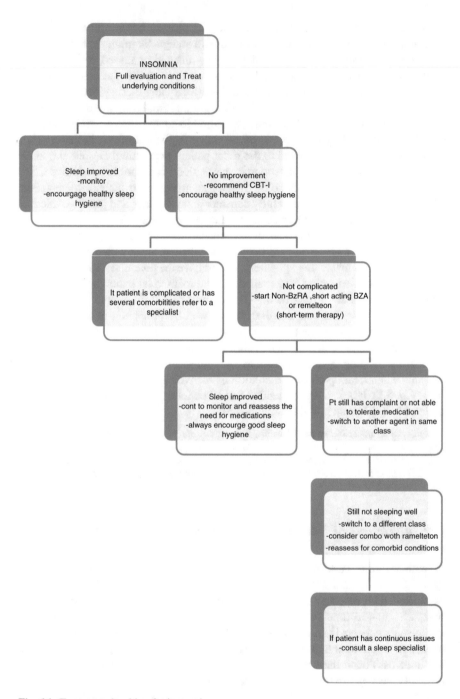

Fig. 6.1 Treatment algorithm for insomnia

Scales

Ford Insomnia in Response to Stress Test

FIRST (Ford Insomnia in Response to Stress Test) is a self-reported measure that may help at predicting initial onset insomnia in individuals without history of insomnia or depression. It consists of questions such as: (1) "In the past year, have you experienced difficulty falling asleep and/or staying asleep?" (2) On average, how long does it take you to fall back asleep after waking up (during the past month)?" and (3) "To what extent do you consider your sleep problem to interfere with your daily functioning (e.g. daytime fatigue, ability to function at work/daily chores, concentration, memory, mood, etc.)?" [89].

The Pittsburgh Sleep Quality Index (PSQI) is a self-rated questionnaire which assesses sleep quality and disturbances over a 1-month time interval. There are 19 individual items that measure 7 components of sleep: subjective sleep quality, sleep latency, sleep duration, habitual sleep efficiency, sleep disturbances, use of sleeping medication, and daytime dysfunction. The higher the score indicates greater sleep dysfunction [90].

Conclusion

Pharmacologic treatment of sleeplessness continues to increase with the formal diagnosis of insomnia, suggesting that life problems are being treated with medication solutions, without benefit of formal complaint or diagnosis [91]. This can lead to patients being on multiple hypnotics and or sedatives. We as clinicians, with the aid of self-assessment tools, should be able to screen more efficiently for patients with insomnia. With more accurate delineation of symptoms, we will be able to tailor better treatment options for patients. Good sleep hygiene and the possibility of CBT-I treatment should always be recommended.

References

1. Léger D, Poursain B, Neubauer D, Uchiyama M. An international survey of sleeping problems in the general population. Curr Med Res Opin. 2008;24(1):307–17.
2. Neubauer D, Flaherty K. Chronic insomnia. Semin Neurol. 2009;29(4):340–53.
3. Panossian L, Avidan A. Sleep disorders in neurologic practice: a case-based approach. Neurol Clin. 2016;34(3):565–94.
4. Quigga M, Gharaib S, Rulandb J, Schroeder C, Hodges M, Ingersoll K. Insomnia in epilepsy is associated with continuing seizures and worse quality of life. Epilepsy Res. 2016;122:91–6.
5. Wu M, Lin H, Weng S, Ho C, Wang J, Hsu Y. Insomnia subtypes and the subsequent risks of stroke: report from a nationally representative cohort. Stroke. 2014;45:1349–54.

6. Institute of Medicine (US) Committee on Sleep Medicine and Research. Sleep physiology. In: Altevogt B, Colten HR, editors. Sleep disorders and sleep deprivation: an unmet public health problem. Washington, DC: National Academies Press (US); 2006.
7. Irwin M. Why sleep is important for health: a psychoneuroimmunology perspective. Annul Rev Psychol. 2015;66:143–72.
8. Poyares D, Guilleminault C, Ohayon M, Tufik S. Chronic benzodiazepine usage and withdrawal insomnia patients. J Psychiatr Res. 2004;38(3):327–34.
9. American Academy of Sleep Medicine. In: Darien IL, editor. International classification of sleep disorders. Weschester: American Academy of sleep medicine; 2014.
10. National Institutes of Health. National institutes of health state of the science conference statement on manifestations and management of chronic insomnia in adults. Bethesda: NIH; 2005.
11. Hollister LE. The pre-benzodiazepine era. J Psychoactive Drugs. 1983;15:9–13.
12. Lopez-Munoz F, Ucha-Udabe R, Alamo C. The history of barbiturates a century after their clinical introduction. Neuropsychiatr Dis Treat. 2005;1(4):329–43.
13. Committee NE. Expert committee on addiction-producing drugs. Geneva: World Health Organization; 1956.
14. Wick J. The history of benzodiazepines. Consult Pharm. 2013;28(9):538–48.
15. Rosenbaum J. Attitudes toward benzodiazepines over the years. J Clin Psychiatry. 2005;66:4–8.
16. Hilty D, Young J. Algorithms from assessment and management of insomnia in primary care. Patient Prefer Adherence. 2009;3:9–20.
17. Mitchell M, Gehrman P, Perlis M, Umscheid C. Comparative effectiveness of cognitive behavioral therapy for insomnia: a systematic review. BMC Fam Pract. 2012;13:40.
18. Benca RM. Diagnosis and treatment of chronic insomnia: a review. Psychiatr Serv. 2005;56(3):332–43.
19. Buysse D. Insomia. JAMA. 2013;309(7):706–16.
20. FDA. U.S. Drug and Food Adminstration. 2015. Retrieved Jan 9, 2017, from http://www.fda.gov/drugs/drugsafety/postmarketdrugsafetyinformationforpatientsandproviders/ucm101557.htm
21. Krystal AD. A compendium of placebo-controlled trials of the risks/benefits of pharmacological treatments for insomnia: the empirical basis for U.S. clinical practice. Sleep Med Rev. 2009;13(4):265–74.
22. Mitler M. Evaluation of temazepam as a hypnotic. Pharmacotherapy. 1981;1(1):3–13.
23. Roehrst T, Zorick F, Lord N, Koshorek G, Roth T. Dose-related effects of estazolam on sleep of patients with insomnia. J Clin Psychopharmacol. 1983;3(3):152–6.
24. Pierce M, Shu V. Efficacy of estazolam. The United States clinical experience. Am J Med. 1990;88(3A):6s–11s.
25. Vogel G, Morris D. The effects of estazolam on sleep, performance, and memory: a long-term sleep laboratory study of elderly insomniacs. J Clin Pharmacol. 1992;32(7):647–51.
26. Scharf M, Roth P, Dominguez R, Ware J. Estazolam and flurazepam: a multicenter, placebo-controlled comparative study in outpatients with insomnia. J Clin Pharmacol. 1990;30 (5):461–7.
27. Roehrs T, Zorick F, Kaffeman M, Sicklesteel J, Roth T. Flurazepam for short-term treatment of complaints of insomnia. J Clin Pharmacol. 1982;22(7):290–6.
28. Pakes G, Brogden R, Heel R, Speight T, Avery G. Triazolam: a review of its pharmacological properties and therapeutic efficacy in patients with insomnia. Drugs. 1981;22(2):81–110.
29. Kroboth P, Juhl R. New drug evaluations. Triazolam. Drug Intell Clin Pharm. 1983;17(7):495–500.
30. Kales A. Quazepam: hypnotic efficacy and side effects. Pharmacotherapy. 1990;10(1):1–10. discussion 10-2.
31. Dündar Y, Boland A, Strobl J, Dodd S, Haycox A, Bagust A. Newer hypnotic drugs for the short-term management of insomnia: a systematic review and economic evaluation. Health Technol Assess. 2004;8(24):1–125.
32. Mohler H, Fritschy J, Rudolph U. A new benzodiazepine pharmacology. J Pharmacol ExperTher. 2002;300(1):2–8.

33. Hoehns J, Perry P. Zolpidem: a benzodiazepine hypnotic for treatment of insomnia. Clin Pharmacol. 1993;12(11):814–28.
34. Merlotti L, Roehrs T, Koshorek G, Zorick F, Lamphere J, Roth T. The dose effects of zolpidem on the sleep of healthy normals. J Clin Pharm Ther. 1989;9:9–14.
35. MacFarland J, Morin C. Hypnotics and insomnia: the experience of zolpidem. Clin Ther. 2014;36(11):1676–701.
36. Paulke A, Wunder C, Toennes S. Sleep self-intoxication and sleep driving as rare zolpidem-induced complex behaviour. Int J Legal Med. 2015;129(1):85–8.
37. Poceta J. Zolpidem ingestion, automatisms, and sleep driving: a clinical and legal case series. J Clin Sleep Med. 2011;7(6):632–8.
38. Noble S, Langtry H, Lamb H. Zopiclone. An update of its pharmacology, clinical efficacy and tolerability in the treatment of insomnia. Drugs. 1998;55(2):277–302.
39. Zammit GK, McNabb L. Efficacy and safety of eszopiclone across six weeks of treatment for primary insomnia. Curr Med Res Opin. 2004;20(12):1979–91.
40. Walsh J, Krystal A, Amato D, Rubens R, Caron J, Wessel T. Nightly treatment of primary insomnia with eszopiclone for six months: effect on sleep, quality of life, and work limitations. Sleep. 2007;30(8):959–68.
41. Najib J. Eszopiclone, a nonbenzodiazepine sedative-hypnotic agent for the treatment of transient and chronic insomnia. Clin Ther. 2006;28(4):491–516.
42. Pinto L Jr, Bittencourt L, Treptow E, Braqa LR, Tufik S. Eszopiclone versus zopiclone in the treatment of insomnia. Clinics (Sao Paulo). 2016;71(1):5–9.
43. Elie R, Ruther E, Farr I, Emilien G, Salinas E. Sleep latency is shortened during 4 weeks of treatment with zaleplon, a novel nonbenzodiazepine hypnotic. J Clin Psychiatry. 1999;60:536–44.
44. Israel A, Kramer J. Safety of zaleplon in the treatment of insomnia. Ann Pharmacother. 2002;36(5):852–9.
45. Roth T, Walsh J, Krystal A, Wessel T, Roehrs TA. An evaluation of the efficacy and safety of eszopiclone over 12 months in patients with chronic primary insomnia. Sleep Med. 2005;6(6):487–95.
46. Krystal A, Walsh J, Laska E, Caron J, Amato DA, Wessel T. Sustained efficacy of eszopiclone over 6 months of nightly treatment: results of a randomized, double-blind, placebo-controlled study in adults with chronic insomnia. Sleep. 2003;26(7):793–9.
47. Randall S, Roehrs T, Roth T. Efficacy of eight months of nightly zolpidem: a prospective placebo-controlled study. Sleep. 2012;35(11):1551–7.
48. Stahl S. Awakening to the psychopharmacology of sleep and arousal: novel neurotransmitters and wake-promoting drugs. J Clin Psychiatry. 2002;63(6):467–8.
49. Coleman PJ, Gotter A. Tthe discovery of suvorexant, the first Orexin receptor drug for insomnia. Ann Rev Psychopharmacol Toxicol. 2016;57:509–33.
50. Sutton EL. Profile of suvorexant in the management of insomnia. Drug Des Devel Ther. 2015;9:6035–42.
51. Merck, Sharp, & Dohme. Belsomra (Survorexant): full prescribing information. 2014. Retrieved Jan 2017, from https://www.merck.com/product/usa/pi_.pdf.
52. Michelson D, Snyder E. Safety and efficacy of suvorexant during 1-year treatment of insomnia with subsequent abrupt treatment discontinuation: a phase 3 randomize, double-blind, placebo-controlled trial. Lancet Neurol. 2014;13(5):461–71.
53. Zhdanova I, Lynch H, Wurtman R. Melatonin: a sleep-promoting hormone. Sleep. 1997;20(10):899–907.
54. Buscemi N, Vandermeer B, Friesen C, Bialy L, Tubman M, Ospina M. The efficacy and safety of drug treatments for chronic insomnia in adults: a meta-analysis of RCTs. J Gen Interl Med. 2007;22(9):1335–50.
55. Kato K, Hirai K, Nishiyama K, Uchikawa O, Fukatsu K, Ohkawa S. Neurochemical properties of ramelteon (TAK-375), a selective MT1/MT2 receptor agonist. Neuropharmacology. 2005;48(2):301–10.
56. Erman M, Seiden D, Zammit G, Sainati, Zhang J. An efficacy, safety, and dose-response study of Ramelteon in patients with chronic primary insomnia. Sleep Med. 2006;7(1):17–24.

57. Miyata A, Iwamoto K, Kawano N, Kohmura K, Yamamoto M, Aleksic B. The effects of acute treatment with ramelteon, triazolam, and placebo on driving performance, cognitive function, and equilibrium function in healthy volunteers. Psychopharmacology. 2015;232(12):2127–37.
58. McCall C, McCall W. What is the role of sedating antidepressants, antipsychotics, and anticonvulsants in the management of insomnia? Curr Psychiatry Rep. 2012;14:494–502.
59. Mendelson W. A review of the evidence for the efficacy and safety of trazodone in insomnia. J Clin Psychiatry. 2005;66(4):469–76.
60. Roth A, McCall W, Liguori A. Cognitive, psychomotor and polysomnographic effects of trazodone in primary insomniacs. J Sleep Res. 2011;20(4):552–8.
61. Hajak G, Rodenbeck A, Voderholzer U, Reimann D, Cohrs S, Hohagen F. Doxepin in the treatment of primary insomnia: a placebo-controlled, double-blind, polysomnographic study. J Clin Psychiatry. 2001;62(2):453–63.
62. Weber J, Siddiqui M, Wagstaff A, McCormack P. Low-dose doxepin: in the treatment of insomnia. CNS Drugs. 2010;24(8):713–20.
63. de Boer T. The effects of mirtazapine on central noradrenergic and serotonergic neurotransmission. Int Clin Psychopharmacol. 1995;10(4):19–23.
64. Aslan S, Isike E, Cosar B. The effects of mirtazapine on sleep: a placebo controlled, double-blind study in young healthy volunteers. Sleep. 2002;25(6):677–9.
65. Schmid D, Wichniak A, Uhr M, M I, Brunner H, Held K. Changes of sleep architecture, spectral composition of sleep EEG, the nocturnal secretion of cortisol, ACTH, GH, prolactin, melatonin, ghrelin, and leptin, and the DEX-CRH test in depressed patients during treatment with mirtazapine. Neuropsychopharmacology. 2006;31(4):832–44.
66. Schittecatte M, Dumont F, Machowski R. Effects of mirtazapine on sleep polygraphic variables in major depression. Neuropsychobiology. 2002;46(4):197–201.
67. Ivgy-Maya N, Ruweb F, Krystalc A, Roth T. Esmirtazapine in non-elderly adult patients with primary insomnia: efficacy and safety from a randomized, 6-week sleep laboratory trial. Sleep Med. 2015;16(7):838–44.
68. Merck & Co., I. 2010. http://www.merck.com/investors/financials/form-10-K-2009-final.pdf. Retrieved Jan 2017.
69. Asnis M, Thomas GM, Henderson M. Pharmacotherapy treatment options for insomnia: a primer for clinicians. Int J Mol Sci. 2015;17(1):50.
70. Vermeeren A. Residual effects of hypnotics: epidemiology and clinical implications. CNS Drugs. 2004;18:297–328.
71. Roth T, Hartse K, Saab P. The effects of flurazepam, lorazepam, and triazolam on sleep and memory. Psychopharmacology. 1980;70(3):231–7.
72. Mets M, Volkerts E, Olivier B, Verste J. Effect of hypnotic drugs on body balance and standing steadiness. Sleep Med Rev. 2010;14:259–67.
73. Weaver MF. Prescription sedative misuse and abuse. J Biol Med. 2015;88:247–56.
74. Zhabenko N, Wojnar M. Prevalence and correlates of insomnia and a polish sample of alcohol dependent patients. Alcohol Clin Exp Res. 2012;36:1600–7.
75. Brower KJ, Perron B. Prevalence and correlates of withdrawal-related insomnia among adults with alcohol dependence: results from a national survey. Am J Addict Tab 201023. 2010;19(3):238–44.
76. Brower KJ. Assessment and treatment of insomnia and adult patients with alcohol use disorder. Alcohol. 2015;49:417–27.
77. Friedmann PD, Rose J. Trazodone sleep disturbance after alcohol detoxification: a double-blind, placebo-controlled trial. Alcohol: Clin Exp Res. 2008;32(9):1652–60.
78. Rodriguez J, Dzierzewski J, Alessi CA. Sleep problems in the elderly. Med Clin N Am. 2015;99(2):431–9.
79. Foley D, Monjan A, Brown S, Simonsick EM, Wallace RB, Blazer D. Sleep complaints among elderly persons: an epidemiologic study of three communities. Sleep. 1995;18(6):425–32.
80. Perlis M, Smith L, Lyness JM, Matteson SR, Pigeon WR, Jungquist C. Insomnia as a risk factor for onset of depression in the elderly. Behav Sleep Med. 2006;4(2):104–13.

81. Wang P, Bohn R, Glynn R, Mogun H, Avorn J. Zolpidem use and hip fractures in older people. J Am Geriatr Soc. 2001;49(12):1685–90.
82. Kang D, Park S, Rhee C, Kim Y, Choi NK, Lee J. Zolpidem use and risk of fracture in elderly insomnia patients. J Prev Med Public Health. 2012;45(4):219–26.
83. Ilomäki J, Paljärvi T, Korhonen M, Enlund H, Alderman CP, Kauchanen J. Prevalence of concomitant use of alcohol and sedative-hypnotic drugs in middle and older aged persons: a systematic review. Ann Pharmacother. 2013;47:257–68.
84. Schutte-Rodin S, Broch L, Buysse D, Dorsey C, Sateia M. Clinical guideline for the evaluation and management of chronic insomnia in adults. J Clin Sleep Med. 2008;4(5):487–504.
85. Qaseem A, Kansagara D, Forciea M, Cooke M, Denberg T, Physicians, C. G. Management of chronic insomnia disorder in adults: a clinical practice guideline from the American College of Physicians. Ann Internl Med. 2016;165(2):125–33.
86. Chung S, Bohnen N, Albin R, Frey KA, Müller ML, Chervin R. Insomnia and sleepiness in Parkinson disease: associations with symptoms and comorbidities. J Clin Sleep Med. 2013;9(11):1131–7.
87. Ylikoski A, Martikainen K, Sieminski M, Partinen M. Parkinson's disease and insomnia. Neurol Sci. 2015;36:2003–10.
88. Gudin J, Mogali S, Jones J, Comer S. Risks, management, and monitoring of combination opioid, benzodiazepines, and/or alcohol use. Postgrad Med. 2013;125(4):115–30.
89. Kalmbach D, Pillai V, Arnedt J, Drake C. Identifying at-risk individuals for insomnia using the ford insomnia response to stress test. Sleep. 2016;39(2):449–4546.
90. Buysse D, Reynolds C 3rd, Monk T, Berman SR, Kupler DJ. The Pittsburgh sleep quality index: a new instrument for psychiatric practice and research. Psychiatry Res. 1989;28(2):193–213.
91. Moloney M, Konrad T, Zimmer C. The medicalization of sleeplessness: a public health concern. Am J Public Health. 2011;101(8):1429–33.
92. Heel R, Brogden R, Speight T, Avery G. Temazepam: a review of its pharmacological properties and therapeutic efficacy as an hypnotic. Drugs. 1981;21(5):321–40.
93. Cohn J, Wilcox C, Bremner J, Ettinger M. Hypnotic efficacy of estazolam compared with flurazepam in outpatients with insomnia. J Clin Pharmacol. 1991;31(8):747–50.
94. Stahl SM. Essential psychopharmacology: neuroscientific basis and practical applications. 2nd ed. New York: Cambridge University Press; 2000.

Chapter 7
Treating the Behavioral Symptoms of Dementia

Brianne M. Newman

Dementia is a term that includes multiple etiologies of cognitive impairment that significantly diminishes an individual's level of daily functioning. Alzheimer's disease (AD) is the most common form of dementia. AD is a progressive neurodegenerative disorder affecting memory and other cognitive domains interfering with daily functioning. Other dementias, such as vascular dementia, Lewy body dementia, and frontotemporal dementia, are less common but also cause considerable distress to patients and caregivers. With all dementias, behavior and mood changes often manifest as the neurodegenerative disorder progresses. These behavior and mood changes are either referred to as the behavioral and psychological symptoms of dementia (BPSD) or the neuropsychiatric symptoms of dementia (NPS). This chapter focuses on the treatment of BPSD, as these symptoms frequently facilitate caregiver stress and nursing home placement [1, 2].

There are three main categories of BPSD, including agitation/aggression, psychosis, and mood disorders. Greater than 90% of patients with dementia develop at least one of these behavioral symptoms in a 5-year period, with 85% of the symptoms rising to the level of clinical significance [3]. Thus, it is imperative that physicians who frequently diagnose and treat patients with dementia are aware of the non-pharmacological and pharmacological treatments available for BPSD. This chapter will first present data for non-pharmacologic treatments of BPSD, as they are the recommended first-line interventions [4–6] (Figs. 7.1 and 7.2). However, the majority of the chapter will review the pharmacological options available to treat BPSD that fail to respond to non-pharmacological interventions.

B. M. Newman, MD (✉)
Adult Psychiatry Training Program, Department of Psychiatry and Behavioral Neuroscience,
Saint Louis University School of Medicine, St. Louis, MO, USA
e-mail: brianne.newman@health.slu.edu

© Springer International Publishing AG, part of Springer Nature 2018   117
G. T. Grossberg, L. J. Kinsella (eds.), *Clinical Psychopharmacology for Neurologists*, https://doi.org/10.1007/978-3-319-74604-3_7

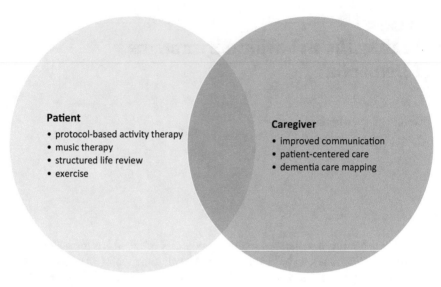

Fig. 7.1 Non-pharmacological interventions for BPSD

Treatment of Agitation in Dementia

Agitation in individuals with dementia manifests in a variety of ways including restlessness, pacing, fidgeting, repetitive motor activities, and abnormal vocalizations. Physicians should first consider the etiology of the agitation; for example, does the patient have an infection such as a UTI and is the patient in pain, delirious, and frustrated by apraxia or word-finding difficulties? Addressing the etiology of the agitation is the most useful first step. However, the symptom of agitation itself may require direct treatment, while the underlying etiology is under investigation.

Non-pharmacological Interventions

There are few randomized, controlled trials examining non-pharmacological treatments of agitation in settings other than care home placement. A recent systematic meta-analysis of non-pharmacological interventions for agitation [7] found significant improvement with caregiver training. Specifically, improving communication, person-centered care, and dementia care mapping within the care home each significantly reduced agitation. Follow-up showed that improvement continued 3–6 months after intervention, demonstrating efficacy with paid caregiver training even months after the intervention ceased. Protocol-based activity and music therapy were also beneficial interventions. However, the benefits persisted only during the therapeutic intervention, with no sustained benefit at follow-up [7–10]. In contrast, interventions such as touch therapy were not beneficial, even during the therapeutic

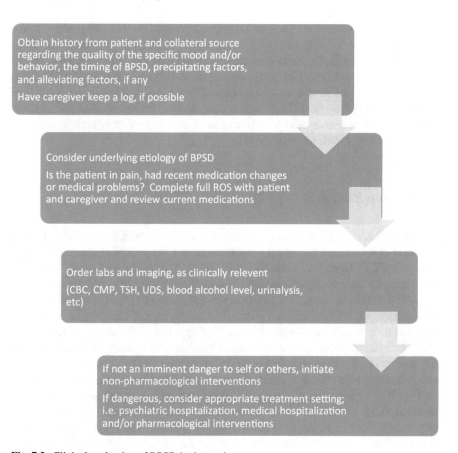

Fig. 7.2 Clinical evaluation of BPSD in dementia

intervention [7]. Aromatherapy has shown some benefit in select studies, but the benefits were not replicated in blinded trials [7, 11, 12]. Similarly, there is insufficient evidence regarding the efficacy of exercise for agitation in dementia [7].

Pharmacological Interventions

Pharmacological interventions for agitation and aggression in dementia are at times necessary based on potential danger to the patient and/or caregivers, despite the lack of FDA-approved medications for these indications. In these situations, treating physicians must delicately weigh the risks versus benefits of available pharmacological interventions. Antipsychotic medications are commonly used to treat agitation and aggression in the elderly with dementia [13]. In 2005, the US Food and Drug Administration (FDA) released a warning that both typical and atypical antipsychotics are associated with increased mortality in the elderly with dementia. The

FDA's announcement was based on 17 placebo-controlled trials (15 positive trials) showing a 1.6- to 1.7-fold mortality increase in the elderly with behavioral disturbances and dementia. Increased mortality was related to both cardiac and noncardiac causes of death [14]. Currently, the American Geriatrics Society (AGS) Beers Criteria 2015 recommends that physicians "avoid antipsychotics for behavioral problems of dementia or delirium unless nonpharmacological options (e.g., behavioral interventions) have failed or are not possible and the older adult is threatening substantial harm to self or others" [15].

Medication Selection

Once physicians, patients, and/or surrogate decision-makers have jointly decided that an antipsychotic is necessary, which one should the prescriber choose? There is a large body of literature examining this question. A recent systematic review of meta-analyses addressing antipsychotic use in dementia provides considerable guidance for prescribing physicians [6]. One meta-analysis of typical antipsychotics for the treatment of BPSD concluded that typical antipsychotics were significantly more effective than placebo at treating symptoms of agitation in dementia, with a modest effect size (0.18). There was no difference in efficacy comparing haloperidol, thioridazine, or other typical antipsychotics [16]. However, other side effects, such as the anticholinergic side effects of thioridazine, must be considered in medication choice.

The 2016 review of meta-analyses included ten studies examining atypical antipsychotics for BPSD. The authors concluded that risperidone, olanzapine, and aripiprazole have significant benefit in treating agitation and aggression in dementia, with a modest effect size. Quetiapine did not significantly improve BPSD in dementia when compared to placebo [6]. Table 7.1 provides guidance on initiation, titration, and dosage recommendations for antipsychotic use in individuals with dementia, adapted from the APA's practice guidelines for Alzheimer's disease and other dementias [17] and guideline watch update from 2014 [18].

Adverse Events/Side Effects

Prescribing physicians must also consider the potential adverse effects related to antipsychotic use. Side effects such as akathisia, Parkinsonism, sedation, anticholinergic effects, cardiac conduction abnormalities, postural hypotension, urinary incontinence and urinary tract infections, and falls must be monitored in the elderly treated with antipsychotic medications [6, 17]. As discussed previously, increased risk of death, as well as an increased risk of cerebrovascular events, in elderly with dementia who are treated with antipsychotics (typical or atypical) is a significant risk that limits their use. Other serious adverse events include tardive dyskinesia, neuroleptic malignant syndrome, and metabolic syndrome [17].

Table 7.1 Common medications for the behavioral and psychological symptoms of dementia

Medication	Formulations	Starting dose	Effective dose	Monitoring
Antipsychotics				
Risperidone	Tablet	0.25–0.5 mg	1–1.5 mg daily	AIMS
	Disintegrating tablet			Metabolic monitoring
	LAI			
Olanzapine	Tablet	2.5–5 mg daily	Up to 10 mg daily	AIMS
	Disintegrating tablet			Metabolic monitoring
	IM			
	LAI			
Aripiprazole	Tablet	2.5–5 mg daily	Up to 15 mg daily	AIMS
	LAI			
Haloperidol	Tablet	0.25–0.5 mg daily	Up to 2 mg daily	AIMS
	Liquid			*IV highest risk of prolonged QTc interval
	IM			
	IV			
	LAI			
Antidepressants				
Sertraline	Tablet	12.5–25 mg daily	50–200 mg daily	Electrolytes
	Liquid			
Citalopram	Tablet	5–10 mg daily	10–20 mg daily	*FDA max dose for age >60 is 20 mg daily
	Liquid			QTc interval
Venlafaxine	Immediate release tablet	IR: 25 mg daily	IR: up to 300 mg in divided doses	Blood pressure (specifically diastolic)
	Extended release tablet	XR: 37.5 mg daily	XR: up to 300 mg daily	
Mirtazapine	Tablet	7.5 mg daily	15–60 mg daily	Weight
	Disintegrating tablet			Falls with sedation
Bupropion	Immediate release	IR: 37.5 BID	IR: up to 100 mg TID	Seizures in anorexia or neurologic abnormalities
	Sustained release (SR)	SR: 100 mg daily	SR: 150 mg BID	
	Extended release (XL)	XL: 150 mg daily	XL: 300 mg daily	

AIMS Abnormal Involuntary Movement Scale, *IM* intramuscular, *IV* intravenous, *LAI* long-acting injectable
*Refers to the source 4, 5 & 6

Length of Treatment

How long should physicians prescribe an antipsychotic medication for agitation or aggression in individuals with dementia? Two meta-analyses [19, 20] are available to help guide this decision, as well as the American Psychiatric Association (APA) guideline on the use of antipsychotics for the treatment of agitation and psychosis in dementia [20]. Mortality rates were lower in individuals for whom antipsychotic discontinuation occurred, as opposed to those who continued treatment [20]. Discontinuation of antipsychotic medications can be well tolerated but has been shown to further aggravate BPSD in those with severe behavioral symptoms [6, 19, 20]. The APA recommends discontinuing antipsychotic medications after 4 weeks if there is limited efficacy at an adequate dose [21]. If there is clinically significant treatment efficacy, physicians should consider tapering and/or discontinuing the antipsychotic within 4 months of initiation, unless there has been a failed attempt at withdrawal. Symptoms should be monitored every month during the taper and for 4 months after discontinuing an antipsychotic medication. Another study looking specifically at subjects who had a significant clinical response to risperidone concluded that in those patients with dementia whose agitation and/or psychosis responded to risperidone which was continued for 4–8 months, discontinuation of the medication worsened relapse [22].

Are there other medication classes that are effective at treating agitation/aggression in individuals with dementia? Considering the increased risk of severe adverse events with antipsychotic medications, there is interest in identifying other medication classes with safer side-effect profiles for treatment of BPSD. Antidepressants have some data supporting their use. A Cochrane review of antidepressants for treating agitation and psychosis in dementia concluded that there is a paucity of high-quality data regarding efficacy of the antidepressants for this indication. They note that there is some evidence that sertraline, citalopram, and trazodone may help treat agitation and psychosis for some individuals with dementia [23]. The more recent Citalopram for Agitation in Alzheimer Disease Study (CitAD), a randomized, double-blind, placebo-controlled, parallel study, examined the use of citalopram (10 mg titrated to a max of 30 mg daily) for BPSD in probable AD individuals. The authors concluded that in combination with a psychosocial intervention, citalopram showed a significant benefit in the treatment of agitation and reduced caregiver distress. However, there were significant cognitive side effects and prolonged QT intervals in the citalopram-treated individuals [24]. It is important to note that the FDA revised prescribing recommendation for citalopram in March 2012 to include the maximum recommended dosage for patients 60 years and older is now 20 mg daily, while the maximum dosage prescribed in the CitAD study was 30 mg daily [25]. Other medications, such as acetylcholinesterase inhibitors (e.g., galantamine 24 mg/day) and the NMDA receptor antagonist memantine, show very modest benefits in the treatment of agitation in dementia [26, 27]. There are other novel treatment investigations ongoing but remain investigational at this time [28]. The use of medications such as carbamazepine, valproate, beta blockers, and lithium for the treatment of agitation in dementia is not recommended at this time by the APA [17, 18].

In conclusion, the most data exists for using antipsychotic medications for the treatment of agitation and aggression in dementia. However, physicians, in consultation with patients and/or surrogate decision-makers, must carefully weigh the following options when non-pharmacological interventions are ineffective: the risks of treatment, the risks of untreated agitation/aggression, and the potential modest benefits of medication treatment. During this deliberation, other less-studied options, such as antidepressants, acetylcholinesterase inhibitors, and memantine, may be considered based on individual clinical factors.

Treatment of Psychosis in Dementia

Psychotic symptoms are common in the course of dementia, with 75% of patients experiencing some form of psychosis during the disease process [29]. Psychotic symptoms are part of the neurodegenerative progression of dementing illnesses and include delusions and hallucinations.

Similar to recommendations for agitation and aggression in dementia, pharmacological treatment of psychosis is appropriate if the symptoms are causing clinically significant distress and/or impacting the patient's quality of life [21]. Although psychotic symptoms are common at some point in the course of dementia, if the symptoms are not causing significant consequences, they can be addressed with non-pharmacological interventions.

Medication Selection

It is helpful to consider the underlying type of dementia when tailoring interventions for individual patients. In patients with AD, antipsychotic medications are again the mainstay of treatment, with the most data supporting the use of risperidone for psychosis in dementia [6, 21]. Meta-analyses also demonstrate modest efficacy with the atypical antipsychotic medications, olanzapine and aripiprazole, with no significant efficacy seen with quetiapine [6]. Patients with Lewy body dementia or Parkinson's dementia are more sensitive to the adverse effects of antipsychotic medications, in particular, extrapyramidal symptoms [30, 31]. Clinically, physicians most often prescribe quetiapine or clozapine in individuals with these particular types of dementia; however, there is very little evidence supporting this practice [21, 31]. Pimavanserin, a selective serotonin$_{2A}$ receptor inverse agonist, is a newer medication now FDA approved specifically for the treatment of hallucinations and delusions due to psychosis in patients with Parkinson's disease. Further research and clinical experience will provide more information on the utility of this medication for the behavioral disturbances with specific dementias.

Adverse events and length of treatment for psychosis with antipsychotic medications are the same as discussed previously for agitation and aggression. There is not enough evidence supporting alternative medication classes for the treatment of psychosis in dementia [6, 32]. There is not sufficient evidence to support prescribing antidepressants specifically to address psychotic symptoms, despite the modest benefits noted when addressing agitation.

Treatment of Mood Disorders in Dementia

The relationship between mood disorders, specifically depression, and dementia is very complex. However, it is clear that depressive symptoms, which include mood changes, irritability, apathy, social isolation, thoughts of death, and suicidal ideation, are very common manifestations of neurodegenerative disorders. In the literature, rates of mood symptoms in individuals with dementia are between 10% and 86%, with 20–40% meeting full criteria for depression [33–36]. Thus, physicians commonly treating older adults with dementia must be familiar with the literature regarding current treatment for mood in this specific population.

Non-pharmacological Interventions

Non-pharmacological interventions for mood symptoms are also first line for patients with dementia. Unlike treatment of cognitively unimpaired older adults, beneficial therapeutic interventions require caregiver participation. Cognitive behavioral therapy (CBT) is an effective treatment modality for non-cognitively impaired older adults with depression and anxiety; however, adaptations are required for the cognitively impaired individual. For individuals with dementia, data support the efficacy of behavioral management techniques such as increased pleasant activities, behavioral problem-solving therapy, and structured life review [37–40]. For caregivers, CBT techniques targeting communication, caregiver stress, and reinforcement of the behavioral techniques helpful for the patient are effective psychosocial treatment modalities [7, 38, 40]. Thus, non-pharmacological interventions for mood disorders can be very effective, particularly when they incorporate caregivers into the treatment.

Pharmacological Interventions

Data for the efficacy of antidepressants in dementia show mixed results. However, SSRI antidepressants remain the mainstay of pharmacological treatment of depression in dementia with data supporting sertraline and citalopram [17, 41–43]. APA guidelines recommend avoiding cyclic antidepressants (such as amitriptyline) in the elderly with dementia, as they are less effective than other antidepressant medications and/or have more intolerable side effects. There is some evidence that psychostimulants such as methylphenidate (20 mg/day) can be an effective treatment for apathy in patients with dementia [17, 43–45]. Modafinil was not effective in treating apathy in a randomized, double-blind placebo-controlled study [46]. Electroconvulsive therapy (ECT) is another effective treatment strategy for elderly patients with depression, but there are limited data specifically studying ECT in elderly individuals with dementia [47–49]. Clinically, individuals with dementia and depression receive ECT if he or she has life-threatening symptoms (i.e., not eating) or has refractory depression to multiple antidepressant trials.

Adverse Events/Side Effects

SSRI antidepressants are the first-line pharmacological treatment in depressed elderly as they have less side effects than other antidepressant categories, such as the cyclic antidepressants and monoamine oxidase inhibitors (MAOIs), which have significant anticholinergic and cardiovascular side effects. Physicians prescribing SSRI antidepressants to elderly with dementia need to monitor for side effects including gastrointestinal side effects (nausea/vomiting), neurological side effects (Parkinsonism, akathisia), and sexual side effects, weight loss, and hyponatremia. There is an increased risk for falls in elderly individuals treated with SSRI medications [50]. Also, SSRIs and other antidepressants are metabolized through the cytochrome P450 system; thus, the prescriber must consider possible drug-drug interactions when prescribing antidepressants in the elderly [17].

Other antidepressants with less data in the elderly with dementia have specific side effects. Mirtazapine, a noradrenergic/specific serotonergic antidepressant, causes weight gain (which may be desirable in older adults with dementia) and sedation, with rare but serious side effects of liver toxicity and neutropenia. Venlafaxine, a serotonin-norepinephrine reuptake inhibitor (SNRI), can cause increased blood pressure during both treatment and discontinuation of the medication. Duloxetine, another SNRI, has no specific data supporting its use in the elderly population but is often used with depression and pain in older adults. Bupropion, a norepinephrine-dopamine reuptake inhibitor, lowers seizure threshold more than other antidepressants and would not be a good choice for older adults with known seizure disorder or other risk factors for seizures. Trazodone, a serotonin-2 antagonist/reuptake inhibitor, has common side effects of sedation and may be used at low doses for insomnia and/or agitation in this population; however, higher doses are required for depression and may cause sedation and orthostatic hypotension, increasing the risk of falls [17].

Length of Treatment

Based on the literature review while preparing this chapter, the recommendations were unclear regarding the length of treatment for depression in the elderly with dementia. According to the APA's guidelines for the treatment of major depressive disorder in the elderly, the same length of treatment for the general adult population is recommended. Specifically, treatment with an effective antidepressant, at the full therapeutic dose, should be continued for 4–9 months, up to 12 months, after remission. If the individual has had three or more recurrent depressive episodes, or other factors that would warrant long-term treatment, medication should be continued indefinitely at the same dose that got the patient well. In the elderly population with dementia, mood symptoms can fluctuate; thus, determining the length of treatment depends on the specific clinical situation [17].

Case Report

Ms. A was a 51-year-old female with no past psychiatric history that self-presented with increased anxiety, irritability, and memory concerns. She reported using no alcohol or other illicit substances. Her family history was notable only for her maternal grandmother having AD and her mother having an unknown dementia in her 60s. Mental status exam was notable for a well-groomed female, good eye contact, very cooperative, increased psychomotor activity, very mild word-finding difficulty, logical thought process, no suicidal ideation, but perseverative concern with her memory and change in mood. She was visibly anxious, but alert and oriented, with good attention but poor recall, some repeating within 5–10 min. Labs (TSH, CBC, CMP, vitamin B12, folate, RPR) were within normal limits. We decided to first treat mood symptoms and then look at memory if not improved. We initiated fluoxetine 20 mg and CBT.

Visit 2: Ms. A's anxiety and irritability were better but no change in memory. Her brain MRI was normal. We sent her for neuropsychological testing.

Visit 3: Ms. A developed myoclonic jerks while sleeping, possibly related to fluoxetine. Since she continued with some residual mood and anxiety symptoms, we changed fluoxetine to citalopram. Neuropsychological testing showed profound anterograde memory deficit, also visual memory and naming deficits. Her executive functioning was mildly impaired, though her anxiety did not fully account for the severity.

Ms. A was sent to a memory clinic, considering her very young age. PET imaging demonstrated biparietal hypometabolism, and CSF biomarkers were consistent with AD. She was diagnosed with Alzheimer's disease and started on donepezil 10 mg daily. She was also continued on citalopram 20 mg daily. Her memory decline slowed over the next few months, and her mood and anxiety improved significantly.

At her last psychiatric visit, her AD was in moderate stage, so memantine was added, donepezil was continued, and her surrogate decision-maker requested a trial off citalopram (tapered 10 mg for 2 weeks, then discontinued). Her neuropsychiatric symptoms remained stable with this regimen.

Clinical Pearls

- Behavioral and psychological symptoms of dementia occur in all dementia subtypes.
- Non-pharmacological interventions are first-line treatments for BPSD.
- Document a thorough risk/benefit discussion with the family in the patient's chart if antipsychotics are the best option and if time permits (not emergency situation).
- If medications are warranted, start at a low dose and titrate slowly, but the patient may require doses typical of other adults to have symptomatic relief.
- Monitor carefully for side effects which are seen more frequently in the elderly with dementia.
- At each visit, consider if the patient needs to continue BPSD medications.

Conclusion

Behavioral and psychological symptoms of dementia are common and part of the clinical presentation of any individual with dementia of any type. Physicians can best guide treatment strategies by considering the differential diagnosis of the emotion or behavior (i.e., is this agitation, aggression, psychosis, or a mood change?) and considering and treating any underlying etiology of that particular symptom. Non-pharmacological interventions should be first-line treatment for any BPSD. Pharmacological treatment initiation should ideally occur only after a full risk/benefit analysis is considered with the patient and/or surrogate decision-maker. When pharmacological treatment is warranted, close monitoring of side effects and regular consideration regarding the need for continued treatment are imperative.

References

1. Steele C, Rovner B, Chase BA, et al. Psychiatric symptoms and nursing home placement of patients with Alzheimer's disease. Am J Psychiatr. 1990;147:1049–51.
2. Balestreri L, Grossberg A, Grossberg GT. Behavioral and psychological symptoms of dementia as a risk factor for nursing home placement. Int Psychogeriatr. 2000;12(Supplement 1):59–62.
3. Ballard CG, et al. Management of agitation and aggression associated with Alzheimer disease. Nat Rev Neurol. 2009;5(5):245–55.

4. Kales H, Gitlin L, Lyketsos C. Management of neuropsychiatric symptoms of dementia in clinical settings: recommendations from a multidisciplinary expert panel. J Am Geriatr Soc. 2014;62:762–9.
5. Kales H. Common sense: addressed to geriatric psychiatrists on the subject of behavioral and psychological symptoms of dementia. Am J Geriatr Psychiatry. 2015;23:1209–13.
6. Tampi RR, Tampi DJ, Balachandran S, Srinivasan S. Antipsychotic use in dementia: a systematic review of benefits and risks from meta-analyses. Ther Adv Chronic Dis. 2016;7(5):229–45.
7. Livingston G, Kelly L, Lewis-Holmes E, Baio G, Morris S, Patel N, Omar RZ, Katona C, Cooper C. Non-pharmacological interventions for agitation in dementia: systematic review of randomised controlled trials. Br J Psychiatry. 2014;205(6):436–42.
8. Cooke ML, Moyle W, Shum DH, Harrison SD, Murfield JE. A randomized controlled trial exploring the effect of music on agitated behaviours and anxiety in older people with dementia. Aging Ment Health. 2010;14:905–16.
9. Lin Y, Chu H, Yang CY, Chen CH, Chen SG, Chang HJ, et al. Effectiveness of group music intervention against agitated behavior in elderly persons with dementia. Int J Geriatr Psychiatry. 2011;26:670–8.
10. Sung HC, Lee WL, Li TL, Watson R. A group music intervention using percussion instruments with familiar music to reduce anxiety and agitation of institutionalized older adults with dementia. Int J Geriatr Psychiatry. 2012;27:621–7.
11. Ballard CG, O'Brien JT, Reichelt K, Perry EK. Aromatherapy as a safe and effective treatment for the management of agitation in severe dementia: the results of a double-blind, placebo-controlled trial with Melissa. J Clin Psychiatry. 2002;63:553–8.
12. Burns A, Perry E, Holmes C, Francis P, Morris J, Howes MJ, et al. A double-blind placebo-controlled randomized trial of Melissa officinalis oil and donepezil for the treatment of agitation in Alzheimer's disease. Dement Geriatr Cogn Disord. 2011;31:158–64.
13. Zuidema S, Johansson A, Selbaek G, Murray M, Burns A, Ballard C, et al. A consensus guideline for antipsychotic drug use for dementia in care homes. Bridging the gap between scientific evidence and clinical practice. Int Psychogeriatr. 2015;27:1849–59.
14. FDA public health advisory: deaths with antipsychotics in elderly patients with behavioral disturbances. 2005. https://www.fda.gov/Drugs/DrugSafety/PostmarketDrugSafetyInformationforPatientsandProviders/ucm053171.htm. Accessed 20 Feb 2017.
15. By the American Geriatrics Society 2015 Beers Criteria Update Expert Panel. American Geriatrics Society 2015 updated beers criteria for potentially inappropriate medication use in older adults. J Am Geriatr Soc. 2015;63(11):2227–46.
16. Schneider L, Pollock V, Lyness S. A meta-analysis of controlled trials of neuroleptic treatment in dementia. J Am Geriatr Soc. 1990;38:553–63.
17. Practice guideline for the treatment of patients with Alzheimer's disease and other dementias. American Psychiatric Association. 2007.
18. Guideline watch (October 2014): practice guideline for the treatment of patients with Alzheimer's disease and other dementias. American Psychiatric Association. 2014.
19. Declercq T, Petrovic M, Azermai M, Vander SR, De Sutter A, Van Driel M, et al. Withdrawal versus continuation of chronic antipsychotic drugs for behavioural and psychological symptoms in older people with dementia. Cochrane Database Syst Rev. 2013;3:CD007726.
20. Pan Y, Wu C, Gau S, Chan H, Banerjee S. Antipsychotic discontinuation in patients with dementia: a systematic review and meta-analysis of published randomized controlled studies. Dement Geriatr Cogn Disord. 2014;37:125–40.
21. Reus VI, Fochtmann LJ, Evan Eyler A, Hilty DM, Horvitz-Lennon M, Jibson MD, Lopez OL, Mahoney J, Pasic J, Tan ZS, Wills CD, Rhoads R, Yager J. The American Psychiatric Association practice guideline on the use of antipsychotics to treat agitation or psychosis in patients with dementia. Am J Psychiatr. 2016;173(5):543–6.
22. Devanand DP, Mintzer J, Schultz SK, et al. Relapse risk after discontinuation of risperidone in Alzheimer's disease. N Engl J Med. 2012;367(16):1497–507.

23. Seitz D, Adunuri N, Gill S, Gruneir A, Herrmann N, Rochon P. Antidepressants for agitation and psychosis in dementia. Cochrane Database Syst Rev. 2011;2:CD008191.
24. Porsteinsson AP, Drye LT, Pollock BG, Devanand DP, Frangakis C, Ismail Z, et al., CitAD Research Group. Effect of citalopram on agitation in Alzheimer's disease – the CitAD randomized controlled trial. JAMA: J Am Med Assoc. 2014;311(7):682–91.
25. FDA Drug Safety Communication: revised recommendations for Celexa (citalopram hydrobromide) related to a potential risk of abnormal heart rhythms with high doses. https://www.fda.gov/Drugs/DrugSafety/ucm297391.html. Accessed 27 Nov 2017.
26. Birks J. Cholinesterase inhibitors for Alzheimer's disease. Cochrane Database Syst Rev. 2006;(1).
27. McShane R, Areosa Sastre A, Minakaran N. Memantine for dementia. Cochrane Database Syst Rev. 2006;(2).
28. Panza F, Solfrizzi V, Seripa D, Imbimbo B, Santamato A, Lozupone M, et al. Progresses in treating agitation: a major clinical challenge in Alzheimer's disease. Expert Opin Pharmacother. 2015;16:2581–8.
29. Sadock BJ, Kaplan VA. Kaplan and Sadock's concise textbook of clinical psychiatry. Philadelphia: Lippincott, Williams and Wilkins; 2008.
30. Aarsland D, Perry R, Larsen JP, et al. Neuroleptic sensitivity in Parkinson's disease and parkinsonian dementias. J Clin Psychiatry. 2005;66(5):633–7.
31. Stinton C, McKeith I, Taylor JP, et al. Pharmacological management of Lewy body dementia: a systematic review and meta-analysis. Am J Psychiatry. 2015;172(8):731–42.
32. Lochhead JD, Nelson MA, Maguire GA. The treatment of behavioral disturbances and psychosis associated with dementia. Psychiatr Pol. 2016;50(2):311–22.
33. Garre-Olmo J, López-Pousa S, Vilata-Franch J, Turon-Estrada A, Hernàndez-Ferràndiz M, Lozano-Gallego M, et al. Evolution of depressive symptoms in Alzheimer's disease: one-year follow-up. Alzheimer Dis Assoc Disord. 2003;17(2):77–85.
34. Zubenko GS, Zubenko WN, McPherson S, Spoor E, Marin DB, Farlow MR, Sunderland T. A collaborative study of the emergence and clinical features of the major depressive syndrome of Alzheimer's disease. Am J Psychiatr. 2003;160(5):857–66.
35. Lyketsos CG, Olin JT. Depression in Alzheimer's disease: overview and treatment. Biol Psychiatry. 2002;52(3):243–52.
36. García-Alberca JM. Cognitive-behavioral treatment for depressed patients with Alzheimer's disease. An open trial. Arch Gerontol Geriatr. 2017;71:1–8.
37. Teri L, Logsdon RG, Uomoto J, McCurry SM. Behavioral treatment of depression in dementia patients: a controlled clinical trial. J Gerontol B Psychol Sci Soc Sci. 1997;52(4):159–66.
38. Teri L, Gibbons LE, McCurry SM, Logsdon RG, Buchner DM, Barlow WE, et al. Exercise plus behavioral management in patients with Alzheimer disease: a randomized controlled trial. J Am Med Assoc. 2003;290:2015–22.
39. Woods B, Spector A, Jones C, Orrell M, Davies S. Reminiscence therapy for dementia. Cochrane Database Syst Rev. 2005;18(2):CD001120.
40. Forstmeier S, Maercker A, Savaskan E, Roth T. Cognitive behavioural treatment for mild Alzheimer's patients and their caregivers (CBTAC): study protocol for a randomized controlled trial. Trials. 2015;16:526.
41. Nyth AL, Gottfries CG, Lyby K, Smedegaard-Andersen L, Gylding-Sabroe J, Kristensen M, Refsum HE, Ofsti E, Eriksson S, Syversen S. A controlled multicenter clinical study of citalopram and placebo in elderly depressed patients with and without concomitant dementia. Acta Psychiatr Scand. 1992;86:138–45.
42. Lyketsos CG, DelCampo L, Steinberg M, Miles Q, Steele CD, Munro C, Baker AS, Sheppard JM, Frangakis C, Brandt J, Rabins PV. Treating depression in Alzheimer disease: efficacy and safety of sertraline therapy, and the benefits of depression reduction: the DIADS. Arch Gen Psychiatry. 2003;60:737–46.
43. Rabins P, Rovner BW, Rummans T, et al. Guideline watch (October 2014): practice guideline for the treatment of patients with Alzheimer's disease and other dementias. Am J Psychiatry. 2007 Dec;164(12 Suppl):5–56.

44. Galynker I, Ieronimo C, Miner C, Rosenblum J, Vilkas N, Rosenthal R. Methylphenidate treatment of negative symptoms in patients with dementia. J Neuropsychiatry Clin Neurosci. 1997;9:231–9.
45. Rosenberg PB, Lanctôt KL, Drye LT, Herrmann N, Scherer RW, Bachman DL, Mintzer JE. ADMET Investigators: safety and efficacy of methylphenidate for apathy in Alzheimer's disease: a randomized, placebo-controlled trial. J Clin Psychiatry. 2013;74(8):810–6.
46. Frakey LL, Salloway S, Buelow M, Malloy P. A randomized, double-blind, placebo-controlled trial of modafinil for the treatment of apathy in individuals with mild-to-moderate Alzheimer's disease. J Clin Psychiatry. 2012;73(6):796–801.
47. Tew JD Jr, Mulsant BH, Haskett RF, Prudic J, Thase ME, Crowe RR, Dolata D, Begley AE, Reynolds CF III, Sackeim HA. Acute efficacy of ECT in the treatment of major depression in the old-old. Am J Psychiatry. 1999;156:1865–70.
48. Rao V, Lyketsos CG. The benefits and risks of ECT for patients with primary dementia who also suffer from depression. Int J Geriatr Psychiatry. 2000;15:729–35.
49. O'Connor MK, Knapp R, Husain M, Rummans TA, Petrides G, Smith G, Mueller M, Snyder K, Bernstein H, Rush AJ, Fink M, Kellner C. The influence of age on the response of major depression to electroconvulsive therapy: a C.O.R.E. report. Am J Geriatr Psychiatry. 2001;9:382–90.
50. Thapa PB, Gideon P, Cost TW, Milam AB, Ray WA. Antidepressants and the risk of falls among nursing home residents. N Engl J Med. 1998;339:875–82.

Chapter 8
Antipsychotics

Alexander Chen and Henry A. Nasrallah

Neurological disorders are almost always associated with psychiatric symptoms because disrupting neural pathways disrupt the circuitry that underlies mental processes. Of all the psychiatric symptoms that neurological lesions can trigger, psychosis is perhaps the most confusing to the patient and alarming to the neurologist due to the seriousness of the symptoms that can range from delusions and hallucinations to bizarre behavior or harm to self or others. While some neurologists refer patients who develop psychotic symptoms to psychiatrists for management, others treat such patients themselves. However, as psychiatrists know well, the management of psychotic disorders goes beyond pharmacotherapy and requires a team approach that can provide the necessary psychosocial interventions and therapies. However, pharmacologic treatment of poor reality testing in psychosis is the most essential initial step toward restoring mental and functional stability to a patient. In this chapter, an overview of the three generations of antipsychotics is provided for neurologists to enable them to initiate the treatment of psychosis in their neurological practice and refer the patient as needed for longer-term management in a psychiatric setting.

Treatment for psychosis, prior to the serendipitous discovery of the first antipsychotic chlorpromazine, represented the dark scientific era of psychiatry. Patients with psychotic disorders spent their lives confined to large institutions known as state hospitals or asylums, which were the psychiatric equivalent of the

A. Chen, MD (✉)
Department of Psychiatry and Behavioral Neuroscience, Saint Louis University
School of Medicine, St. Louis, MO, USA
e-mail: chena@slu.edu

H. A. Nasrallah, MD
Department of Psychiatry and Behavioral Neuroscience, SSM Health Saint Louis University
Hospital, St. Louis, MO, USA

© Springer International Publishing AG, part of Springer Nature 2018   131
G. T. Grossberg, L. J. Kinsella (eds.), *Clinical Psychopharmacology for Neurologists*, https://doi.org/10.1007/978-3-319-74604-3_8

leprosariums of the Middle Ages, where afflicted individuals received useless treatments akin to snake oil remedies. The advent of antipsychotics heralded a new era in psychiatric brain disorders and was monumental in demystifying psychiatric illnesses, especially severe psychotic disorders like schizophrenia which were believed to be untreatable. Antipsychotics validated the medical and neurochemical nature of mental and behavioral disorders and helped to inspire scientific research into the neurobiological underpinnings of psychiatric pathologies, launching the neuroscience revolution of the past half century. This chapter will review the history, efficacy, tolerability, safety, and dosages of antipsychotics, starting with the first-generation antipsychotics (FGA) that paved the way for a revolution in treating psychosis and leading to the second-generation antipsychotics (SGA) that have largely supplanted FGA in modern practice. An exciting third-generation antipsychotic was introduced in mid-2016 for psychosis in Parkinson Disease, with a completely different mechanism of action from the FGA and SGA. Neurologists are loathe to use the FGA due to their well-known neurological side effects (movement disorders) that are no longer acceptable in clinical practice now that less neurotoxic agents have been developed and are widely available. Thus, the section on FGA is included for historical reasons as the foundation of modern antipsychotic therapy.

First-Generation Antipsychotics

First-generation antipsychotics are also referred to as major tranquilizers, neuroleptics, typical antipsychotics, conventional antipsychotics, or classic antipsychotics. The forefather of antipsychotics is chlorpromazine, first discovered in 1952 by a happy coincidence during studies for synthetic antimalarial treatment near the height of World War 2. Paul Charpentier of Rhone-Poulenc, a French chemical and pharmaceutical company, synthesized chlorpromazine as a sedative for surgical patients to induce temporary "chemical lobotomy." It was subsequently found to be efficacious in treating psychotic patients by Jean Delay and Pierre Deniker, leading to open-label studies published in *The New England Journal of Medicine* and widespread use. Pharmaceutical companies attempted to capitalize on the success of chlorpromazine by synthesizing other phenothiazine-derived antipsychotics through side chain substitutions. Six classes of FGAs were developed from 1952 to 1975 (Table 8.1), with 12 of them still available for use in the United States [1]. All the FGA are associated with intolerable movement disorders such as akathisia, dystonia, dyskinesia, hypokinesia, and tardive dyskinesia. Most patients did not adhere to the FGA due to their poor tolerability, resulting in frequent psychotic relapses and readmissions (known as the revolving-door syndrome).

Table 8.1 Classes of FGAs with their representative drugs and potency

Class	Representative drug	Potency
Phenothiazines		
Aliphatic	Chlorpromazine (Thorazine)	Low
Piperazine	Trifluoperazine (Stelazine)	High
Piperidine	Thioridazine (Mellaril)	Low
Butyrophenones	Haloperidol (Haldol)	High
Thioxanthines	Thiothixene (Navane)	Medium
Dibenzoxazepines	Loxapine (Loxitane)	Medium
Dihydroindolones	Molindone (Moban)	Medium
Diphenylbutylpiperidine	Pimozide (Orap)	High

Pharmacology

The FGAs can be further categorized based on potency, ranging from high to low (Table 8.1). High-potency FGAs have strong antidopaminergic effects relative to other neurotransmitter pathways. Medium-potency FGAs have relatively equivalent effects on dopaminergic and other neurotransmitter pathways. Low-potency FGAs have relatively low antidopaminergic effects relative to other neurotransmitter pathways, leading to an increased risk for non-EPS adverse effects such as sedation, weight gain, and anticholinergic adverse effects [1, 2].

FGAs have a variety of formulations and routes of administration including oral tablet, liquid suspension, intramuscular, intravenous, and long-acting injectables (LAIs) formerly known as "depot" antipsychotics. Oral peak plasma levels are typically within 1–4 h of administration, and parenteral peak plasma levels are reached faster, typically within 30–60 min, as it circumvents first-pass metabolism. Long-acting depot injections are administered every 2–4 weeks and are released slowly into the bloodstream and require several weeks to reach steady-state levels. Even though serum concentrations have been studied extensively in research, they have been found to be unreliable for predicting efficacy and adverse effects due to high degrees of variability between individuals [2]. FGAs are highly lipophilic, and 85–90% are bound to protein as they travel in the bloodstream. Consideration must be given when using other medications that are also highly protein bound, as displacement would increase the serum-free concentration of both [3].

The elimination half-lives for oral, intramuscular, and intravenous administration range from 16 to 45 h, and LAIs range from 2 to 6 weeks. The long half-life of LAIs can be attributed to their formulation by esterification of the hydroxyl moiety to an enanthate or decanoate suspension. The longer half-life of LAIs is very beneficial in treating noncompliant patients as the physician only needs to administer a dose every 2–4 weeks. This is especially significant in psychotic disorders like schizophrenia where poor adherence is particularly prevalent and a major cause of relapse [3].

Most are metabolized by the liver through glucuronidation, oxidation, reduction, methylation, or hydroxylation. The cytochrome P450 (CYP450) system also plays

Table 8.2 Common CYP450 inhibitors and inducers

CYP450 enzyme	3A4	2D6	1A2
Inhibitors	Cimetidine	Bupropion	Caffeine
	Diltiazem	Clomipramine	Ciprofloxacin
	Fluoxetine	Duloxetine	Fluvoxamine
	Fluvoxamine	Fluoxetine	
	Nefazodone	Haloperidol	
	Verapamil	Paroxetine	
Inducers	Modafinil		Omeprazole
	Carbamazepine		Phenobarbital
	Phenobarbital		Phenytoin
	Phenytoin		Tobacco
	St. John's wort		

a role in the metabolism of FGAs, especially CYP2D6, with more minor roles from CYP1A2 and CYP3A4. Variations in CYP450 metabolism (slow vs. fast) and inhibition or induction of the CYP450 system by other medications or foods (Table 8.2) can influence FGA plasma levels and efficacy. The final FGA metabolites are then eliminated through the kidneys or gastrointestinal tract [1].

Mechanism of Action (MOA)

The MOA for FGAs was largely unknown during their initial discovery, and it was the extrapyramidal side effects, like pseudoparkinsonism, that ultimately clued researchers in to the possibility of FGAs interfering with dopaminergic neurotransmission [3]. This led to the simplistic notion that positive symptoms (hallucinations, delusions, thought disorders, and bizarre behavior) of schizophrenia are the result of increased dopaminergic activity in the *mesolimbic* pathways of the brain and that FGAs treat these symptoms through antagonism of postsynaptic dopamine (D_2) receptors. The revised dopamine hypothesis includes hypo- (not hyper-)dopaminergic activity in mesocortical dopamine tract, where the reduction of dopamine activity can lead to worsening of cognition and negative and mood symptoms. Blockade of dopamine in the nigrostriatal pathways results in iatrogenic Parkinsonism and other movement disorders [4].

Recent studies using positron-emission topography (PET) have demonstrated that postsynaptic D_2 receptor occupancy only needs to reach saturation levels of 65% for antipsychotics to exert clinical efficacy. The same studies showed that EPS doesn't appear until saturation levels of 78% or more, which is significantly in excess of the level necessary for clinical efficacy [3]. Thus, the old dogma in the 1960s and 1970s that EPS is necessary for antipsychotic efficacy has been debunked. Further, the proper management of EPS is to reduce the dose by 10–15% instead of adding an anticholinergic medication which can cause dry mouth, constipation, blurry vision, and memory loss, worsening the patient's quality of life.

Efficacy and Indications

When antipsychotics were first discovered in the 1950s, no regulatory agency had yet been established to govern their official uses, and FGAs saw clinical applications in a wide variety of psychotic illnesses. Currently, the Food and Drug Administration (FDA) has granted FGA approval for acute and maintenance treatment of schizophrenia. Some FGAs are also approved by the FDA for use in Tourette syndrome, bipolar mania, generalized nonpsychotic anxiety, and agitation/ behavioral problems. Off-label use of FGAs is also common in disorders such as schizoaffective disorder, psychotic depression, and psychosis secondary to general medical conditions [3].

When FGAs initially became available, it was believed that they would "cure" psychosis, but physicians soon realized that the FGA efficacy was limited to the positive symptoms (delusions and hallucinations), and had no therapeutic efficacy on the negative symptoms (flat affect, alogia, avolition, amotivation) or cognitive impairment (memory dysfunction and executive dysfunction) [3].

Neurological Adverse Effects

FGAs have a myriad of adverse effects, and they can be primarily separated into those that affect the central nervous system (CNS) and those that affect non-CNS organ systems. Of the CNS side effects, FGAs are most prominently known for their neurological movement disorders that result from D_2 blockade in the nigrostriatal pathway.

The acute movement disorders typically occur within hours to weeks of initiating treatment and include akathisia, dystonia, and Parkinsonism. Akathisia can develop within 12 h of initiating therapy and is characterized by motor agitation and subjective feelings of restlessness, predominantly in the limbs. Clinical presentation often involves inability to sit or lie still and constant fidgeting. The symptoms of acute movement disorders can often be reduced by lowering the dose of the FGA by 10–20% or preferably switching to a second-generation antipsychotic (SGA). Propranolol, clonidine, benzodiazepines, and mirtazapine have also been shown to be efficacious in managing akathisia, but none of them have been approved by the FDA. Acute dystonia usually peaks around 24–48 h after initiation of therapy and is characterized by involuntary muscle contractions that can be intermittent or sustained. It most commonly affects the muscles of the head and neck, which can lead to a compromised airway if laryngeal or pharyngeal muscles are involved. Treatment involves airway protection and intramuscular (IM) or intravenous (IV) benztropine or diphenhydramine in severe cases or oral benztropine in mild cases. Parkinsonism develops slowly over the course of days after initiating therapy and is characterized by lead pipe or cogwheel rigidity of the limbs. Tremor, bradykinesia, shuffling gait, postural abnormalities, cognitive decline, and restricted affect can

Table 8.3 Differential diagnosis of tardive dyskinesia

Drug-induced disorders
Anticholinergics
Anticonvulsants
Heavy metal poisoning
Levodopa and other dopamine agents
Lithium
Stimulants
Genetic neurological disorders
Basal ganglia calcifications
Familial dystonia
Huntington disease
Wilson disease
Acquired neurological disorders
Age-related orobuccal movements
Brain tumors
Postanoxic movement disorders
Postencephalitic movement disorders
Naturally occurring choreiform movement disorder (never-medicated schizophrenia)

also be observed but are less common. Short-term anticholinergic medications like benztropine and trihexyphenidyl can be helpful acutely in reducing antipsychotic-induced Parkinsonism, and amantadine can be used to supplement in persistent cases.

The long-term movement disorders typically occur after months or years of consistent treatment and include tardive dystonia, tardive dyskinesia, and tardive akathisia. Tardive dystonia is the chronic form of acute dystonia and presents with identical symptoms. It is far less likely to occur, with an estimated prevalence of 1.5–4%, and is more difficult to treat. Tardive dyskinesia is characterized by involuntary choreiform movements of the face, mouth, and tongue. It typically occurs after chronic antipsychotic treatment for 6 months or more and presents clinically as protrusions of the tongue, smacking of the lips, and/or grimacing of the face. Patients may also develop choreiform movements of the trunk or limbs. Laryngeal TD may manifest as repetitive grunting. Patients on antipsychotics should be screened at least every 3 months for tardive disorders using the Abnormal Involuntary Movement Scale (AIMS). There are currently no therapies that have demonstrated consistent efficacy in treating tardive disorders, but two new drugs (deuterated tetrabenazine and valbenazine) have shown efficacy in FDA trials and are expected to be approved by the FDA soon. Tardive dyskinesia is often irreversible, but there are several other disorders that can mimic tardive dyskinesia (Table 8.3) and should be considered in the differential diagnosis [3].

Neuroleptic malignant syndrome (NMS) is another serious side effect associated with antipsychotic use and is a risk of both FGAs and SGAs. It presents as extreme muscle rigidity, hyperthermia, elevated creatine kinase, elevated white blood cell count, autonomic instability, and fluctuating consciousness. While uncommon, with an incidence of 0.21–3%, NMS can be deadly in approximately 10% of the cases unless the antipsychotic is immediately discontinued and a muscle relaxant (like dantrolene) is administered. Essential steps to minimizing the risk of NMS include avoiding the rapid titration of the antipsychotic and maintaining adequate hydration. Immediate discontinuation of the antipsychotic and medical stabilization upon onset of NMS are essential.

Other CNS side effects of FGAs include hyperprolactinemia, poikilothermia, lowered seizure thresholds, and cognitive dysfunction. Hyperprolactinemia results from D_2 receptor blockade in the tuberoinfundibular pathway that leads to a loss of tonic inhibition of prolactin by hypothalamic dopamine. Hyperprolactinemia can cause reduced libido, anorgasmia, erectile dysfunction, gynecomastia, galactorrhea, oligomenorrhea, or amenorrhea. Effective management strategies include reducing antipsychotic dosage, switching to an SGA, or supplementing with bromocriptine (a dopamine agonist). Antipsychotics can also lower seizure threshold, with low-potency phenothiazines (such as chlorpromazine and thioridazine) presenting the most risk. Close monitoring is suggested in patients with a history of seizure disorder and those that are at increased risk of developing seizures. Lastly, FGAs can worsen cognitive functioning through increased sedation, confusion, memory impairment, and delirium. Careful consideration and low doses must be given to especially high-risk populations, such as the elderly and patients with neurocognitive decline [3].

Peripheral Side Effects

Antipsychotics also have a plethora of non-CNS side effects that stem from non-brain pathways including metabolic, gastrointestinal (GI), genitourinary (GU), ophthalmological, cardiovascular, hematological, and dermatological systems.

Metabolic side effects are attributed to antiserotonergic (5HT) and antihistaminic (H_1) properties of antipsychotics. They can present as weight gain, obesity, hyperlipidemia, insulin resistance, and diabetes. Low-potency FGAs carry a greater risk for metabolic dysregulation than their high-potency counterparts, but psychotic disorders such as schizophrenia and bipolar disorder are also independently associated with an increased risk for diabetes and glucose dysregulation even before the advent of the SGA [4].

Anticholinergic properties of FGA are associated with GI, GU, and ophthalmological side effects. GI symptoms may include constipation, nausea, vomiting, dry mouth, cholestatic jaundice, and paralytic ileus. GU symptoms include urinary hesitancy, urinary retention, increased risk of urinary tract infections (UTI), erectile dysfunction, and retrograde ejaculation. Ophthalmological side effects include blurred vision, dry eyes, narrow-angle glaucoma, and lenticular opacities. Schizophrenia also independently carries an increased risk for lenticular opacities, and thioridazine in high doses can cause permanent retinal pigmentation that may lead to visual impairment as well [1].

Cardiovascular side effects include arrhythmias (QTc prolongation, PR prolongation, T wave blunting, ST depression, heart block, ventricular tachycardia, and torsades de pointes), orthostatic hypotension, and reflex tachycardia. Thioridazine has the most associated cardiac side effects and has had a bolded black box warning since 2002, but care must also be given in using other FGAs as they all carry a risk for cardiac arrhythmias. Screening electrocardiograms (ECG) and thorough cardiac history are important before starting antipsychotics that are associated with arrhythmias. Orthostatic hypotension can result from α_1-adrenergic blockade and is especially significant in elderly patients as they are at increased risk for falls and subsequently increased mortality. Reflex tachycardia can also result from the α_1 blockade and can lead to increased myocardial oxygen demand and risk of arrhythmias. Precautions with adequate hydration, bedtime medication administration, and patient education all help to mitigate these risks [4].

Additionally FGAs have been associated with some hematological and dermatological side effects. Some of the associated blood dyscrasias include leukopenia, agranulocytosis, pancytopenic purpura, and thrombocytopenic purpura. FGAs can also cause photosensitivity, maculopapular rash, and cutaneous discolorations (chlorpromazine) [3].

Second-Generation Antipsychotics (SGA)

As much of a breakthrough as the FGAs were in the treatment of psychosis, they also created new problems. While patients' positive symptoms were controlled, it came at the price of worsened negative and cognitive symptoms along with a gamut of additional side effects, some equally severe as any psychotic illness. FGAs clearly demonstrated that while hallucinations and delusions may be the most salient aspects of psychosis, the functional impairment caused by psychosis extended beyond the positive symptoms. Patients treated with FGAs still had significant difficulties integrating into society and achieving satisfaction in life. Mood symptoms also persisted, and suicide rates in schizophrenia continued to be 50-fold higher than the general population.

Given the significant neurological side effect profiles of FGAs and their inadequate efficacy on negative and cognitive domains of schizophrenia, an alternate class of drugs was obviously necessary. The main goal was a class of medications that would have minimal EPS and would reverse negative and cognitive symptoms. The pharmaceutical companies stopped introducing FGA in the early 1970s with molindone being the last first-generation antipsychotic introduced in 1972. The clue for developing a "better mousetrap" antipsychotic was clozapine, a drug synthesized in 1959 but ignored because it has no EPS whatsoever. In that era of ignorance it was believed to be an ineffective antipsychotic because of the prevailing dogma that inducing EPS is a pre-requisite for antipsychotic efficacy (Table 8.4).

Table 8.4 Atypical antipsychotics (second-generation antipsychotics)

Generic name	Trade name	Approval year	Formulation	Dose range
Clozapine	Clozaril®	1989	Oral	300–900 mg/day
Risperidone	Risperdal®	1993	Oral	4–16 mg/day
	Risperdal Consta®	2003	Long-acting IM	25, 37.5, or 50 mg/2 weeks or 410 mg/4 weeks
Olanzapine	Zyprexa®	1996	Oral	10–20 mg/day (higher doses in treatment refractory)
	Zyprexa Relprevv®	2009	Long-acting IM	150–300 mg/2 weeks and 400 mg/4 weeks
Quetiapine	Seroquel®, Seroquel XR®	1997 2007	Oral	150–800 mg/day (higher doses in treatment refractory)
Ziprasidone	Geodon®	2001	Oral	80–160 mg/day
Aripiprazole	Abilify®	2002	Oral	10–30 mg/day
	Abilify Maintena®	2013	Long-acting IM	160, 200, 300, or 405 mg/month
Aripiprazole Lauroxil	Aristada®	2015	Long-acting IM	441 mg/4 weeks, 662 mg/4 weeks, or 882 mg/4 or 6 weeks
Paliperidone	Invega®	2006	Oral	6–12 mg/day
	Invega Sustenna®	2009	Long-acting IM	39, 78, 117, 156, or 234 mg/month
	Invega Trinza®	2015	Long-acting IM	273, 410, 546, or 819 mg/q3 months
Iloperidone	Fanapt®	2010	Oral	6–12 mg/twice daily
Asenapine	Saphris®	2010	Sublingual	5–10 mg/twice daily
Lurasidone	Latuda®	2011	Oral	40–160 mg/day
Brexpiprazole	Rexulti®	2015	Oral	1–4 mg/day
Cariprazine	Vraylar®	2015	Oral	1.5–6 mg/day

Clozapine

In 1972, clozapine was finally introduced in Europe and launched, but it was promptly withdrawn in 1974 when dozens of fatalities due to agranulocytosis were reported. However, emboldened by the potential that clozapine had shown, researchers persisted in their clinical trials and used clozapine in severe cases of psychosis where patients were unresponsive to all FGAs. It was its efficacy in treating the most refractory psychotic patients that gave clozapine a second life when the FDA approved it in 1988 for refractory schizophrenia but with very strict weekly white blood count (WBC) monitoring. In 2002, the FDA additionally approved clozapine as the only antipsychotic indicated for the treatment of suicidality in schizophrenia.

Weekly WBC checks were required of all patients on clozapine, and after 1–2 years of stable therapy, the checks can be reduced to monthly, with further reductions permissible after 5 years of stable therapy. The incidence of agranulocytosis has been estimated as 1% or less. Also, strong CYP1A2 inhibitors, such as fluvoxamine, could not be used in conjunction as clozapine is predominantly metabolized by CYP1A2 and inhibiting that cytochrome could lead to toxicity and death. However, despite clozapine's nonexistent risk of EPS, it still shared many other side peripheral effects with FGAs [3].

SGA Mechanism of Action (MOA)

Modeled after clozapine, SGAs have much stronger affinity to serotonin 5HT-2A receptors than to dopamine D_2 receptors (by four to tenfold) and are more specific in targeting mesolimbic rather than mesocortical and nigrostriatal pathways. Clozapine and many SGAs (especially quetiapine) also disassociate more rapidly from D_2 receptors than FGAs and maintain a lower occupancy rate, which might contribute to their improved tolerability [5]. 5HT-2A blockade at the cerebral cortex leads to a decrease in glutamate release from cortical glutamate projections in the ventral tegmental area (VTA) with a subsequent decrease in dopamine excitation and reduction in positive symptoms. 5HT-2A blockade also increases mesocortical dopamine release as it reduces tonic serotonergic inhibition of frontal cortex dopamine, leading to less iatrogenic EPS and avoidance of *secondary* negative symptoms, cognitive dysfunction, and affective symptoms [4]. MOA unique to specific SGAs will be discussed in later sections of this chapter.

Efficacy and Indications

Based on large placebo-controlled clinical trials, several SGAs have been approved for schizophrenia, as well as bipolar mania and depression, and adjunctive treatment of major depression. Clozapine is also the only antipsychotic approved for suicidality in schizophrenic patients. Paliperidone is the only antipsychotic officially approved for schizoaffective disorder. SGAs are also all approved for acute mania and mixed episode in bipolar disorder. Some are additionally approved for maintenance of bipolar mania (quetiapine) and bipolar depression (quetiapine, lurasidone, and olanzapine with fluoxetine). Quetiapine is approved by FDA as add-on therapy for treatment-resistant major depressive disorder (MDD), and aripiprazole is approved as an adjunctive therapy to antidepressants in MDD that is partially responsive to antidepressants. SGAs have a multitude of off-label uses including psychotic depression (as an adjunct with antidepressants), Parkinson disease psychosis, Huntington psychosis, delusional disorder, delirium, PTSD, and transient psychosis associated with personality disorders [4].

Adverse Effects

Like FGA, all SGAs have a bolded warning in their label for increased mortality in patients with dementia-related psychosis. This warning was based on a meta-analysis of 17 clinical trials where SGAs were found to have an absolute risk increase of 2% in mortality compared to placebo (4.5% vs. 2.5%). None of the SGAs have been approved by the FDA for psychosis emergent in the context of dementia, but nursing home physicians often use small doses temporarily to control the delusions and hallucination of dementia patients with the family's consent.

Many of the other adverse effects encountered in SGAs are similar to those found in FGAs, with differences primarily in their prevalence. Weight gain and metabolic dysregulation (hyperglycemia, insulin resistance, diabetes, and hyperlipidemia) are some of the more common adverse effects of SGAs. Olanzapine and clozapine have the highest risk for metabolic dysregulation, while aripiprazole, ziprasidone, and lurasidone have the lowest risk [6]. In 2003, the FDA required routine pre- and post-treatment monitoring of waist circumference, fasting glucose, triglycerides, HDL, and blood pressure for patients receiving SGAs [2].

SGAs overall have lower risks of EPS and tardive dyskinesia compared to FGAs, with clozapine and quetiapine carrying almost no risk of EPS even at relatively high doses. The other SGAs tend to have a dose-dependent curve for EPS risk, and SGAs are more likely to present with akathisia than acute dystonias or tardive disorders. Clozapine additionally carries a risk of inducing seizures (particularly with doses greater than 600 mg per day), and care should be taken in populations with increased seizure risks [7].

Some FGAs and SGAs share a commonality in their cardiovascular side effects, particularly arrhythmias and orthostatic hypotension. Some SGAs, such as ziprasidone, may carry some risk of QTc prolongation, so caution is warranted in patients with histories of arrhythmia or elevated baseline QTc, but the QTc prolongation from SGAs has not been shown to be clinically significant after large-scale use for over many years. Some SGAs like iloperidone also carry some risk of orthostatic hypotension secondary to α_1-adrenergic antagonism, with clozapine being the most prominent. The risk for postural hypotension can be mitigated with hydration, nighttime dosing, and psychoeducation. Clozapine is also associated with a risk of myocarditis and cardiomyopathy, and patients should receive routine cardiovascular screening prior to drug initiation.

Hyperprolactinemia secondary to D_2 blockade in the tuberoinfundibular pathway has a class warning for SGAs with risperidone and paliperidone having the highest increases. Symptoms of hyperprolactinemia include reduced libido, amenorrhea, gynecomastia, galactorrhea, and erectile dysfunction. The adolescent and young adult population are particularly susceptible, but prolactin levels do not necessarily correlate with severity of sexual dysfunction. Some SGAs (clozapine, olanzapine, and quetiapine) can also have anticholinergic side effects that include constipation, dry mouth, and blurry vision. Ileus can be a serious side effect of clozapine. Clozapine, olanzapine, and quetiapine are the most sedating of the SGAs, while aripiprazole is the least sedating [3].

Short-Acting Atypical Antipsychotics

The following is a brief description of the oral SGAs that were modeled as serotonin-dopamine antagonists like clozapine and presented in the chronological order in which they were introduced. Each section includes unique facts about their history, formulations, pharmacodynamics, and adverse effects.

Risperidone (Risperdal)

Risperidone was launched in 1993 by Janssen and is a benzisoxazole derivative. It is available in immediate-release oral, rapid melt tablets and liquid formulations and is dosed once daily. It is rapidly absorbed without being affected by food, and peak plasma level is reached within 1 h. It is metabolized by CYP2D6 with an elimination half-life around 20 h. It has the strongest affinity for D_2 out of all the SGAs and thus has dose-related EPS. It has minimal anticholinergic, some H_1, and potent α-adrenergic effects. It is also one of two SGAs (other is paliperidone) that produces the highest prolactin levels and has increased risks of sexual dysfunction [8]. Dose range is 1–8 mg/day with the higher doses for schizophrenia.

Olanzapine (Zyprexa)

Olanzapine was launched in 1996 by Eli Lilly and Company and is a thiobenzodiazepine. It is available in immediate-release oral, rapid melt tablets and IM injections and is dosed once daily, preferably at bedtime due to its sedative effects. It is well absorbed without being affected by food, and peak plasma level is reached around 30 min for IM injection and 6 h for oral. It is metabolized by CYP1A2 and CYP2D6 with elimination half-life around 30 h. It has strong affinity for H_1, α_1, and M_1 receptors. Primary side effects include weight gain, hyperglycemia, diabetes, hyperlipidemia, orthostatic hypotension, anticholinergic effects, sedation, and liver enzyme elevation [9]. Dose range is 5–20 mg/day with the higher doses for schizophrenia.

Quetiapine (Seroquel)

Quetiapine was launched in 1997 by Zeneca and is a dibenzothiazepine derivative. It is available in immediate-release oral tablets and extended-release (XR) gel caps. It is dosed twice daily for immediate-release and once daily for extended-release. It is rapidly absorbed without being affected by food, and peak plasma level is reached around 1.5 h for immediate-release and 6 h for extended-release. It is metabolized by CYP3A4 with an elimination half-life around 6 h. Its metabolite, norquetiapine, is a norepinephrine reuptake inhibitor and exerts antidepressant effects, which is why it was later approved for bipolar depression based on FDA trials. It has affinity for H_1 and α_1. Primary side effects include weight gain, hyperglycemia, diabetes, hyperlipidemia, sedation (the extended-release formulation has less sedation), and orthostatic hypotension [10]. Dose range is 50 mg/day for anxiety, 100–300 mg/day for depression, 500–600 mg/day for mania, and 600–800 mg/day for schizophrenia. Some neurologists use it off-label for migraine as well.

Ziprasidone (Geodon)

Ziprasidone was launched in 2002 by Pfizer and is a benzoisothiazol derivative. It is available in immediate-release oral tablets and IM injections and is dosed twice daily with meals. Its absorption is enhanced with food (500 calories or greater), and peak plasma level is within 1 h for IM injection and 6–8 h for oral. It is metabolized through the liver primarily by reduction via glutathione and aldehyde oxidase with an elimination half-life of 2–5 h for IM and 7 h for oral. It has QTc prolongation with no clinically relevant torsades de pointes in studies, but FDA warning was still included on the label. It has low affinity for H_1 (low sedation and benign metabolic profile) and α_1 (low orthostatic hypotension). Primary side effects include dysphoria, akathisia, nausea, EPS, and dizziness [11]. Dose range is 80–160 mg/day.

Aripiprazole (Abilify)

Aripiprazole, the first dopamine partial agonist, was discovered by Otsuka and was launched in 2003 and is a dihydroquinoline. It is available in immediate-release rapid-melting oral tablets, liquid formulation, and IM injection and is dosed once daily. It is well absorbed without being affected by food, and peak plasma level is reached around 1–3 h for IM and 3–5 h for oral. It is metabolized by CYP2D6 and CYP3A4 with an elimination half-life around 75 h. It is a dopamine and serotonin partial agonist, which gives it a milder side effect profile compared to other SGAs. It has a benign metabolic profile overall but is associated with significant weight gain in first-break psychosis and adolescents. Primary side effects include akathisia, insomnia, and nausea [12]. Dose range is 5–30 mg/day with the higher doses for schizophrenia. 5–10 mg/day is the dose range for adjunctive therapy with antidepressants for treatment-resistant depression.

Paliperidone (Invega)

Paliperidone, or 9-hydroxy risperidone, is the final metabolite of risperidone. It was launched in 2006 by Janssen and is a benzisoxazole derivative. It is available only in oral extended-release tablets and is dosed daily, preferably in the mornings because it is released during peristalsis all day. It is absorbed better with food and peak plasma level is around 24 h. It is primarily excreted unchanged by the kidneys with minimal liver metabolism, so it is the only antipsychotic that can be used for patients with liver failure but needs extra monitoring for those with serious renal disease. Its elimination half-life is around 23 h. Unlike risperidone, it binds minimally to H_1 (low sedation) and is well tolerated with less EPS because of the extended-release. Primary side effects include dizziness, fatigue, dry mouth, EPS, and hyperprolactinemia-related sexual dysfunction [8]. Dose range is 3–12 mg/day with the higher doses for schizophrenia.

Iloperidone (Fanapt)

Iloperidone was launched in 2009 by Novartis and is a piperidinyl-benzisoxazole. It is available only in oral immediate-release tablets and is dosed twice daily. It is well absorbed regardless of food and peak plasma level is 2–4 h. It is metabolized by CYP2D6 and CYP3A4 with an elimination half-life around 18–33 h. It requires gradual titration over 4 days (1 mg bid, 2 mg bid, 4 mg bid, and 6 mg bid) and has strong affinity for alpha1 receptors that may result in orthostatic hypotension if rapidly titrated. It has very low levels of EPS and akathisia risk. Primary side effects include dizziness, orthostasis, tachycardia, fatigue, dry mouth, nasal congestion, somnolence, and weight gain [3]. Dose range for schizophrenia is 6 mg bid to 12 mg bid.

Asenapine (Saphris)

Asenapine was launched in 2010 by Merck and is a dibenzo-oxepino pyrrole. It is available only in sublingual formulation and is dosed twice daily. It is rapidly absorbed from mucous membranes regardless of food, and peak plasma level is 0.5–1.5 h. It is metabolized by CYP1A2 and glucuronidation with an elimination half-life around 24 h. Sublingual tablets have to be absorbed without chewing, splitting, crushing, or swallowing, and food and drink should be avoided for 10 min after administration. It is impossible to overdose on asenapine due to poor GI absorption. It produces better negative symptom reduction than other SGAs and has very benign side effect profile. Primary side effects include somnolence, oral hypoesthesia, and akathisia [3]. Dose range is 5–10 mg bid, with the higher doses for schizophrenia or bipolar mania.

Lurasidone (Latuda)

Lurasidone was launched in 2011 by Sunovion and is a benzoisothiazol. It is only available in immediate-release oral tablets. It is better absorbed in the presence of food and is dosed once daily. It is metabolized by CYP3A4, and the dose should be lowered in the presence of strong inhibitors and increased in the presence of strong inducers of that enzyme. Lurasidone's major advantage is its relatively benign metabolic profile with low weight gain, glucose, and lipid levels even after months of treatment according to safety follow-up studies. Its common side effects (5% or more and twice the placebo rate) are akathisia, EPS, and somnolence. Lurasidone was initially approved for schizophrenia but was subsequently approved for bipolar 1 depression as monotherapy or as adjunctive therapy with a mood stabilizer. Dose range is 20–40 mg/day with food for bipolar depression and 40–160 mg/day for schizophrenia.

Brexpiprazole (Rexulti)

Brexpiprazole was launched in 2015 by Otsuka and Lundbeck and is a serotonin and dopamine partial agonist like aripiprazole, but its receptor profile is quite different and has a lower intrinsic agonist effect. It is available only in oral immediate-release tablets and is dosed once daily. It is well absorbed regardless of food and peak plasma level is 4 h. It is metabolized by CYP3A4 and CYP2D6 with an elimination half-life of around 91 h. It needs to be titrated up in dosage for efficacy and has a relatively benign side effect profile due to its partial agonist activity. Primary side effects include weight gain and akathisia [13]. Dose range is 1–4 mg/day.

Cariprazine (Vraylar)

Cariprazine was launched in 2015 by Gedeon Richter and Allergan and is a serotonin and dopamine partial agonist like aripiprazole and brexpiprazole. It is available only in oral immediate-release tablet and is dosed once daily. It is well absorbed regardless of food and peak plasma level is 3–6 h. It is metabolized by CYP3A4 and CYP2D6 with an elimination half-life around 2–4 days. However, one of its two active metabolites (didesmethylcariprazine) has a half-life of 2 weeks, which may lessen the risk of relapse in case of discontinuation by patients. It has stronger affinity for dopamine receptors than aripiprazole and brexpiprazole, giving it an increased risk for EPS, although it has stronger affinity for D_3 than D_2 receptors, but the clinical implications of that distinction is currently unclear. Primary side effects include EPS and akathisia [13]. Dose range is 1.5–6 mg/day for schizophrenia or mania.

Third-Generation Antipsychotic

In mid-2016, a new atypical antipsychotic, pimavanserin (Nuplazid), was approved for Parkinson disease psychosis. This novel antipsychotic is a selective inverse agonist of serotonin 5HT-2A receptor with some affinity to serotonin 5HT-2C receptor, but no binding affinity at all to dopaminergic, histaminergic, muscarinic, or alpha receptors. It represents a major paradigm shift because it is the first antipsychotic in history that does not block dopamine receptors and is therefore the first of a new third-generation of antipsychotics. The absence of dopamine antagonism makes it an ideal agent to treat Parkinson disease psychosis, which is characterized mainly by visual hallucinations, paranoid delusions, and delusions of marital infidelity. Unlike dopamine antagonists, pimavanserin does not worsen the motor symptoms of Parkinson disease at all by virtue of not blocking dopamine receptors in this dopamine deficiency syndrome. FDA clinical trials led to its approval in May 2016, and it is currently being tested in schizophrenia as well as psychosis in Alzheimer disease. The dose of pimavanserin is two tablets of 17 mg (34 mg/day) with or without food. Its side effects are low with the most common being peripheral edema (7%) and confusional state (6%). It is metabolized by CYP 3A4, and thus the dose should be titrated down to 17 mg/day in the presence of a strong inhibitor and increased to 51 mg/day in the presence of a strong inducer.

Long-Acting Injectable Atypical Antipsychotics

Long acting injectables are invaluable tools for managing non-adhering psychotic patients to prevent relapses by simplifying the medication regiment for patients and providing healthcare providers with reliable tracking for adherence. Five atypical long-acting injectables (LAIs) are currently available.

1. The first LAI introduced was risperidone microspheres (Risperdal Consta) in 2003 by Janssen. It requires oral supplementation with oral risperidone for 4–6 weeks after the initial biweekly injection in order to achieve steady state. After steady state is reached, maintenance therapy consists of biweekly injections administered by a trained healthcare provider such as a nurse. Dose range is 25–50 mg IM q 2 weeks.

2. The second LAI introduced was olanzapine palmitate (Relprevv), which was brought to market in 2010 by Lilly. Patients had to be established on a stable dose of oral olanzapine prior to LAI use. Injections can only be administered in the gluteal region and must be administered by a healthcare provider in a registered facility adjacent to emergency services due to a black box warning by the FDA for a possible (low) risk of severe sedation and delirium syndrome. It can be dosed monthly or biweekly for maintenance therapy. Dose range is 100–400 mg IM every 2 or 4 weeks.

3. Paliperidone palmitate (Invega Sustenna) was introduced by Janssen in 2010. It is released immediately into the bloodstream upon administration and can be used in acute episodes without oral supplementation. First and second doses (234 mg and 156 mg, respectively) should be injected into the deltoid 4–12 days apart, after which maintenance is monthly and may be administered in the deltoid or gluteal region. For patients that have never tried risperidone or paliperidone, an oral trial should be provided prior to LAI to check for allergic reactions [3].

The maintenance dose range is 39–234 mg IM every month after the two initiation doses. In 2015 paliperidone palmitate became available in 3-monthly injections (Invega Trinza) which can be started after 4–5 months of stabilization on the monthly Invega Sustenna formulation. The switch to the maintenance doses of Invega Trinza (273, 410, 546 and 819 mg q 3 months) is roughly 3.5 times the Invega Sustenna doses (78, 117, 156 and 234 mg, respectively).

4. Aripiprazole monthly injection (Abilify Maintena) is the long-acting formulation of aripiprazole. Two weeks of oral supplementation (10–20 mg/day) is started at the time of the first injection, after which it is discontinued. The standard dose is 400 mg IM/month, but lower doses are available (300, 200, and 160 mg) for patients who are poor metabolizers of CYP2D6 or are receiving an inhibitor of CYP2D6 and/or CYP3A4 or both. The main side effects are akathisia and weight gain.

5. The latest long-acting injectable antipsychotic prior to the development of Invega Trinza was aripiprazole lauroxil, which is a prodrug of aripiprazole. Three weeks of oral supplementation with aripiprazole (10–20 mg/day) is given after the first injection. The available doses are 441 mg/month, 662 mg/month, and 882 mg every 6 weeks. A higher dose of about 1000 mg is being developed for injection every 2 months. The main side effect is akathisia.

Effectiveness Comparison of FGA and SGA

Effectiveness is the combination of efficacy, safety, and tolerability. Two large-scale studies compared the effectiveness of FGAs with SGAs. The first study, Clinical Antipsychotic Trials of Intervention Effectiveness (CATIE), funded by NIMH, randomly assigned 1460 ambulatory subjects with schizophrenia to treatment with one FGA (perphenazine) and four SGAs (risperidone, olanzapine, quetiapine, or ziprasidone) over an 18-month period. At the conclusion of the study, there were no significant differences found in the all-cause discontinuation (measure of effectiveness), symptomology, cognition, social functioning, or EPS. However, clozapine was found to have the best efficacy, and olanzapine was found to have the worst metabolic profile among the SGAs. The CATIE study was criticized for its low mean dose for all drugs except olanzapine.

The second study, Cost Utility of the Latest Antipsychotic Drugs in Schizophrenia Study (CUtLASS), funded by the UK government, randomly assigned subjects with psychotic illnesses to treatment with 1 of 11 different FGAs or one of four different SGAs for 12 months. The primary effectiveness parameter was quality of life. No significant differences were noted between groups, but the study was underpowered, and recruitment flaws were noted (patients with good quality of life while taking SGAs did not accept to be in the study).

The World Psychiatric Association section on pharmacotherapy provided a consensus statement that summarized several large-scale meta-analysis of antipsychotic studies. It concluded that the efficacy of all FGAs and SGAs were essentially similar, with the exception of clozapine that showed superiority in the treatment of refractory schizophrenia. They found that the varying challenges with different antipsychotics, like problems with titration, side effect profile, and tolerability, may lead to medication switching. SGAs were deemed to have broader efficacy than FGAs and had less EPS. Lastly, side effect differences among the SGAs are more prominent than the side effect differences across SGAs and FGAs [3].

SGAs have also been shown in recent studies to provide neuroprotective effects and induce neurogenesis. Animal studies have demonstrated new neuronal production in key regions of the brain, like the hippocampus dentate gyrus and the subventricular zone [14]. Haloperidol and other FGAs have been shown in numerous studies to be neurotoxic, causing neuronal death, while the SGAs have been shown to have multiple neuroprotective effects [15, 16]

Special Populations

Pregnant Women

All antipsychotics currently in production have received FDA Category C assignment (animal reproduction studies have shown an adverse effect on the fetus, and there are no adequate and well-controlled studies in humans, but potential benefits may warrant use of the drug in pregnant women despite the risk) with the exception of lurasidone's assignment as Category B (animal reproduction studies have failed to demonstrate a risk to the fetus, and there are no adequate and well-controlled studies in pregnant women). Current consensus among psychiatrist is that the benefits of antipsychotic therapy in managing psychotic symptoms far outweigh the relatively minor risks of teratogenicity. Further data is necessary to determine a more accurate rate of teratogenicity with antipsychotic use, and clinicians are encouraged to contribute to the database by reporting to the FDA regarding the health of newborns with mothers that received antipsychotics during pregnancy [3]. Recent studies reported that the rate of birth defects in women receiving SGAs was the same as the general population [17].

Children

A large pool of published data is available regarding the use of antipsychotics in adolescents (13–18 years of age), and several of the SGAs have received FDA approval for adolescents in treating schizophrenia and bipolar disorder. Comparatively, data on antipsychotic use in the prepubescent population is more scarce, and none of the antipsychotics have received FDA approval for patients under 12 years of age due to lack of controlled studies. However, many SGAs have been used off-label by child psychiatrists for a variety of psychotic and nonpsychotic disorders, due to the severity of childhood psychopathology, demonstrating a significant need for more research in this population group [3].

Parkinson Disease Psychosis

This special population, characterized by severe motor symptoms due to dopamine deficiency, is perhaps the most vulnerable group of patients to dopamine antagonism, which is the mechanism of action of all antipsychotics, until recently when a novel antipsychotic (pimavanserin/Nuplazid), whose mechanism of action is entirely non-dopaminergic and purely serotonergic, was discovered (see Third-Generation Antipsychotic). Given that over 50% of Parkinson disease patients develops psychosis (hallucinations and delusions), the availability of an antipsychotic that does not reduce dopamine activity is most welcome and represents a major advance in antipsychotic pharmacotherapy. The possibility that pimavanserin may also help reduce the psychosis of Alzheimer or Lewy body dementia, where no drug has been approved and where mortality is higher with FGA and SGA, would be a major advance, and clinical trials have been launched.

The future of antipsychotic therapy looks exciting due to the paradigm shift that is taking place, and other approaches (glutamatergic and GABAergic) may also lead to innovative interventions in the heterogeneous primary and secondary psychosis syndromes.

References

1. Nasrallah HA, Tandon R. Classic antipsychotic medications. In: Schatzberg AF, Nemeroff CB, editors. The American Psychiatric Publishing textbook of psychopharmacology. 4th ed. Arlington: American Psychiatric Publishing; 2009. p. 533–54.
2. Rosenbaum JF, Arana GW, Hymann SE, et al. Handbook of psychiatric drug therapy. 5th ed. Philadelphia: Lippincott Williams & Wilkins; 2005.
3. Nasrallah HA, Smeltzer DJ. Contemporary diagnosis and management of schizophrenia. Newtown: Hand- books in Healthcare Co; 2011.
4. Stahl SM. Antipsychotics. Carlsbad: NEI Press; 2008.
5. Kapur S, Seeman P. Does fast dissociation from dopamine D2 receptor explain the action of atypical antipsychotics? A new hypothesis. Am J Psychiatry. 2001;158:360–9.
6. American Diabetes Association, American Psychiatric Association, American Association of Clinical Endocrinologists, North American Association for the Study of Obesity. Consensus development conference on antipsychotic drugs and obesity and diabetes. J Clin Psychiatry. 2004;65:267–72.
7. Marder SR, Wirshing DA. Clozapine. In: Schatzberg AF, Nemeroff CB, editors. The American Psychiatric Publishing textbook of psychopharmacology. 4th ed. Arlington: American Psychiatric Publishing; 2009. p. 555–72.
8. Goff DC. Risperidone and paliperidone. In: Schatzberg AF, Nemeroff CB, editors. The American Psychiatric Publishing textbook of psychopharmacology. 4th ed. Arlington: American Psychiatric Publishing; 2009. p. 627–40.

9. Ballon JS, Wirshing DA, Schultz SC. Olanzapine. In: Schatzberg AF, Nemeroff CB, editors. The American Psychiatric Publishing textbook of psychopharmacology. 4th ed. Arlington: American Psychiatric Publishing; 2009. p. 573–98.

10. Buckley PF, Foster AE. Quetiapine. In: Schatzberg AF, Nemeroff CB, editors. The American Psychiatric Publishing textbook of psychopharmacology. 4th ed. Arlington: American Psychiatric Publishing; 2009. p. 599–612.

11. Newcomer JW, Fallucco EM. Ziprasidone. In: Schatzberg AF, Nemeroff CB, editors. The American Psychiatric Publishing textbook of psychopharmacology. 4th ed. Arlington: American Psychiatric Publishing; 2009. p. 641–68.

12. Sharif Z, Lieberman JA. Aripiprazole. In: Schatzberg AF, Nemeroff CB, editors. The American Psychiatric Publishing textbook of psychopharmacology. 4th ed. Arlington: AmericanPsychiatric Publishing; 2009. p. 613–26.

13. Citrome L. The ABC's of dopamine receptor partial agonists – aripiprazole, brexpiprazole, and cariprazine: the 15-min challenge to sort these agents out. Int J Clin Pract. 2015;11:1211–20.

14. Pillai A, Terry A, Mahadik SP. Differential effects of long-term treatment with typical and atypical antipsychotics on NGF and BDNF levels in rat striatum and hippocampus. Schizophr Res. 2006;82:95–106.

15. Nasrallah HA. Haloperidol is clearly neurotoxic: should it be banned. Curr Psychiatr Ther. 2013;12:7–9.

16. Nasrallah HA. A decade after the CATIE study, the focus has shifted to neuroprotection. Curr Psychiatr Ther. 2015;14:19–21.

17. Cohen LS, Viguera AC, McInerny KA, et al. Reproductive safety of second generation antipsychotics: current data from the Massachusetts General Hospital Pregnancy registry for atypical antipsychotics. Am J Psychiatr. 2016;173:263–70.

Chapter 9
Cognitive Enhancers

William James Deardorff and George T. Grossberg

Cognitive Enhancers in Mild Neurocognitive Disorders

Case Vignette Part 1

Mr. Jones is a 72-year-old man who was referred to a neurologist by his primary care physician for further evaluation of memory loss. His wife and children report that Mr. Jones has had some difficulty with his memory for the past year. He reports some problems remembering specific details about prior conversations and frequently misplaces his car keys and reading glasses. He admits that he once became lost while driving in a familiar neighborhood. He still manages his finances without any significant errors, although he says these tasks now require more effort. He has no difficulties with activities of daily living (ADLs), such as feeding, dressing, and toileting. His past medical history is significant only for hypertension, for which he takes amlodipine. Physical examination is unremarkable. His score on the Mini-Mental State Examination (MMSE) is 26/30, where he lost two points for only recalling one of three objects and lost two points for errors when performing serial sevens.

W. J. Deardorff, MD (✉)
Department of Psychiatry and Behavioral Neuroscience, Saint Louis University
School of Medicine, St. Louis, MO, USA
e-mail: deardorff@slu.edu

G. T. Grossberg, MD
Division of Geriatric Psychiatry, Department of Psychiatry & Behavioral Neuroscience,
St. Louis University School of Medicine, St. Louis, MO, USA

© Springer International Publishing AG, part of Springer Nature 2018   151
G. T. Grossberg, L. J. Kinsella (eds.), *Clinical Psychopharmacology for Neurologists*, https://doi.org/10.1007/978-3-319-74604-3_9

Therapeutic Options

Based on his symptoms, Mr. Jones would meet diagnostic criteria for a mild neuro-cognitive disorder provided that reversible causes of cognitive decline are ruled out, such as another mental disorder (major depressive disorder, schizophrenia), delir-ium, medications, infections, and metabolic causes. Mr. Jones demonstrates evi-dence of modest cognitive decline in several cognitive domains (particularly complex attention and memory) based on feedback from the patient and family members as well as modest impairment in cognitive performance on the MMSE. The key feature that differentiates a mild neurocognitive disorder from a major neuro-cognitive disorder in this patient is that the cognitive deficits do not appear to signifi-cantly interfere with independence in everyday activities. He is still able to perform all his ADLs and instrumental ADLs, even though they now require more effort.

Once the diagnosis is established, many patients will ask what they can poten-tially do to enhance their cognition and prevent the progression to a major neuro-cognitive disorder. While some patients with mild cognitive impairment (MCI) will revert back to a cognitively normal status, the estimated annual conversion rate to a major neurocognitive disorder is likely between 3% and 15% per year [1, 2]. With regard to modifiable risk factors that increase the risk of dementia, the Alzheimer's Association concluded that there was strong evidence for traumatic brain injury; moderate evidence for midlife obesity, midlife hypertension, current smoking, and diabetes; and unclear evidence for history of depression, sleep disturbances, and hyperlipidemia [3]. For risk factors that decrease the risk of dementia, there was strong evidence for years of formal education, moderate evidence for physical activity, lower evidence for Mediterranean diet and cognitive training, and unclear evidence for moderate alcohol consumption and social engagement.

Table 9.1 presents select examples of clinical trials examining pharmacologic and non-pharmacologic interventions for the management of MCI [4–16]. The cho-linesterase inhibitors (ChEIs) donepezil, galantamine, and rivastigmine have been approved by the Food and Drug Administration (FDA) for the symptomatic treat-ment of Alzheimer's disease (AD). These medications inhibit the enzyme acetylcho-linesterase, which normally functions to degrade the neurotransmitter acetylcholine. This ameliorates the cholinergic deficit seen in patients with AD. Several clinical trials of ChEIs, ranging from 6 to 48 months, have been performed in patients with MCI. These trials have mostly failed to either demonstrate significant benefits on cognition and functioning or to decrease the time to conversion to AD.

One of these trials, the Investigation into Delay to Diagnosis of Alzheimer's Disease with Exelon (InDDEx) study, involved 1018 patients with MCI randomly assigned to rivastigmine or placebo for up to 48 months [13]. Over the study's dura-tion, 17.3% ($n = 88$) of patients on rivastigmine and 21.4% ($n = 109$) of patients on placebo progressed to AD (hazard ratio (HR) = 0.85; 95% confidence interval (CI) = 0.64, 1.12; $p = 0.225$). Mean time to AD progression was 1318 days in the rivastig-mine group and 1289 days in the placebo group. No significant benefits with regard to cognitive, global, functional, or neuropsychiatric outcomes were seen with riv-astigmine therapy compared to placebo. Another study evaluating 10 mg of donepezil daily for 3 years reported lower rates of progression to AD during the first 12 months

Table 9.1 Select examples of interventions tested in patients with mild cognitive impairment

	Intervention studied	Duration	Results on primary end point	Other notable results
Nutrition	Vitamin E (2000 IU daily) [4]	36 months	No significant difference in probability of progression from MCI to AD at 36 months (HR = 1.02; 95% CI = 0.74, 1.41; $p = 0.91$)	No significant difference at 36 months on ADLs, CDR-SB, GDS, or ADAS-cog
	B vitamins (B6, B9, B12) [5]	24 months	Significantly slower rate of brain atrophy per year by 29.6% with active treatment (0.76%; 95% CI = 0.63, 0.90) compared to placebo (1.08%; 95% CI = 0.94, 1.22; $p = 0.001$)	
	DHA (2 g/day) [6]	12 months	Significant difference in full-scale intelligence quotient at 12 months ($p = 0.039$)	Significant differences in volumes of hippocampus and global cerebrum
	Cocoa flavanol [7]	8 weeks	Significant changes on cognitive z score (from 4 cognitive tests) at 8 weeks ($p < 0.0001$) with high and intermediate flavanol	Effects possibly mediated by improvement in insulin sensitivity
Cognition/ exercise	Multicomponent exercise [8]	6 months	No (group × time) interaction on cognitive tests (MMSE, ADAS-cog) and brain atrophy in MCI patients	Significant (group × time) interaction on MMSE ($p = 0.04$) and reduction in cortical atrophy ($p < 0.05$) in a MCI subgroup
	Cognitive activity training [9]	5 weeks	No significant difference in CAMCOG-R scores at 2-year follow-up	Mostly negative results on secondary outcomes
Pharmacological	Antihypertensives (lisinopril, candesartan, or HCTZ) [10]	12 months	Significant improvement on TMT-B with candesartan ($p = 0.008$)	

(continued)

Table 9.1 (continued)

Intervention studied	Duration	Results on primary end point	Other notable results
NSAID (rofecoxib) [11]	4 years	Significantly higher annual AD diagnosis rate with rofecoxib (14.8%) compared to placebo (11.2%, HR = 1.46; $p = 0.011$)	No significant difference on ADAS-cog and CDR
NSAID (triflusal) [12]	13 months	No significant difference on ADAS-cog (mean difference = 0.89; 95% CI = −0.3, 2.1; $p = 0.139$). Prematurely stopped due to slow recruitment	Significantly lower risk of progression to AD with triflusal (HR = 2.10; 95% CI = 1.10, 4.01; $p = 0.024$)
Donepezil [4]	36 months	No significant difference in progression from MCI to AD at 36 months (HR = 0.80; 95% CI = 0.57, 1.13; $p = 0.42$)	Lower risk of AD progression for first 12 months ($p = 0.04$). Benefits on secondary measures (CDR-SB, GDS, ADAS-cog) confined to first 18 months
Rivastigmine [13]	48 months	No significant difference on progression to AD in rivastigmine group (17.3%) compared with placebo group (21.4%; HR = 0.85; 95% CI = 0.64, 1.12; $p = 0.225$)	No significant difference on co-primary outcome of z score for cognitive test battery (−0.10; 95% CI = −0.63, 0.44; $p = 0.726$)
Galantamine [14]	24 months	No significant difference between galantamine and placebo in conversion rate to AD at 24 months (study 1, 22.9% for galantamine vs. 22.6% for placebo, $p = 0.146$; study 2, 25.4% for galantamine vs. 31.2% for placebo, $p = 0.619$)	Mean decline in CDR-SB was significantly less with galantamine compared with placebo at 24 months in study 1 ($p = 0.028$) but not in study 2 ($p = 0.056$)

(continued)

Table 9.1 (continued)

	Intervention studied	Duration	Results on primary end point	Other notable results
	Galantamine and memantine [15]	52 weeks	No significant difference on ADAS-cog score at 6 months. Stopped early due to safety concerns with galantamine in MCI	Significant difference on ADAS-cog in subgroup of MCI with presumed AD etiology
	Metformin [16]	12 months	Nonsignificant advantage with placebo on ADAS-cog at 12 months; nonsignificant advantage with metformin on SRT	Significant advantage with metformin on SRT after adjusting for baseline ADAS-cog ($p = 0.02$)

Abbreviations: *AD* Alzheimer's disease, *ADAS-cog* Alzheimer's Disease Assessment Scale-Cognitive subscale, *ADLs* activities of daily living, *aMCI* amnestic mild cognitive impairment, *CAMCOG* cognitive and self-contained part of the Cambridge Examination for Mental Disorders of the Elderly, *CDR-SB* Clinical Dementia Rating Scale Sum of Boxes, *CI* confidence interval, *DHA* docosahexaenoic acid, *GDS* Global Deterioration Scale, *HCTZ* hydrochlorothiazide, *HR* hazard ratio, *MCI* mild cognitive impairment, *MMSE* Mini-Mental State Examination, *NSAID* nonsteroidal anti-inflammatory drug, *SRT* Selective Reminding Test, *TMT* Trail Making Test

of treatment compared to placebo, most prominently among APOEε4 carriers [4]. However, this benefit was not significant at the 36-month time point, which was the primary end point. Differences on cognitive, global, and functional measures with donepezil compared with placebo were also not significant at 36 months. A Cochrane meta-analysis involving nine studies from eight published reports concluded that there was little evidence that ChEIs affect progression to dementia or scores on measures of cognition (Alzheimer's Disease Assessment Scale-Cognitive subscale (ADAS-cog)), global impression (Clinical Dementia Rating (CDR)), or functioning (Alzheimer's Disease Cooperative Study-Activities of Daily Living Inventory (ADCS-ADL)) [17]. There were significantly more adverse events (AEs) in patients receiving ChEIs, predominantly diarrhea, nausea, and vomiting.

Other pharmacologic agents that have been tested in clinical trials include antihypertensives, nonsteroidal anti-inflammatory drugs (NSAIDs), statins, and *Ginkgo biloba*. Antihypertensives may play a protective role through their blood pressure lowering effects or by altering angiotensin II-mediated processes in the central nervous system [18]. The results from both epidemiologic studies and clinical trials suggest some benefit in patients with hypertension, and the ongoing Systolic Blood Pressure Intervention Trial-MIND (SPRINT-MIND) study will provide more definitive data [10, 19].

While epidemiologic evidence suggests that NSAIDs may protect against the development of AD, clinical trials have failed to replicate these findings. The largest of these trials in patients with MCI was a randomized, double-blind study in 1457 patients randomized to rofecoxib or placebo treatment for up to 4 years [11]. At the trial's end point, rofecoxib was associated with a significantly higher estimated annual AD diagnosis rate compared to placebo. No significant difference was seen on secondary measures of cognition and global functioning. The authors felt the higher risk of AD progression with rofecoxib was likely not a true effect given the lack of significant difference on secondary measures and may have been due to differential discontinuation rates in the two groups. The AD Anti-inflammatory Prevention Trial (ADAPT) study compared naproxen or celecoxib to placebo in 2528 cognitively normal volunteers over the age of 70 with at least one first-degree relative with AD [20–22]. This trial was stopped early due to safety concerns with celecoxib, and the overall results suggested that neither naproxen nor celecoxib reduced the risk of AD or attenuated decline in cognitive functioning. While NSAIDs cannot be recommended specifically for the purpose of preventing AD, the data from epidemiologic studies is reassuring in that patients requiring NSAIDs for other purposes likely do not have an increased risk of dementia and may derive some benefit.

Ginkgo biloba is a dietary supplement that may prevent cognitive decline via reduction of oxygen free radicals and cerebral vasorelaxation [23]. Results from three prominent randomized controlled trials (RCTs) have been negative in demonstrating a benefit in preventing dementia [24]. One RCT involving 3069 community volunteers aged 75 years or older with either normal cognition ($n = 2587$) or MCI ($n = 482$) studied a twice-daily dose of 120 mg extract of Ginkgo biloba compared with placebo [25]. Over a median follow-up of 6.1 years, the overall dementia rate was 3.3 per 100 person-years in the Ginkgo biloba group compared to 2.9 per 100 person-years in the placebo group (HR = 1.12; 95% CI = 0.94, 1.33; $p = 0.21$). No significant effect was seen in the subgroup of participants with MCI. Another RCT failed to show a reduction in the risk of progression to AD in participants with spontaneously reported memory complaints [26]. A Cochrane meta-analysis found inconsistent evidence for any benefit in patients with MCI [27]. No excess side effects were seen with Ginkgo biloba treatment compared with placebo.

Dietary supplements, such as vitamin B12 (cobalamin), vitamin B9 (folic acid), vitamin B6 (pyridoxine), vitamin E (alpha tocopherol), selenium, and omega-3 fatty acids, have also been studied in various clinical trials. Elevated plasma homocysteine may be a risk factor for the development of dementia, and supplementation with B vitamins appears to lower plasma homocysteine levels [28, 29]. The VITACOG trial demonstrated that supplementation with B vitamins (vitamins B6, B9, and B12) may slow the mean rate of brain atrophy per year in patients with MCI, particularly those with elevated levels of homocysteine at baseline [5]. However, a meta-analysis of 11 trials involving B vitamins did not demonstrate any significant effect on cognitive domains or global cognitive functioning [30].

Vitamin E and selenium have been proposed to protect against the development of AD primarily through their antioxidant effects. One 3-year trial of 2000 IU/day of vitamin E failed to show any significant effect on progression to AD in patients with MCI [4]. The Prevention of Alzheimer's Disease with Vitamin E and Selenium (PREADVISE) trial enrolled patients between 60 and 90 years of age to one of four groups: vitamin E and selenium, vitamin E and placebo, selenium and placebo, or placebo [31, 32]. The study failed to show a difference among the four study arms in dementia incidence, although it was underpowered due to limited recruitment.

Due to an epidemiologic link between increased dietary omega-3 fatty acids and reduction in the risk of AD, supplementation with omega-3 fatty acids, such as eicosapentaenoic acid (EPA), docosahexaenoic acid (DHA), and alpha-linolenic acid, has been proposed to improve memory function [33]. In a study involving healthy older adults with age-related cognitive decline, supplementation with DHA improved learning and memory [34]. However, these results were not replicated in two other studies [35, 36]. Similarly, a Cochrane review failed to show any benefit of omega-3 supplementation on cognitive function in cognitively healthy older people [37]. Other dietary interventions, such as a Mediterranean diet supplemented with either extra-virgin olive oil or mixed nuts, have been shown to improve cognition in patients at high vascular risk [38].

Some exercise interventions have demonstrated modest cognitive improvements in patients with MCI [39–41]. However, the trials are generally small and have low statistical power [42]. The majority (92%) of outcomes in these studies were not statistically significant. Interventions such as home-based and center-based tai chi training sessions have also improved cognitive functioning in patients with MCI [43].

A variety of multimodal approaches have shown benefit in either patients with MCI or cognitively normal patients at higher risk of cognitive decline [44, 45]. Three of the largest studies include the Finnish Geriatric Intervention Study to Prevent Cognitive Impairment and Disability (FINGER), the French Multi-Domain Alzheimer's Prevention Trial (MAPT), and the Prevention of Dementia by Intensive Vascular care (preDIVA) study.

FINGER enrolled 1260 individuals aged 60–77 years who had a higher risk of dementia based on the Cardiovascular risk factors, Aging, and Incidence of Dementia (CAIDE) risk score [46]. The intervention group participated in nutritional education sessions, a physical exercise training program guided by physiotherapists involving aerobic activities and strength training, cognitive training involving group sessions led by psychologists and individual computer-based training sessions, and management of metabolic and vascular risk factors. At the 2-year end point, a significant difference favoring the intervention group was seen on the primary outcome (change in cognitive performance on a neuropsychological test battery (NTB) composed of 14 tests). The control group also experienced an increased risk of cognitive decline, defined as any decline on the NTB total score, compared to the intervention group (odds ratio (OR) = 1.31; 95% CI = 1.01, 1.71; $p = 0.04$).

MAPT was a 36-month study involving patients aged 70 years or older with frailty, defined as either a subjective memory complaint, inability to perform one of instrumental ADLs, or a slow walking speed. Patients were divided into four groups: omega-3 supplementation (800 mg/day of DHA), omega-3 supplementation and multi-domain intervention, placebo and multi-domain intervention, and placebo without any intervention. The multi-domain intervention involved training sessions focused on nutrition, physical activity, and cognition and individualized preventive outpatient visits exploring risk factors for cognitive decline such as hypertension, diabetes, and hypercholesterolemia [47]. At the 36-month end point, no significant group differences were observed for the primary outcome, defined as change in cognitive function at 36 months based on a composite z score which combined four cognitive tests [48].

preDIVA was a 6-year nurse-led study involving 3526 community-dwelling individuals aged 70–78 without dementia randomized to an intervention or control group [49]. The intervention consisted of visits to a nurse every 4 months in which cardiovascular risk factors such as smoking habits, diet, and physical activity were assessed. Drug treatment was initiated or optimized if indicated, and lifestyle advice was given in accordance with guidelines on cardiovascular risk management. No significant differences were seen on either primary outcome: cumulative incidence of dementia or disability score based on the Academic Medical Center Linear Disability Score at the 6-year follow-up. Dementia developed in 121 (7%) of 1853 participants in the intervention group and in 112 (7%) of 1601 participants in the control group (HR = 0.92; 95% CI = 0.71, 1.19; p = 0.54). Among participants with untreated hypertension who were adherent to the intervention, the intervention did significantly reduce the risk of dementia (HR = 0.54; 95% CI = 0.32, 0.92; p = 0.02), suggesting that interventions should be focused on those with significant risk factors [50].

Cognitive Enhancement in Mild Alzheimer's Disease

Case Vignette Part 2

Two years after his initial diagnosis, Mr. Jones and his wife return to the neurologist reporting worsening symptoms. His wife reports that he often repeats the same question, and she no longer feels that he is safe to drive. He has made several mistakes when handling their finances, frequently forgets to take his blood pressure medication, and is beginning to forget certain appointments. His children report that he is more impulsive. His MMSE score is now 22/30.

Therapeutic Options

This patient's continued decline in multiple cognitive domains and difficulty with independence in daily activities suggest a diagnosis of a major neurocognitive disorder, likely due to AD. The only pharmacologic agents FDA approved and available for the treatment of mild AD are the ChEIs donepezil, galantamine, and rivastigmine. Table 9.2 summarizes the formulations, dosages, and titration schemes for the ChEIs. These agents are generally considered equivalent in efficacy and demonstrate modest benefits (Cohen's d effect sizes in the range of 0.2–0.3) across cognitive, functional, and neuropsychiatric domains. For example, one meta-analysis found a difference of −2.37 points (95% CI = −2.73, −2.02) on the

Table 9.2 Summary of the formulations, dosages, and titration schemes for the cholinesterase inhibitors and memantine

Drug	Mechanism	Formulation	Dosages	FDA recommended titration scheme
Donepezil	Noncompetitive and reversible ChEI	Tablet	5, 10, 23 mg	Start at 5 mg/day. Increase to 10 mg/day after 4–6 weeks. Increase to 23 mg/day after at least 3 months on 10 mg/day. The 23 mg/day tablet should not be split, crushed, or chewed. 10 and 23 mg/day dosing FDA approved for moderate-to-severe AD
		Orally disintegrating tablet	5, 10 mg	
Rivastigmine	Pseudo-irreversible ChEI	Capsule	1.5, 3, 4.5, 6 mg	Start with 1.5 mg BID. Increase to 3 mg BID after 2–4 weeks. Increase to 4.5 mg BID then to 6 mg BID at 2–4 week intervals. Not approved for severe AD
		Oral solution	2 mg/mL	
		Transdermal patch	4.6 (5 cm^2), 9.5 (10 cm^2), 13.3 (15 cm^2) mg/24 h	Start with 4.6 mg/24 h patch. Increase to 9.5 mg/24 h patch after 4 weeks. Increase to 13.3 mg/24 h after 4 weeks. 13.3 mg/24 h dose FDA approved for severe AD. Switching from capsules to patch: if total oral dose is <6 mg/day, switch to 4.6 mg/24 h patch; if total oral dose is 6–12 mg/day, switch to 9.5 mg/24 h patch
Galantamine	Competitive and reversible ChEI and nAChR modulator	Extended-release capsule	8, 16, 24 mg	Start at 8 mg/day. Increase to 16 mg/day after 4 weeks. May increase to 24 mg/day after 4 weeks. Not approved for severe AD
		Tablet	4, 8, 12 mg	Start at 4 mg BID. Increase to 8 mg BID after 4 weeks. May increase to 12 mg BID after 4 weeks. Not approved for severe AD
		Oral solution	4 mg/mL	

(continued)

Table 9.2 (continued)

Drug	Mechanism	Formulation	Dosages	FDA recommended titration scheme
Memantine	NMDA receptor antagonist	Extended-release capsule	7, 14, 21, 28 mg	Start at 7 mg/day. Increase in 7 mg increments to 28 mg/day in 1 week intervals. FDA approved for moderate-to-severe AD. Can switch directly from 10 mg BID tablets to 28 mg/day ER capsule the day after last dose of tablets
		Tablet	5, 10 mg	Start at 5 mg once daily.
		Oral solution	2 mg/mL	Increase in 5 mg increments to 20 mg/day (10 mg BID) in 1 week intervals. FDA approved for moderate-to-severe AD
Memantine and donepezil FDC	NMDA receptor antagonist and ChEI	Memantine extended-release and donepezil capsule	7/10, 14/10, 21/10, 28/10 mg	Patients stabilized on memantine (10 mg BID or 28 mg/day ER) and 10 mg/day donepezil may be switched directly to 28/10 mg. Patients stabilized on 10 mg/day donepezil start at the 7 mg/10 mg tablet and increase weekly in 7 mg increments to maximum dose of 28/10 mg daily. FDA approved for moderate-to-severe AD

Abbreviations: *AD* Alzheimer's disease, *ChEI* cholinesterase inhibitor, *ER* extended release, *FDA* Food and Drug Administration, *FDC* fixed-dose combination, *nAChR* nicotinic acetylcholine receptor, *NMDA* N-methyl-D-aspartate

ADAS-cog at 6 months for ChEIs compared with placebo, which represents a modest improvement on this 70-point scale [51]. The effect size on global clinical scales is similar to that seen with cognition, and there does appear to be a dose response with regard to improved cognition and global impression [52]. ChEIs are symptomatic in nature and do not prevent the progression of disease. Side effects are predominantly cholinergic and related to GI symptoms, such as nausea, vomiting, and diarrhea (Table 9.3) [51, 53–59].

First approved by the FDA in 1996, donepezil is available as oral or orally disintegrating tablets and comes in three dosages (5, 10, and 23 mg/day). In a Cochrane review of donepezil in mild-to-moderate AD, the 5 mg and 10 mg/day dosages showed significant benefits on cognition, global clinical state, ADLs, and behavior [60]. Significant differences from placebo at 24 weeks on the ADAS-cog were slightly smaller with the 5 mg/day dose (−2.01 points, 95% CI = −2.69, −1.34) than the 10 mg/day (−2.80 points, 95% CI = −3.74, −2.12). Significantly

Table 9.3 Common side effects of cholinesterase inhibitors and memantine in clinical trials and population studies

		ChEIs as a group [51]	Donepezil 5 mg [53]	Donepezil 10 mg [53]	Galantamine 24 mg [53]	Rivastigmine 12 mg [53]	Memantine 20 mg [53]
Clinical trials (frequency versus placebo)	Withdrawals (any reason)	29% vs. 18% (OR = 1.76; 95% CI = 1.54, 2.02)	14.1 vs. 19.9	25.9 vs. 19.7[a]	20.4 vs. 16.4[a]	21.6 vs. 11.4[a]	18.0 vs. 21.2
	Withdrawals due to AEs	18% vs. 8% (OR = 2.32; 95% CI = 1.95, 2.76)	7.8 vs. 9.1	15.3 vs. 8.4[a]	10.9 vs. 8.3	13.4 vs. 6.7[a]	10.0 vs. 8.4
	Nausea	31.5% vs. 9.1% (OR = 4.87; 95% CI = 4.13, 5.74)	5.5 vs. 4.6	12.5 vs. 4.2[a]	18.2 vs. 6.0[a]	39.1 vs. 9.0[a]	2.2 vs. 5.9
	Vomiting	21.4% vs. 5.4% (OR = 4.82; 95% CI = 3.91, 5.94)	3.8 vs. 3.4	11.6 vs. 4.6[a]	13.0 vs. 4.8[a]	26.2 vs. 5.0[a]	
	Diarrhea	14.4% vs. 7.9% (OR = 1.91; 95% CI = 1.59, 2.30)	7.9 vs. 4.5[a]	13.7 vs. 5.1[a]	7.3 vs. 8.6	12.3 vs. 6.7[a]	6.1 vs. 7.0
	Anorexia	12.2% vs. 3.6% (OR = 3.75; 95% CI = 2.89, 4.87)	2.6 vs. 1.5	7.2 vs. 2.5[a]	7.2 vs. 2.0[a]	11.5 vs. 1.7[a]	

(continued)

Table 9.3 (continued)

	ChEIs as a group [51]	Donepezil 5 mg [53]	Donepezil 10 mg [53]	Galantamine 24 mg [53]	Rivastigmine 12 mg [53]	Memantine 20 mg [53]
Dizziness	14.8% vs. 7.8% (OR = 1.99; 95% CI = 1.64, 2.42)	6.8 vs. 4.8	8.2 vs. 5.0[a]	14.1 vs. 3.1[a]	14.3 vs. 5.2[a]	5.9 vs. 5.8
Headache	14.5% vs. 9.7% (OR = 1.56; 95% CI = 1.27, 1.91)	2.9 vs. 0.8	10.8 vs. 7.7	5.7 vs. 4.3	13.0 vs. 6.0[a]	5.0 vs. 4.3
Population studies	ChEIs as a group: Increased frequency of hospital visits for syncope, bradycardia, pacemaker insertion, and hip fracture [54]. Increased risk of hospitalization for bradycardia [55]. Increased risk of syncope, but not falls, fracture, or accidental injury [56]. Increased risk of 10 lb weight loss at 1 year [57]. Conflicting data on risk of pneumonia with rivastigmine compared to donepezil [58, 59]					

[a]Indicates $p < 0.05$

Abbreviations: AEs adverse events, *ChEIs* cholinesterase inhibitors, *CI* confidence interval, *OR* odds ratio more patients receiving 10 mg/day compared to placebo withdrew before the end of treatment. Donepezil is typically started at the 5 mg/day dose and may be titrated to the 10 mg/day dose after a period of 4–6 weeks. Clinicians should warn patients of a potential increase in cholinergic-related AEs (vomiting, diarrhea) that occur during uptitration.

First approved by the FDA in 2000, rivastigmine is available as a capsule, oral solution, or transdermal patch. A Cochrane review of clinical trials involving rivastigmine reported modest benefits on cognitive function, ADLs, and global functioning, with a weighted mean difference from placebo on the ADAS-cog of −1.79 points (95% CI = −2.21, −1.37) and a standardized mean difference on measures of ADLs of 0.20 (95% CI = 0.13, 0.27) [61]. Rivastigmine is the only ChEI currently available as a transdermal patch, with the 9.5 mg/24 h (10 cm^2) patch considered equivalent to the 6 mg BID capsule dosing. The 13.3 mg/24 h (15 cm^2 patch) was approved for severe AD in 2013. Potential advantages of the patch compared to oral administration include reduced caregiver burden, improved adherence, and a better tolerability profile possibly related to decreased peak-trough fluctuations and slower rate of drug release [62]. Disadvantages include application site reactions, such as pruritus, erythema, and dermatitis and increased cost. The patch may be beneficial in patients prone to GI side effects of medications as well as those who have difficulty swallowing capsules. In the Investigation of Transdermal Exelon in Alzheimer's disease (IDEAL) study, use of the 10 cm^2 patch compared to 6 mg BID capsules was associated with a decreased frequency of nausea (7.2% vs. 23.1%) and vomiting (6.2% vs. 17.0%) [63]. More patients in the 10 cm^2 patch group reached the target dose compared with patients in the capsule group (95.9% vs. 64.4%, respectively). Efficacy was similar between the 10 cm^2 patch and the capsules. Clinicians should make sure to review with patients and caregivers the proper administration of the patch as some deaths have been reported owing to the administration of multiple patches at once [64]. The patch should be removed after 24 h before placing a new patch, and only one patch should be applied per day [65].

First approved by the FDA in 2001, galantamine is available as once-daily extended-release capsules, twice-daily immediate-release tablets, and an oral solution. Similar to donepezil and rivastigmine, galantamine produces modest benefits on cognition, functioning, and global impression. One unique study involving galantamine was a 2-year RCT of galantamine in patients with mild-to-moderate AD (MMSE 10–26) randomly assigned to galantamine (n = 1024) or placebo (n = 1021) [66]. This study reported a significantly lower mortality rate in patients receiving galantamine compared to placebo (HR = 0.58; 95% CI = 0.37, 0.89) as well as significant benefits on cognition (MMSE scores) and functional impairment (Disability Assessment in Dementia score). While the effective dosage in clinical trials was 16–24 mg/day, the 16 mg/day dosing may be more favorable in a mild AD population given that it displays a similar efficacy to the 24 mg/day dose and was associated with a trend toward fewer discontinuations due to AEs in one post hoc analysis [67]. In a trial involving galantamine extended release and galantamine immediate release, both forms produced statistically significant differences from placebo at week 26 on the ADAS-cog but not the Clinician's

Interview-Based Impression of Change Plus Caregiver Input (CIBIC-plus) [68, 69]. AE profiles were similar between the ER and IR forms. In clinical practice, galantamine immediate release is typically initiated at the 8 mg/day dose (4 mg BID) and increased to a maintenance dose of 16 mg/day (8 mg BID) after a period of 4 weeks. Patients who begin to decline on the 16 mg/day dose may be titrated to a 24 mg/day dose (12 mg tablets BID) with the caveat that this dose has not been shown to be significantly better than the 16 mg/day dose.

Despite belonging to the same general class, patients who are unable to tolerate one ChEI or do not demonstrate any treatment response may benefit from a therapeutic trial with an alternative ChEI owing to different pharmacologic properties [70, 71]. Interestingly, one open-label study reported that lack of efficacy or presence of intolerable side effects with donepezil therapy was not predictive of similar problems when switched to rivastigmine [72]. Greater than half (54.5%) of patients who discontinued donepezil due to lack of efficacy responded to rivastigmine by the end of 6 months on a global measure of disease severity. Patients and their families should also be reminded that mild improvement or a lack of significant decline is considered a positive treatment response based on the nature of disease progression. Given that most of the clinical trials involving ChEIs were performed for a period of 6 months, a therapeutic trial of this duration is often necessary to determine if there is a clinical response. When considering a switch of ChEI due to intolerance, clinicians should generally wait until the initial symptoms have fully resolved before initiating and titrating the new ChEI according to the package insert. In the case of lack of benefit (i.e., unsatisfactory response within the first year of treatment), clinicians may safely switch between ChEIs immediately [73].

Memantine is an N-methyl-D-aspartate (NMDA) receptor antagonist that is FDA approved for the treatment of moderate-to-severe AD. Clinical trials involving memantine in mild AD have not shown a significant benefit, and its use is not recommended at this stage [74, 75]. Use of vitamin E (alpha tocopherol) supplements in patients with diagnosed AD is controversial. One trial randomized Veterans Affairs (VA) patients (>95% male) with mild-to-moderate AD (MMSE between 12 and 26 inclusive) who were currently taking a ChEI to receive either 2000 IU/day alpha tocopherol (given as 1000 IU twice a day), 20 mg/day memantine, memantine and alpha tocopherol, or placebo [76]. Over a mean follow-up period of 2.27 years, participants receiving alpha tocopherol demonstrated a slower rate of decline compared with placebo as measured by the ADCS-ADL (primary outcome) (mean difference = 3.15; 95% CI = 0.92, 5.39; $p = 0.03$). No significant difference on the primary outcome was seen with the memantine only or the alpha tocopherol plus memantine groups compared with placebo. Secondary outcomes that measured cognition (ADAS-cog, MMSE) and neuropsychiatric symptoms (Neuropsychiatric Inventory) were not significantly different from placebo with any treatment group after adjustment for multiple comparisons. Based on the results of this study and an earlier trial (using a dose of 1000 IU twice a day), vitamin E supplementation may be offered to patients, especially men based on the results of the VA study, looking for other options [77]. While early meta-analyses suggested that high-dosage vitamin E supplements may increase all-cause mortality, this finding was not replicated in a recent meta-analysis which included mortality data from additional large-scale studies [78, 79]. Since vitamin E may induce vitamin K deficiency, it should be used with caution in patients taking warfarin [80].

NSAIDs, statins, and omega-3 fatty acids have been studied in multiple trials in mild-to-moderate AD populations without much success. Both simvastatin and atorvastatin failed to show any effect on cognition, as measured by ADAS-cog scores, or global functioning, as measured by the ADCS-CGIC [81, 82]. Trials involving *Ginkgo biloba* in the treatment of AD have demonstrated inconsistent effects on cognition and were limited due to small sample size, considerable heterogeneity, and poor methodological quality [83–86]. As a supplement, patients wishing to take *Ginkgo biloba* should be aware of the considerable variability in quality control among companies producing this supplement. Addition of omega-3 fatty acids has generally not demonstrated a statistically significant slowing in the rate of cognitive or functional decline in mild-to-moderate AD [87–89]. Of the few studies that reported adverse events, no significant differences in frequency of all AEs or serious AEs were seen [90]. Huperzine A, a natural cholinesterase inhibitor derived from the Chinese herb *Huperzia serrata*, did not demonstrate any cognitive, global, or functional benefit in an RCT involving patients with mild-to-moderate AD [91].

Non-pharmacologic approaches that have been shown to delay functional decline and improve quality of life in people with dementia include exercise and dyadic interventions [92, 93]. Dyadic interventions are psychosocial programs that involve both the patient with dementia and care partner. These interventions may include support components, with educational tools that focus on communication skills and planning pleasant activities. These interventions have minimal side effects and should be recommended for interested patients.

Cognitive Enhancement in Moderate-to-Severe Alzheimer's Disease

Case Vignette Part 3

Mr. Jones was started on 5 mg/day donepezil by his neurologist, which was titrated up to 10 mg/day after 4 weeks. He experienced some nausea during the first week, but his symptoms subsided. He and his family noticed some improvement in his cognition during the first several months. However, over the next 2 years, he begins to require more assistance with dressing and personal hygiene. He is no longer oriented to month or year, and his wife reports that he has trouble recognizing his grandchildren. His MMSE is 14/30.

Therapeutic Options

Several different methods can be used to assess the severity of Alzheimer's disease. Clinical trials will typically use various MMSE cutoffs as inclusion criteria that can vary between individual studies. For example, MMSE scores between 21 and 26 may indicate a mild AD population, 10–20 as moderate AD, and less than 10 as severe AD. The Global Deterioration Scale (GDS) and the CDR are additional tools used for staging AD [94, 95]. The GDS is broken into seven stages with characteristics listed that are typical of each stage. The CDR is a five-point scale that encompasses six domains of cognitive and functional performance, including memory, orientation, judgment and problem solving, community affairs, home and hobbies, and personal care. Characteristics typical of moderate dementia include inability to remember names of close family members, disorientation to time and sometimes place, impairment in problem solving and social judgment, restricted interests, and requiring assistance in dressing and hygiene. This patient has now entered the moderate stages of AD given his MMSE score and impairments in cognition and functioning.

If patients continue to deteriorate on the 10 mg/day donepezil dose, one option is to escalate to the 23 mg/day dose which was approved in 2012 for patients with moderate-to-severe AD. The approval of this dose was based on a 24-week RCT involving patients with MMSE scores 0–20 who were stabilized on donepezil 10 mg/day for ≥12 weeks [96]. The 23 mg/day dose demonstrated a statistically significant benefit over the 10 mg/day dose on the SIB (LSMD = 2.2; $p < 0.001$). No significant difference was seen on the co-primary outcome measure, CIBIC-plus, which is a measure of global functioning. No significant difference was seen on the secondary measures (MMSE and ADCS-ADL). While a post hoc analysis suggested a significant benefit on the CIBIC-plus in patients with more impairment at baseline (MMSE 0–16) ($p = 0.028$), the FDA statistical reviewers demonstrated that many subgroups did not reach statistical significance [97]. For example, in a subgroup of patients with MMSE scores of 0–14, there was no statistical significance on the CIBIC-plus ($p = 0.1663$). AEs with the 23 mg/day dose that occurred at >5% and >2× the frequency of the 10 mg/day dose included nausea (11.8% vs. 3.4%), vomiting (9.2% vs. 2.5%), and anorexia (5.3% vs. 1.7%). The mean duration of vomiting was 5.61 days in the 23 mg/day group and 1.25 days in the donepezil 10 mg/day group, with most vomiting classified as moderate in severity [98]. Most withdrawals due to AEs occurred within the first 2 weeks during the uptitration phase. Due to the uncertain clinical benefit and higher incidence of adverse events, the medical and statistical reviewers recommended against approval of the 23 mg/ day dose. However, the summary reviewer recommended approval based on the superiority on the cognitive measure and the recognition that the 23 mg/day dose was likely as effective as the 10 mg/day dose on global functioning. Donepezil 23 mg/day may be an option in patients with moderate-to-severe AD who have been stabilized on the 10 mg/day dose for at least 3–6 months. Clinicians should monitor patients for side effects during the first few weeks after the dose increase. Patients in the clinical trial who were particularly prone to AEs and may not be appropriate candidates for the 23 mg/day dose include those with low body weight (e.g., <55 kg), poor appetite, history of GI bleeding, and bradycardia [99, 100].

Patients who are on the 10 cm^2 (9.6 mg/24 h) rivastigmine patch may benefit from an increase to the 15 cm^2 patch (13.3 mg/24 h), which is indicated by the FDA only for severe AD. In a mild-to-moderate (MMSE scores ≥10 and ≤24) AD population, the Optimizing Transdermal Exelon in Mild-to-Moderate Alzheimer's disease (OPTIMA) trial failed to demonstrate a significant difference on the ADAS-cog between the 15 and 10 cm^2 patch at 48 weeks ($p = 0.227$) [101]. However, there was a significant difference at week 48 on functioning as measured by the Instrumental Activities of Daily Living domain of the ADCS-ADL scale (co-primary outcome) as well as a significant difference at week 24 on the ADAS-cog ($p = 0.027$). Given that the population was more in the moderate-to-severe AD range (mean MMSE of 14.2), the ADAS-cog might not have been able to detect differences at week 48 due to floor effects seen in more severe AD populations. Notable adverse events that occurred at higher rates with the 15 cm^2 patch compared to the 10 cm^2 patch included nausea (12.1% vs. 4.9%), vomiting (10.4% vs. 4.6%), weight decrease (6.9% vs. 2.8%), and decreased appetite (6.4% vs. 2.5%).

Approval of the 15 cm^2 patch for severe AD was based on the ACTivities of daily living and cognitION (ACTION) study, which compared the 15 cm^2 (13.3 mg/24 h) patch to the 5 cm^2 (4.6 mg/24 h) patch in patients with severe AD (MMSE scores ≥3 and ≤12) [102]. Treatment with the 15 cm^2 patch resulted in significantly less deterioration on both primary outcomes, the Severe Impairment Battery and ADCS-ADL-severe impairment version compared with the 5 cm^2 patch at 24-week end point. In clinical practice, the rivastigmine patch is initiated at the 4.6 mg/24 h (5 cm^2) dose and titrated up to the 9.5 mg/24 h (10 cm^2) dose after a minimum of 4 weeks. Patients with mild-to-moderate AD may be titrated to the 13.3 mg/24 h (15 cm^2) dose based on the results of the OPTIMA trial. The rivastigmine patch displays a more linear dose-response curve compared to the capsules which means that there is a potentially greater benefit at higher doses compared to up-titrating the capsules, although this has not been proven in clinical trials. Based on clinical experience, titration is generally better tolerated with the patch than the capsules due to lower GI side effects. However, the OPTIMA trial results still demonstrated higher rates of nausea, vomiting, and decreased appetite in the 15 cm^2 patch group which may be of concern in certain patients.

Memantine is FDA approved for moderate-to-severe AD and may be used as monotherapy or in combination with ChEIs. Immediate-release tablets and once-daily extended-release capsules are available. Clinical trials involving memantine have generally shown statistically significant improvements over placebo across broad clinical domains, with one meta-analysis reporting effect sizes of 0.26 for a cognitive domain ($p < 0.001$), 0.22 for a global domain ($p < 0.001$), 0.18 for a functional domain ($p < 0.001$), and 0.12 for a behavioral domain ($p = 0.03$) [103, 104]. Combination therapy involving memantine and a ChEI appears to show significant benefits compared to ChEI monotherapy on some but not all domains [105, 106]. A recent scientific panel concluded that combination therapy provided modestly significant benefits on behavior, cognitive function, and global assessment compared to monotherapy [107]. No benefit was seen on functioning. This is similar to another analysis, which concluded that combination therapy provides additive benefits that continue to accumulate through 6-month treatment periods compared to monotherapy [108]. Memantine is generally well tolerated, with fewer discontinuations due to AEs compared with placebo in clinical trials (odds ratio = 0.80; 95% CI = 0.59, 1.09) [101]. Potential side effects include dizziness, headache, and somnolence.

Patients with moderate-to-severe AD who were not on any medication previously may be started on combination therapy directly. Typically, one drug is initiated and titrated to the effective dosage before starting the second medication. There is a theoretical advantage to starting memantine before a ChEI because it is a 5-HT3 antagonist, which may decrease the rates of nausea and vomiting during titration with a ChEI [109]. Patients can also be titrated on a fixed-dose combination of memantine extended release and donepezil, which was approved by the FDA in 2014 [110]. Advantages of the combination include a simplified medication regimen and the ability to sprinkle the capsule onto soft foods. While it remains a more expensive option, it may be beneficial in patients with significant dysphagia or a history of poor compliance.

Treatment Duration and Discontinuation in Alzheimer's Disease

Case Vignette Part 4

The patient was continued on donepezil 10 mg/day and started on memantine, which was gradually titrated to 10 mg BID. Over the next 2 years, Mr. Jones begins to forget the name of his wife and becomes more dependent on her for dressing, bathing, and feeding. He eventually becomes incontinent and is no longer able to walk. He was admitted to a nursing home a few months ago. On physical exam, he exhibits generalized rigidity. His MMSE is 7/30.

Therapeutic Options

A common question in managing patients with AD revolves around the duration of pharmacotherapy. Because most RCTs are only performed for 6 months to a year, long-term observational controlled studies (LTOCs) provide complementary data to RCTs regarding long-term therapy [111]. These trials are performed in a real-world setting and involve patients who often have multiple comorbidities, take multiple medications, and may not always be adherent with treatment regimens. One important finding from these studies was that greater treatment persistence, defined as total years of drug use divided by the total years of disease symptoms, was associated with significantly slower rates of decline on the MMSE, instrumental ADL scale, Physical Self-Maintenance Scale (PSMS), and CDR-SB [112]. Compared with untreated patients, maximally treated patients would have less decline in the range of 1 point per year on the MMSE and 0.6 points per year on the CDR-SB. After 5 years, maximally treated patients would retain 4 more points on the MMSE and 1.6 fewer points on the CDR-SB. In another study, combination therapy significantly slowed cognitive and functional decline compared to ChEI monotherapy, with effect sizes that increased with treatment duration [113]. A third study found that use of ChEIs delayed admission to nursing homes compared to patients never receiving a ChEI (relative HR = 0.37; 95% CI = 0.27, 0.49) [114]. In addition, patients receiving memantine and a ChEI were significantly less likely to be admitted to a nursing home versus those receiving only ChEI therapy (relative HR = 0.29; 95% CI = 0.11, 0.72). Combined data from these studies suggests that greater persistence with therapy can slow cognitive and functional decline and may delay admission to nursing homes.

Decisions regarding discontinuing AD pharmacotherapy are difficult and must be individualized based on careful assessment of risks versus benefits [115]. AD can be broken into four major stages: mild, moderate, severe, and terminal. The terminal stage occurs when patients become hospice eligible and is characterized by a loss of all verbal abilities, incontinence, inability of walk, and assistance with most ADLs. It is our opinion that AD pharmacotherapy should be discontinued when patients enter this stage. Only medications indicated for comfort should be continued. Other potential indications for treatment discontinuation include intolerable side effects and comorbidities that make continued use of these agents futile. Discontinuation may lead to worsening of cognition and neuropsychiatric symptoms and increased risk of admission to a nursing home in community-dwelling patients [116–118]. However, at least one study demonstrated that ChEI discontinuation was safe and well tolerated in the majority of patients with moderate-to-severe AD in an institutionalized setting [119]. Particular caution should be given to discontinuing these medications in patients with baseline hallucinations and delusions, as discontinuation might lead to worsening of symptoms. Ultimately, the choice of whether or not to discontinue these medications should be made on a case by case basis, weighing the potential for worsening of cognition and increased neuropsychiatric symptoms with the risk of side effects and drug costs. The dose should be tapered over a period of 2–4 weeks, and the patient should be monitored over the next few months.

Cognitive Enhancers in Other Disorders

Table 9.4 presents a survey of other disorders that are associated with cognitive decline. Treatment of cognitive symptoms in these disorders is often limited, and many clinical trials have been performed demonstrating little benefit.

Table 9.4 Examples of cognitive enhancers tested in other neurologic and psychiatric disorders

Disorder	Intervention
Vascular dementia	Inconclusive evidence for ChEIs and memantine based on several randomized trials with considerable heterogeneity. Small, positive effect on cognition; limited effect on function, behavior, and global impression; increase in adverse events [120, 121]
	Benefit with galantamine in mixed population of vascular dementia or AD [122]
Frontotemporal dementia	No benefit of rivastigmine on cognition, but some benefit on behavior [123]
	No benefit of memantine on cognition based on 2 RCTs, but small benefit on global impression [124]
Lewy body dementia	Benefit with rivastigmine on neuropsychiatric inventory (NPI-4) [125]
	Benefit with donepezil and rivastigmine on cognitive and global measures [126]
	Possible benefit with memantine on global impression [127]
Parkinson's disease dementia (PDD)	Rivastigmine FDA approved for mild-to-moderate PDD [128]
	Questionable benefit with memantine [129, 130]
HIV-associated neurocognitive disorders (HAND)	Antiretroviral treatment is mainstay of therapy [131]. For patients with symptoms of HAND, neuroimaging and CSF analysis may be warranted. Patients can be switched to a regimen with higher CNS penetration effectiveness rank based on CSF viral load
	Negative studies with memantine, [132] minocycline, [133] and selegiline [134]
Huntington's disease	No significant effects on cognition with donepezil or rivastigmine in small RCTs [135, 136]
Multiple sclerosis	Treatment with disease-modifying therapies may improve cognition [137]
	ChEIs, memantine, and *Ginkgo biloba* generally show no significant benefits on cognition [138]
	Small benefits with neuropsychological rehabilitation and cognitive training [139]
Depression	SSRIs, SNRIs, and vortioxetine associated with improvements on cognitive measures [140, 141]
	No apparent benefit of galantamine augmentation [142]
Schizophrenia	Mostly negative studies involving ChEIs (donepezil, rivastigmine, galantamine) and glutamatergic agents (glycine, D-cycloserine) [143–145]. Mixed evidence with memantine [146]

Abbreviations: *AD* Alzheimer's disease, *ChEIs* cholinesterase inhibitors, *CNS* central nervous system, *CSF* cerebrospinal fluid, *RCTs* randomized controlled trials, *SNRI* serotonin-norepinephrine reuptake inhibitor, *SSRI* selective serotonin reuptake inhibitor

Clinical Pearls

Patients with MCI should be advised that the best way to prevent or delay the conversion to a major neurocognitive disorder is through a multi-domain approach. An emphasis is placed on lifestyle modification, exercise (both physical and mental), dietary modification such as the Mediterranean diet, mindfulness and stress reduction, and control of cardiovascular risk factors (e.g., hypertension, hyperlipidemia, and smoking). A B complex multivitamin may also be added, although the evidence is mixed. Once a diagnosis of Alzheimer's disease is made, patients should be initiated on a ChEI, with the recognition that most patients will experience either slight improvement or clinical stability. Patients unable to tolerate one ChEI or demonstrate continued cognitive decline at a period of 6 months on a therapeutic dose may be switched to another ChEI. Any attempt to titrate ChEIs to higher doses may result in AEs such as nausea, vomiting, or diarrhea particularly within the first few weeks. In the moderate-to-severe stages of AD, patients can be initiated on combination therapy with a ChEI and memantine. In these stages, patients and their families should be counseled that the goals of care will gradually shift from improving cognition to maintaining function, delaying institutionalization, and managing the behavioral and psychological symptoms of dementia. Evidence from LTOCs suggest that greater persistence with AD pharmacotherapy may slow the rate of cognitive and functional decline and delay admission to a nursing home. When patients become hospice eligible, AD pharmacotherapy may be safely discontinued due to the limited benefits and side effects.

References

1. Roberts RO, Knopman DS, Mielke MM, Cha RH, Pankratz VS, Christianson TJ, et al. Higher risk of progression to dementia in mild cognitive impairment cases who revert to normal. Neurology. 2014;82(4):317–25. https://doi.org/10.1212/WNL.0000000000000055.
2. Mitchell AJ, Shiri-Feshki M. Temporal trends in the long term risk of progression of mild cognitive impairment: a pooled analysis. J Neurol Neurosurg Psychiatry. 2008;79(12):1386–91. https://doi.org/10.1136/jnnp.2007.142679.
3. Baumgart M, Snyder HM, Carrillo MC, Fazio S, Kim H, Johns H. Summary of the evidence on modifiable risk factors for cognitive decline and dementia: a population-based perspective. Alzheimers Dement. 2015;11(6):718–26. https://doi.org/10.1016/j.jalz.2015.05.016.
4. Petersen RC, Thomas RG, Grundman M, Bennett D, Doody R, Ferris S, et al. Vitamin E and donepezil for the treatment of mild cognitive impairment. N Engl J Med. 2005;352(23):2379–88. https://doi.org/10.1056/NEJMoa050151.
5. Smith AD, Smith SM, de Jager CA, Whitbread P, Johnston C, Agacinski G, et al. Homocysteine-lowering by B vitamins slows the rate of accelerated brain atrophy in mild cognitive impairment: a randomized controlled trial. PLoS One. 2010;5(9):e12244. https://doi.org/10.1371/journal.pone.0012244.
6. Zhang YP, Miao R, Li Q, Wu T, Ma F. Effects of DHA supplementation on hippocampal volume and cognitive function in older adults with mild cognitive impairment: a 12-month

randomized, double-blind, placebo-controlled trial. J Alzheimers Dis. 2016;55(2):497–507. https://doi.org/10.3233/JAD-160439.

7. Desideri G, Kwik-Uribe C, Grassi D, Necozione S, Ghiadoni L, Mastroiacovo D, et al. Benefits in cognitive function, blood pressure, and insulin resistance through cocoa flavanol consumption in elderly subjects with mild cognitive impairment: the Cocoa, Cognition, and Aging (CoCoA) study. Hypertension. 2012;60(3):794–801. https://doi.org/10.1161/HYPERTENSIONAHA.112.193060.

8. Suzuki T, Shimada H, Makizako H, Doi T, Yoshida D, Ito K, et al. A randomized controlled trial of multicomponent exercise in older adults with mild cognitive impairment. PLoS One. 2013;8(4):e61483. https://doi.org/10.1371/journal.pone.0061483.

9. Vidovich MR, Lautenschlager NT, Flicker L, Clare L, McCaul K, Almeida OP. The PACE study: a randomized clinical trial of cognitive activity strategy training for older people with mild cognitive impairment. Am J Geriatr Psychiatry. 2015;23(4):360–72. https://doi.org/10.1016/j.jagp.2014.04.002.

10. Hajjar I, Hart M, Chen YL, Mack W, Milberg W, Chui H, et al. Effect of antihypertensive therapy on cognitive function in early executive cognitive impairment: a double-blind randomized clinical trial. Arch Intern Med. 2012;172(5):442–4. https://doi.org/10.1001/archinternmed.2011.1391.

11. Thal LJ, Ferris SH, Kirby L, Block GA, Lines CR, Yuen E, et al. A randomized, double-blind, study of rofecoxib in patients with mild cognitive impairment. Neuropsychopharmacology. 2005;30(6):1204–15. https://doi.org/10.1038/sj.npp.1300690.

12. Gomez-Isla T, Blesa R, Boada M, Clarimon J, Del Ser T, Domenech G, et al. A randomized, double-blind, placebo controlled-trial of triflusal in mild cognitive impairment: the TRIMCI study. Alzheimer Dis Assoc Disord. 2008;22(1):21–9. https://doi.org/10.1097/WAD.0b013e3181611024.

13. Feldman HH, Ferris S, Winblad B, Sfikas N, Mancione L, He Y, et al. Effect of rivastigmine on delay to diagnosis of Alzheimer's disease from mild cognitive impairment: the InDDEx study. Lancet Neurol. 2007;6(6):501–12. https://doi.org/10.1016/S1474-4422(07)70109-6.

14. Winblad B, Gauthier S, Scinto L, Feldman H, Wilcock GK, Truyen L, et al. Safety and efficacy of galantamine in subjects with mild cognitive impairment. Neurology. 2008;70(22):2024–35. https://doi.org/10.1212/01.wnl.0000303815.69777.26.

15. Peters O, Lorenz D, Fesche A, Schmidtke K, Hull M, Perneczky R, et al. A combination of galantamine and memantine modifies cognitive function in subjects with amnestic MCI. J Nutr Health Aging. 2012;16(6):544–8.

16. Luchsinger JA, Perez T, Chang H, Mehta P, Steffener J, Pradabhan G, et al. Metformin in amnestic mild cognitive impairment: results of a pilot randomized placebo controlled clinical trial. J Alzheimers Dis. 2016;51(2):501–14. https://doi.org/10.3233/JAD-150493.

17. Russ TC, Morling JR. Cholinesterase inhibitors for mild cognitive impairment. Cochrane Database Syst Rev. 2012;9:CD009132. https://doi.org/10.1002/14651858.CD009132.pub2.

18. Ashby EL, Kehoe PG. Current status of renin-aldosterone angiotensin system-targeting anti-hypertensive drugs as therapeutic options for Alzheimer's disease. Expert Opin Investig Drugs. 2013;22(10):1229–42. https://doi.org/10.1517/13543784.2013.812631.

19. Forette F, Seux ML, Staessen JA, Thijs L, Babarskiene MR, Babeanu S, et al. The prevention of dementia with antihypertensive treatment: new evidence from the systolic hypertension in Europe (Syst-Eur) study. Arch Intern Med. 2002;162(18):2046–52.

20. ADAPT Research Group, Lyketsos CG, Breitner JC, Green RC, Martin BK, Meinert C, et al. Naproxen and celecoxib do not prevent AD in early results from a randomized controlled trial. Neurology. 2007;68(21):1800–8. https://doi.org/10.1212/01.wnl.0000260269.93245.d2.

21. Breitner JC, Baker LD, Montine TJ, Meinert CL, Lyketsos CG, Ashe KH, et al. Extended results of the Alzheimer's disease anti-inflammatory prevention trial. Alzheimers Dement. 2011;7(4):402–11. https://doi.org/10.1016/j.jalz.2010.12.014.

22. ADAPT-FS Research Group. Follow-up evaluation of cognitive function in the randomized Alzheimer's disease anti-inflammatory prevention trial and its follow-up study. Alzheimers Dement. 2015;11(2):216–25 e1. https://doi.org/10.1016/j.jalz.2014.03.009.
23. Pietri S, Maurelli E, Drieu K, Culcasi M. Cardioprotective and anti-oxidant effects of the terpenoid constituents of *Ginkgo biloba* extract (EGb 761). J Mol Cell Cardiol. 1997;29(2):733–42. https://doi.org/10.1006/jmcc.1996.0316.
24. Snitz BE, O'Meara ES, Carlson MC, Arnold AM, Ives DG, Rapp SR, et al. *Ginkgo biloba* for preventing cognitive decline in older adults: a randomized trial. JAMA. 2009;302(24):2663–70. https://doi.org/10.1001/jama.2009.1913.
25. DeKosky ST, Williamson JD, Fitzpatrick AL, Kronmal RA, Ives DG, Saxton JA, et al. *Ginkgo biloba* for prevention of dementia: a randomized controlled trial. JAMA. 2008;300(19):2253–62. https://doi.org/10.1001/jama.2008.683.
26. Vellas B, Coley N, Ousset PJ, Berrut G, Dartigues JF, Dubois B, et al. Long-term use of standardised *Ginkgo biloba* extract for the prevention of Alzheimer's disease (GuidAge): a randomised placebo-controlled trial. Lancet Neurol. 2012;11(10):851–9. https://doi.org/10.1016/S1474-4422(12)70206-5.
27. Birks J, Grimley EJ. *Ginkgo biloba* for cognitive impairment and dementia. Cochrane Database Syst Rev. 2007;2:CD003120. https://doi.org/10.1002/14651858.CD003120.pub2.
28. de Jager CA, Oulhaj A, Jacoby R, Refsum H, Smith AD. Cognitive and clinical outcomes of homocysteine-lowering B-vitamin treatment in mild cognitive impairment: a randomized controlled trial. Int J Geriatr Psychiatry. 2012;27(6):592–600. https://doi.org/10.1002/gps.2758.
29. Seshadri S, Beiser A, Selhub J, Jacques PF, Rosenberg IH, D'Agostino RB, et al. Plasma homocysteine as a risk factor for dementia and Alzheimer's disease. N Engl J Med. 2002;346(7):476–83. https://doi.org/10.1056/NEJMoa011613.
30. Clarke R, Bennett D, Parish S, Lewington S, Skeaff M, Eussen SJ, et al. Effects of homocysteine lowering with B vitamins on cognitive aging: meta-analysis of 11 trials with cognitive data on 22,000 individuals. Am J Clin Nutr. 2014;100(2):657–66. https://doi.org/10.3945/ajcn.113.076349.
31. Kryscio RJ, Abner EL, Schmitt FA, Goodman PJ, Mendiondo M, Caban-Holt A, et al. A randomized controlled Alzheimer's disease prevention trial's evolution into an exposure trial: the PREADViSE trial. J Nutr Health Aging. 2013;17(1):72–5. https://doi.org/10.1007/s12603-012-0083-3.
32. Kryscio RJ, Abner EL, Caban-Holt A, Lovell M, Goodman P, Darke AK, et al. Association of antioxidant supplement use and dementia in the prevention of Alzheimer's disease by vitamin E and selenium trial (PREADViSE). JAMA Neurol. 2017;74(5):567–73.
33. Morris MC, Evans DA, Bienias JL, Tangney CC, Bennett DA, Wilson RS, et al. Consumption of fish and n-3 fatty acids and risk of incident Alzheimer disease. Arch Neurol. 2003;60(7):940–6. https://doi.org/10.1001/archneur.60.7.940.
34. Yurko-Mauro K, McCarthy D, Rom D, Nelson EB, Ryan AS, Blackwell A, et al. Beneficial effects of docosahexaenoic acid on cognition in age-related cognitive decline. Alzheimers Dement. 2010;6(6):456–64. https://doi.org/10.1016/j.jalz.2010.01.013.
35. Dangour AD, Allen E, Elbourne D, Fasey N, Fletcher AE, Hardy P, et al. Effect of 2-y n-3 long-chain polyunsaturated fatty acid supplementation on cognitive function in older people: a randomized, double-blind, controlled trial. Am J Clin Nutr. 2010;91(6):1725–32. https://doi.org/10.3945/ajcn.2009.29121.
36. van de Rest O, Geleijnse JM, Kok FJ, van Staveren WA, Dullemeijer C, Olderikkert MG, et al. Effect of fish oil on cognitive performance in older subjects: a randomized, controlled trial. Neurology. 2008;71(6):430–8. https://doi.org/10.1212/01.wnl.0000324268.45138.86.
37. Sydenham E, Dangour AD, Lim WS. Omega 3 fatty acid for the prevention of cognitive decline and dementia. Cochrane Database Syst Rev. 2012;6:CD005379. https://doi.org/10.1002/14651858.CD005379.pub3.

38. Martinez-Lapiscina EH, Clavero P, Toledo E, Estruch R, Salas-Salvado J, San Julian B, et al. Mediterranean diet improves cognition: the PREDIMED-NAVARRA randomised trial. J Neurol Neurosurg Psychiatry. 2013;84(12):1318–25. https://doi.org/10.1136/jnnp-2012-304792.

39. Sofi F, Valecchi D, Bacci D, Abbate R, Gensini GF, Casini A, et al. Physical activity and risk of cognitive decline: a meta-analysis of prospective studies. J Intern Med. 2011;269(1):107–17. https://doi.org/10.1111/j.1365-2796.2010.02281.x.

40. Lautenschlager NT, Cox KL, Flicker L, Foster JK, van Bockxmeer FM, Xiao J, et al. Effect of physical activity on cognitive function in older adults at risk for Alzheimer disease: a randomized trial. JAMA. 2008;300(9):1027–37. https://doi.org/10.1001/jama.300.9.1027.

41. Strohle A, Schmidt DK, Schultz F, Fricke N, Staden T, Hellweg R, et al. Drug and exercise treatment of Alzheimer disease and mild cognitive impairment: a systematic review and meta-analysis of effects on cognition in randomized controlled trials. Am J Geriatr Psychiatry. 2015;23(12):1234–49. https://doi.org/10.1016/j.jagp.2015.07.007.

42. Gates N, Fiatarone Singh MA, Sachdev PS, Valenzuela M. The effect of exercise training on cognitive function in older adults with mild cognitive impairment: a meta-analysis of randomized controlled trials. Am J Geriatr Psychiatry. 2013;21(11):1086–97. https://doi.org/10.1016/j.jagp.2013.02.018.

43. Sungkarat S, Boripuntakul S, Chattipakorn N, Watcharasaksilp K, Lord SR. Effects of tai chi on cognition and fall risk in older adults with mild cognitive impairment: a randomized controlled trial. J Am Geriatr Soc. 2016. https://doi.org/10.1111/jgs.14594.

44. Lee KS, Lee Y, Back JH, Son SJ, Choi SH, Chung YK, et al. Effects of a multidomain lifestyle modification on cognitive function in older adults: an eighteen-month community-based cluster randomized controlled trial. Psychother Psychosom. 2014;83(5):270–8. https://doi.org/10.1159/000360820.

45. Han JW, Lee H, Hong JW, Kim K, Kim T, Byun HJ, et al. Multimodal cognitive enhancement therapy for patients with mild cognitive impairment and mild dementia: a multi- center, randomized, controlled, double-blind. Crossover Trial J Alzheimers Dis. 2016;55(2):787–96. https://doi.org/10.3233/JAD-160619.

46. Ngandu T, Lehtisalo J, Solomon A, Levalahti E, Ahtiluoto S, Antikainen R, et al. A 2 year multidomain intervention of diet, exercise, cognitive training, and vascular risk monitoring versus control to prevent cognitive decline in at-risk elderly people (FINGER): a randomised controlled trial. Lancet. 2015;385(9984):2255–63. https://doi.org/10.1016/S0140-6736(15)60461-5.

47. Vellas B, Carrie I, Gillette-Guyonnet S, Touchon J, Dantoine T, Dartigues JF, et al. Mapt study: a multidomain approach for preventing Alzheimer's disease: design and baseline data. J Prev Alzheimers Dis. 2014;1(1):13–22.

48. Kivipelto M, Vellas B. Non-pharmacological intervention in populations at high risk of AD dementia: results of the MAPT and LipiDiDiet studies. Symposium 2, Clinical Trials on Alzheimer's Disease 9th Annual Meeting. San Diego; 2016.

49. Moll van Charante EP, Richard E, Eurelings LS, van Dalen JW, Ligthart SA, van Bussel EF, et al. Effectiveness of a 6-year multidomain vascular care intervention to prevent dementia (preDIVA): a cluster-randomised controlled trial. Lancet. 2016;388(10046):797–805. https://doi.org/10.1016/S0140-6736(16)30950-3.

50. Schneider LS. Reduce vascular risk to prevent dementia? Lancet. 2016;388(10046):738–40. https://doi.org/10.1016/S0140-6736(16)31129-1.

51. Birks J. Cholinesterase inhibitors for Alzheimer's disease. Cochrane Database Syst Rev. 2006;1:CD005593. https://doi.org/10.1002/14651858.cd005593.

52. Rockwood K. Size of the treatment effect on cognition of cholinesterase inhibition in Alzheimer's disease. J Neurol Neurosurg Psychiatry. 2004;75(5):677–85.

53. Tan CC, Yu JT, Wang HF, Tan MS, Meng XF, Wang C, et al. Efficacy and safety of done-pezil, galantamine, rivastigmine, and memantine for the treatment of Alzheimer's disease:

a systematic review and meta-analysis. J Alzheimers Dis. 2014;41(2):615–31. https://doi. org/10.3233/JAD-132690.

54. Gill SS, Anderson GM, Fischer HD, Bell CM, Li P, Normand SL, et al. Syncope and its consequences in patients with dementia receiving cholinesterase inhibitors: a population-based cohort study. Arch Intern Med. 2009;169(9):867–73. https://doi.org/10.1001/ archinternmed.2009.43.

55. Park-Wyllie LY, Mamdani MM, Li P, Gill SS, Laupacis A, Juurlink DN. Cholinesterase inhibitors and hospitalization for bradycardia: a population-based study. PLoS Med. 2009;6(9):e1000157. https://doi.org/10.1371/journal.pmed.1000157.

56. Kim DH, Brown RT, Ding EL, Kiel DP, Berry SD. Dementia medications and risk of falls, syncope, and related adverse events: meta-analysis of randomized controlled trials. J Am Geriatr Soc. 2011;59(6):1019–31. https://doi.org/10.1111/j.1532-5415.2011.03450.x.

57. Sheffrin M, Miao Y, Boscardin WJ, Steinman MA. Weight loss associated with cholinesterase inhibitors in individuals with dementia in a national healthcare system. J Am Geriatr Soc. 2015;63(8):1512–8. https://doi.org/10.1111/jgs.13511.

58. Lai EC, Wong MB, Iwata I, Zhang Y, Hsieh CY, Kao Yang YH, et al. Risk of pneumonia in new users of cholinesterase inhibitors for dementia. J Am Geriatr Soc. 2015;63(5):869–76. https://doi.org/10.1111/jgs.13380.

59. Lampela P, Tolppanen AM, Tanskanen A, Tiihonen J, Lavikainen P, Hartikainen S, et al. Use of antidementia drugs and risk of pneumonia in older persons with Alzheimer's disease. Ann Med. 2016:1–10. https://doi.org/10.1080/07853890.2016.1254349.

60. Birks J, Harvey RJ. Donepezil for dementia due to Alzheimer's disease. Cochrane Database Syst Rev. 2006;1:CD001190. https://doi.org/10.1002/14651858.CD001190.pub2.

61. Birks JS, Chong LY, Grimley EJ. Rivastigmine for Alzheimer's disease. Cochrane Database Syst Rev. 2015;9:CD001191. https://doi.org/10.1002/14651858.CD001191.pub4.

62. Nieto RA, Deardorff WJ, Grossberg GT. Efficacy of rivastigmine tartrate, transdermal system, in Alzheimer's disease. Expert Opin Pharmacother. 2016;17(6):861–70. https://doi. org/10.1517/14656566.2016.1159296.

63. Winblad B, Grossberg G, Frolich L, Farlow M, Zechner S, Nagel J, et al. IDEAL: a 6-month, double-blind, placebo-controlled study of the first skin patch for Alzheimer disease. Neurology. 2007;69(4 Suppl 1):S14–22. https://doi.org/10.1212/01.wnl.0000281847.17519. e0.

64. Lovborg H, Jonsson AK, Hagg S. A fatal outcome after unintentional overdosing of rivastigmine patches. Curr Drug Saf. 2012;7(1):30–2.

65. Important Drug Warning. U.S. Food and Drug Administration. 2010. http://www.fda.gov/ downloads/Safety/MedWatch/SafetyInformation/UCM226090.pdf. Accessed 1 Dec 2016.

66. Hager K, Baseman AS, Nye JS, Brashear HR, Han J, Sano M, et al. Effects of galantamine in a 2-year, randomized, placebo-controlled study in Alzheimer's disease. Neuropsychiatr Dis Treat. 2014;10:391–401. https://doi.org/10.2147/ndt.s57909.

67. Aronson S, Van Baelen B, Kavanagh S, Schwalen S. Optimal dosing of galantamine in patients with mild or moderate Alzheimer's disease: post Hoc analysis of a randomized, double-blind, placebo-controlled trial. Drugs Aging. 2009;26(3):231–9. https://doi. org/10.2165/00002512-200926030-00004.

68. Brodaty H, Corey-Bloom J, Potocnik FC, Truyen L, Gold M, Damaraju CR. Galantamine prolonged-release formulation in the treatment of mild to moderate Alzheimer's disease. Dement Geriatr Cogn Disord. 2005;20(2–3):120–32. https://doi.org/10.1159/000086613.

69. Seltzer B. Galantamine-ER for the treatment of mild-to-moderate Alzheimer's disease. Clin Interv Aging. 2010;5:1–6.

70. Emre M. Switching cholinesterase inhibitors in patients with Alzheimer's disease. Int J Clin Pract Suppl. 2002;127:64–72.

71. Cagnin A, Cester A, Costa B, Ermani M, Gabelli C, Gambina G, et al. Effectiveness of switching to the rivastigmine transdermal patch from oral cholinesterase inhibitors: a natu-

ralistic prospective study in Alzheimer's disease. Neurol Sci. 2015;36(3):457–63. https://doi. org/10.1007/s10072-014-2002-3.

72. Auriacombe S, Pere JJ, Loria-Kanza Y, Vellas B. Efficacy and safety of rivastigmine in patients with Alzheimer's disease who failed to benefit from treatment with donepezil. Curr Med Res Opin. 2002;18(3):129–38. https://doi.org/10.1185/030079902125000471.

73. Massoud F, Desmarais JE, Gauthier S. Switching cholinesterase inhibitors in older adults with dementia. Int Psychogeriatr. 2011;23(3):372–8. https://doi.org/10.1017/s1041610210001985.

74. Porsteinsson AP, Grossberg GT, Mintzer J, Olin JT, Group MM-M-S. Memantine treatment in patients with mild to moderate Alzheimer's disease already receiving a cholinesterase inhibitor: a randomized, double-blind, placebo-controlled trial. Curr Alzheimer Res. 2008;5(1):83–9.

75. Schneider LS, Dagerman KS, Higgins JP, McShane R. Lack of evidence for the efficacy of memantine in mild Alzheimer disease. Arch Neurol. 2011;68(8):991–8. https://doi. org/10.1001/archneurol.2011.69.

76. Dysken MW, Sano M, Asthana S, Vertrees JE, Pallaki M, Llorente M, et al. Effect of vitamin E and memantine on functional decline in Alzheimer disease: the TEAM-AD VA cooperative randomized trial. JAMA. 2014;311(1):33–44. https://doi.org/10.1001/jama.2013.282834.

77. Sano M, Ernesto C, Thomas RG, Klauber MR, Schafer K, Grundman M, et al. A controlled trial of selegiline, alpha-tocopherol, or both as treatment for Alzheimer's disease. N Engl J Med. 1997;336(17):1216–22. https://doi.org/10.1056/NEJM199704243361704.

78. Miller ER, Pastor-Barriuso R, Dalal D, Riemersma RA, Appel LJ, Guallar E. Meta-analysis: high-dosage vitamin E supplementation may increase all-cause mortality. Ann Intern Med. 2005;142(1):37–46.

79. Abner EL, Schmitt FA, Mendiondo MS, Marcum JL, Kryscio RJ. Vitamin E and all-cause mortality: a meta-analysis. Curr Aging Sci. 2011;4(2):158–70.

80. Kim JM, White RH. Effect of vitamin E on the anticoagulant response to warfarin. Am J Cardiol. 1996;77(7):545–6.

81. Sano M, Bell KL, Galasko D, Galvin JE, Thomas RG, van Dyck CH, et al. A randomized, double-blind, placebo-controlled trial of simvastatin to treat Alzheimer disease. Neurology. 2011;77(6):556–63. https://doi.org/10.1212/WNL.0b013e318228bf11.

82. Feldman HH, Doody RS, Kivipelto M, Sparks DL, Waters DD, Jones RW, et al. Randomized controlled trial of atorvastatin in mild to moderate Alzheimer disease: LEADe. Neurology. 2010;74(12):956–64. https://doi.org/10.1212/WNL.0b013e3181d6476a.

83. Yang G, Wang Y, Sun J, Zhang K, Liu J. *Ginkgo biloba* for mild cognitive impairment and Alzheimer's disease: a systematic review and meta-analysis of randomized controlled trials. Curr Top Med Chem. 2016;16(5):520–8.

84. Jiang L, Su L, Cui H, Ren J, Li C. *Ginkgo biloba* extract for dementia: a systematic review. Shanghai Arch Psychiatry. 2013;25(1):10–21. https://doi.org/10.3969/j. issn.1002-0829.2013.01.005.

85. Hashiguchi M, Ohta Y, Shimizu M, Maruyama J, Mochizuki M. Meta-analysis of the efficacy and safety of *Ginkgo biloba* extract for the treatment of dementia. J Pharm Health Care Sci. 2015;1:14. https://doi.org/10.1186/s40780-015-0014-7.

86. Tan MS, Yu JT, Tan CC, Wang HF, Meng XF, Wang C, et al. Efficacy and adverse effects of *ginkgo biloba* for cognitive impairment and dementia: a systematic review and meta-analysis. J Alzheimers Dis. 2015;43(2):589–603. https://doi.org/10.3233/JAD-140837.

87. Quinn JF, Raman R, Thomas RG, Yurko-Mauro K, Nelson EB, Van Dyck C, et al. Docosahexaenoic acid supplementation and cognitive decline in Alzheimer disease: a randomized trial. JAMA. 2010;304(17):1903–11. https://doi.org/10.1001/jama.2010.1510.

88. Mazereeuw G, Lanctot KL, Chau SA, Swardfager W, Herrmann N. Effects of omega-3 fatty acids on cognitive performance: a meta-analysis. Neurobiol Aging. 2012;33(7):1482. e17-29. https://doi.org/10.1016/j.neurobiolaging.2011.12.014.

89. Freund-Levi Y, Eriksdotter-Jonhagen M, Cederholm T, Basun H, Faxen-Irving G, Garlind A, et al. Omega-3 fatty acid treatment in 174 patients with mild to moderate Alzheimer disease:

OmegAD study: a randomized double-blind trial. Arch Neurol. 2006;63(10):1402–8. https://doi.org/10.1001/archneur.63.10.1402.

90. Burckhardt M, Herke M, Wustmann T, Watzke S, Langer G, Fink A. Omega-3 fatty acids for the treatment of dementia. Cochrane Database Syst Rev. 2016;4:CD009002. https://doi.org/10.1002/14651858.CD009002.pub3.

91. Rafii MS, Walsh S, Little JT, Behan K, Reynolds B, Ward C, et al. A phase II trial of huperzine A in mild to moderate Alzheimer disease. Neurology. 2011;76(16):1389–94. https://doi.org/10.1212/WNL.0b013e318216eb7b.

92. Laver K, Dyer S, Whitehead C, Clemson L, Crotty M. Interventions to delay functional decline in people with dementia: a systematic review of systematic reviews. BMJ Open. 2016;6(4):e010767. https://doi.org/10.1136/bmjopen-2015-010767.

93. Van't Leven N, Prick AE, Groenewoud JG, Roelofs PD, de Lange J, Pot AM. Dyadic interventions for community-dwelling people with dementia and their family caregivers: a systematic review. Int Psychogeriatr. 2013;25(10):1581–603. https://doi.org/10.1017/S1041610213000860.

94. Reisberg B, Ferris SH, de Leon MJ, Crook T. The global deterioration scale for assessment of primary degenerative dementia. Am J Psychiatry. 1982;139(9):1136–9. https://doi.org/10.1176/ajp.139.9.1136.

95. Morris JC. The clinical dementia rating (CDR): current version and scoring rules. Neurology. 1993;43(11):2412–4.

96. Farlow MR, Salloway S, Tariot PN, Yardley J, Moline ML, Wang Q, et al. Effectiveness and tolerability of high-dose (23 mg/d) versus standard-dose (10 mg/d) donepezil in moderate to severe Alzheimer's disease: a 24-week, randomized, double-blind study. Clin Ther. 2010;32(7):1234–51. https://doi.org/10.1016/j.clinthera.2010.06.019.

97. Statistical review(s). Donepezil 23 mg tablets drug approval package. U.S. Food and Drug Administration. 2010. https://www.accessdata.fda.gov/drugsatfda_docs/nda/2010/022568Orig1s000StatR.pdf. Accessed 1 Dec 2016.

98. Medical review(s). Donepezil 23 mg tablets drug approval package. U.S. Food and Drug Administration. 2010. Available at: http://www.accessdata.fda.gov/drugsatfda_docs/nda/2010/022568Orig1s000MedR.pdf. Accessed 1 Dec 2016.

99. Cummings JL, Geldmacher D, Farlow M, Sabbagh M, Christensen D, Betz P. High-dose donepezil (23 mg/day) for the treatment of moderate and severe Alzheimer's disease: drug profile and clinical guidelines. CNS Neurosci Ther. 2013;19(5):294–301. https://doi.org/10.1111/cns.12076.

100. Farlow M, Veloso F, Moline M, Yardley J, Brand-Schieber E, Bibbiani F, et al. Safety and tolerability of donepezil 23 mg in moderate to severe Alzheimer's disease. BMC Neurol. 2011;11:57. https://doi.org/10.1186/1471-2377-11-57.

101. Cummings J, Froelich L, Black SE, Bakchine S, Bellelli G, Molinuevo JL, et al. Randomized, double-blind, parallel-group, 48-week study for efficacy and safety of a higher-dose rivastigmine patch (15 vs. 10 cm(2)) in Alzheimer's disease. Dement Geriatr Cogn Disord. 2012;33(5):341–53. https://doi.org/10.1159/000340056.

102. Farlow MR, Grossberg GT, Sadowsky CH, Meng X, Somogyi M. A 24-week, randomized, controlled trial of rivastigmine patch 13.3 mg/24 h versus 4.6 mg/24 h in severe Alzheimer's dementia. CNS Neurosci Ther. 2013;19(10):745–52. https://doi.org/10.1111/cns.12158.

103. Winblad B, Jones RW, Wirth Y, Stöffler A, Möbius HJ. Memantine in moderate to severe Alzheimer's disease: a meta-analysis of randomised clinical trials. Dement Geriatr Cogn Disord. 2007;24(1):20–7. https://doi.org/10.1159/000102568.

104. Rive B, Gauthier S, Costello S, Marre C, Francois C. Synthesis and comparison of the meta-analyses evaluating the efficacy of memantine in moderate to severe stages of Alzheimer's disease. CNS Drugs. 2013;27(7):573–82. https://doi.org/10.1007/s40263-013-0074-x.

105. Farrimond LE, Roberts E, McShane R. Memantine and cholinesterase inhibitor combination therapy for Alzheimer's disease: a systematic review. BMJ Open. 2012;2(3):e000917. https://doi.org/10.1136/bmjopen-2012-000917.

106. Matsunaga S, Kishi T, Iwata N. Combination therapy with cholinesterase inhibitors and memantine for Alzheimer's disease: a systematic review and meta-analysis. Int J Neuropsychopharmacol. 2014. https://doi.org/10.1093/ijnp/pyu115.
107. Schmidt R, Hofer E, Bouwman FH, Buerger K, Cordonnier C, Fladby T, et al. EFNS-ENS/EAN guideline on concomitant use of cholinesterase inhibitors and memantine in moderate to severe Alzheimer's disease. Eur J Neurol. 2015;22(6):889–98. https://doi.org/10.1111/ene.12707.
108. Atri A, Hendrix SB, Pejovic V, Hofbauer RK, Edwards J, Molinuevo JL, et al. Cumulative, additive benefits of memantine-donepezil combination over component monotherapies in moderate to severe Alzheimer's dementia: a pooled area under the curve analysis. Alzheimers Res Ther. 2015;7(1):28. https://doi.org/10.1186/s13195-015-0109-2.
109. Rogawski MA, Wenk GL. The neuropharmacological basis for the use of memantine in the treatment of Alzheimer's disease. CNS Drug Rev. 2003;9(3):275–308.
110. Deardorff WJ, Grossberg GT. A fixed-dose combination of memantine extended-release and donepezil in the treatment of moderate-to-severe Alzheimer's disease. Drug Des Devel Ther. 2016;10:3267–79. https://doi.org/10.2147/DDDT.S86463.
111. Rountree SD, Atri A, Lopez OL, Doody RS. Effectiveness of antidementia drugs in delaying Alzheimer's disease progression. Alzheimers Dement. 2013;9(3):338–45. https://doi.org/10.1016/j.jalz.2012.01.002.
112. Rountree SD, Chan W, Pavlik VN, Darby EJ, Siddiqui S, Doody RS. Persistent treatment with cholinesterase inhibitors and/or memantine slows clinical progression of Alzheimer disease. Alzheimers Res Ther. 2009;1(2):7. https://doi.org/10.1186/alzrt7.
113. Atri A, Shaughnessy LW, Locascio JJ, Growdon JH. Long-term course and effectiveness of combination therapy in Alzheimer disease. Alzheimer Dis Assoc Disord. 2008;22(3):209–21. https://doi.org/10.1097/WAD.0b013e31816653bc.
114. Lopez OL, Becker JT, Wahed AS, Saxton J, Sweet RA, Wolk DA, et al. Long-term effects of the concomitant use of memantine with cholinesterase inhibition in Alzheimer disease. J Neurol Neurosurg Psychiatry. 2009;80(6):600–7. https://doi.org/10.1136/jnnp.2008.158964.
115. Parsons C. Withdrawal of antidementia drugs in older people: who, when and how? Drugs Aging. 2016;33(8):545–56. https://doi.org/10.1007/s40266-016-0384-z.
116. O'Regan J, Lanctot KL, Mazereeuw G, Herrmann N. Cholinesterase inhibitor discontinuation in patients with Alzheimer's disease: a meta-analysis of randomized controlled trials. J Clin Psychiatry. 2015;76(11):e1424–31. https://doi.org/10.4088/JCP.14r09237.
117. Howard R, McShane R, Lindesay J, Ritchie C, Baldwin A, Barber R, et al. Donepezil and memantine for moderate-to-severe Alzheimer's disease. N Engl J Med. 2012;366(10):893–903. https://doi.org/10.1056/NEJMoa1106668.
118. Howard R, McShane R, Lindesay J, Ritchie C, Baldwin A, Barber R, et al. Nursing home placement in the donepezil and memantine in moderate to severe Alzheimer's disease (DOMINO-AD) trial: secondary and post-hoc analyses. Lancet Neurol. 2015;14(12):1171–81. https://doi.org/10.1016/S1474-4422(15)00258-6.
119. Herrmann N, O'Regan J, Ruthirakuhan M, Kiss A, Eryavec G, Williams E, et al. A randomized placebo-controlled discontinuation study of cholinesterase inhibitors in institutionalized patients with moderate to severe Alzheimer disease. J Am Med Dir Assoc. 2016;17(2):142–7. https://doi.org/10.1016/j.jamda.2015.08.019.
120. O'Brien JT, Thomas A. Vascular dementia. Lancet. 2015;386(10004):1698–706. https://doi.org/10.1016/S0140-6736(15)00463-8.
121. Kavirajan H, Schneider LS. Efficacy and adverse effects of cholinesterase inhibitors and memantine in vascular dementia: a meta-analysis of randomised controlled trials. Lancet Neurol. 2007;6(9):782–92. https://doi.org/10.1016/S1474-4422(07)70195-3.
122. Erkinjuntti T, Kurz A, Gauthier S, Bullock R, Lilienfeld S, Damaraju CV. Efficacy of galantamine in probable vascular dementia and Alzheimer's disease combined with cerebrovascular disease: a randomised trial. Lancet. 2002;359(9314):1283–90. https://doi.org/10.1016/S0140-6736(02)08267-3.
123. Moretti R, Torre P, Antonello RM, Cattaruzza T, Cazzato G, Bava A. Rivastigmine in frontotemporal dementia: an open-label study. Drugs Aging. 2004;21(14):931–7.

124. Kishi T, Matsunaga S, Iwata N. Memantine for the treatment of frontotemporal dementia: a meta-analysis. Neuropsychiatr Dis Treat. 2015;11:2883–5. https://doi.org/10.2147/NDT. S94430.
125. McKeith I, Del Ser T, Spano P, Emre M, Wesnes K, Anand R, et al. Efficacy of rivastigmine in dementia with Lewy bodies: a randomised, double-blind, placebo-controlled international study. Lancet. 2000;356(9247):2031–6. https://doi.org/10.1016/S0140-6736(00)03399-7.
126. Stinton C, McKeith I, Taylor JP, Lafortune L, Mioshi E, Mak E, et al. Pharmacological management of Lewy body dementia: a systematic review and meta-analysis. Am J Psychiatry. 2015;172(8):731–42. https://doi.org/10.1176/appi.ajp.2015.14121582.
127. Matsunaga S, Kishi T, Iwata N. Memantine for Lewy body disorders: systematic review and meta-analysis. Am J Geriatr Psychiatry. 2015;23(4):373–83. https://doi.org/10.1016/j. jagp.2013.11.007.
128. Emre M, Aarsland D, Albanese A, Byrne EJ, Deuschl G, De Deyn PP, et al. Rivastigmine for dementia associated with Parkinson's disease. N Engl J Med. 2004;351(24):2509–18. https:// doi.org/10.1056/NEJMoa041470.
129. Emre M, Tsolaki M, Bonuccelli U, Destee A, Tolosa E, Kutzelnigg A, et al. Memantine for patients with Parkinson's disease dementia or dementia with Lewy bodies: a randomised, double-blind, placebo-controlled trial. Lancet Neurol. 2010;9(10):969–77. https://doi. org/10.1016/S1474-4422(10)70194-0.
130. Aarsland D, Ballard C, Walker Z, Bostrom F, Alves G, Kossakowski K, et al. Memantine in patients with Parkinson's disease dementia or dementia with Lewy bodies: a double-blind, placebo-controlled, multicentre trial. Lancet Neurol. 2009;8(7):613–8. https://doi. org/10.1016/S1474-4422(09)70146-2.
131. Sanmarti M, Ibanez L, Huertas S, Badenes D, Dalmau D, Slevin M, et al. HIV-associated neurocognitive disorders. J Mol Psychiatry. 2014;2(1):2. https://doi. org/10.1186/2049-9256-2-2.
132. Schifitto G, Navia BA, Yiannoutsos CT, Marra CM, Chang L, Ernst T, et al. Memantine and HIV-associated cognitive impairment: a neuropsychological and proton magnetic resonance spectroscopy study. AIDS. 2007;21(14):1877–86. https://doi.org/10.1097/ QAD.0b013e32813384e8.
133. Sacktor N, Miyahara S, Deng L, Evans S, Schifitto G, Cohen BA, et al. Minocycline treatment for HIV-associated cognitive impairment: results from a randomized trial. Neurology. 2011;77(12):1135–42. https://doi.org/10.1212/WNL.0b013e31822f0412.
134. Schifitto G, Zhang J, Evans SR, Sacktor N, Simpson D, Millar LL, et al. A multicenter trial of selegiline transdermal system for HIV-associated cognitive impairment. Neurology. 2007;69(13):1314–21. https://doi.org/10.1212/01.wnl.0000268487.78753.0f.
135. Sesok S, Bolle N, Kobal J, Bucik V, Vodusek DB. Cognitive function in early clinical phase huntington disease after rivastigmine treatment. Psychiatr Danub. 2014;26(3):239–48.
136. Cubo E, Shannon KM, Tracy D, Jaglin JA, Bernard BA, Wuu J, et al. Effect of donepezil on motor and cognitive function in Huntington disease. Neurology. 2006;67(7):1268–71. https:// doi.org/10.1212/01.wnl.0000238106.10423.00.
137. Patti F. Treatment of cognitive impairment in patients with multiple sclerosis. Expert Opin Investig Drugs. 2012;21(11):1679–99. https://doi.org/10.1517/13543784.2012.716036.
138. He D, Zhang Y, Dong S, Wang D, Gao X, Zhou H. Pharmacological treatment for memory disorder in multiple sclerosis. Cochrane Database Syst Rev. 2013;12:CD008876. https://doi. org/10.1002/14651858.CD008876.pub3.
139. Rosti-Otajarvi EM, Hamalainen PI. Neuropsychological rehabilitation for multiple sclerosis. Cochrane Database Syst Rev. 2014;2:CD009131. https://doi.org/10.1002/14651858. CD009131.pub3.
140. Bortolato B, Miskowiak KW, Kohler CA, Maes M, Fernandes BS, Berk M, et al. Cognitive remission: a novel objective for the treatment of major depression? BMC Med. 2016;14:9. https://doi.org/10.1186/s12916-016-0560-3.

141. Rosenblat JD, Kakar R, McIntyre RS. The cognitive effects of antidepressants in major depressive disorder: a systematic review and meta-analysis of randomized clinical trials. Int J Neuropsychopharmacol. 2015;19(2). https://doi.org/10.1093/ijnp/pyv082.
142. Holtzheimer PE 3rd, Meeks TW, Kelley ME, Mufti M, Young R, McWhorter K, et al. A double blind, placebo-controlled pilot study of galantamine augmentation of antidepressant treatment in older adults with major depression. Int J Geriatr Psychiatry. 2008;23(6):625–31. https://doi.org/10.1002/gps.1951.
143. Buchanan RW, Javitt DC, Marder SR, Schooler NR, Gold JM, McMahon RP, et al. The cognitive and negative symptoms in schizophrenia trial (CONSIST): the efficacy of glutamatergic agents for negative symptoms and cognitive impairments. Am J Psychiatry. 2007;164(10):1593–602. https://doi.org/10.1176/appi.ajp.2007.06081358.
144. Freudenreich O, Herz L, Deckersbach T, Evins AE, Henderson DC, Cather C, et al. Added donepezil for stable schizophrenia: a double-blind, placebo-controlled trial. Psychopharmacology. 2005;181(2):358–63. https://doi.org/10.1007/s00213-005-2235-1.
145. Buchanan RW, Conley RR, Dickinson D, Ball MP, Feldman S, Gold JM, et al. Galantamine for the treatment of cognitive impairments in people with schizophrenia. Am J Psychiatry. 2008;165(1):82–9. https://doi.org/10.1176/appi.ajp.2007.07050724.
146. Kishi T, Iwata N. NMDA receptor antagonists interventions in schizophrenia: meta-analysis of randomized, placebo-controlled trials. J Psychiatr Res. 2013;47(9):1143–9. https://doi.org/10.1016/j.jpsychires.2013.04.013.

Chapter 10
Drug-Drug Interactions and Psychiatric Medication

Laurence J. Kinsella

Introduction

How many of us in clinical practice have heard the question: "Doctor, will this drug interact with any of my other medications?" This common question has been challenging to answer, often leading to using laborious drug interaction computer programs, smartphone-based programs, or a call to the pharmacist. The purpose of this chapter is to help address this question, assess the likelihood of a drug-drug interaction, and advise the patient on what to expect should they experience an adverse drug effect.

This chapter will discuss serotonin syndrome and other toxicity syndromes, adverse drug events (ADEs), drug-drug interactions (DDIs), the P450 enzymatic system, and the multiple inhibitors and inducers of drug metabolism. It will also address genetic variability of drug metabolism within certain populations and ethnic groups. Finally, we will develop a system for evaluating DDIs that includes a pocket-sized guide that can be used in the office or bedside to determine whether a patient may be at risk for a DDI.

Case Study

A 93-year-old woman presents with a 6-week history of recurrent syncopal events. She had been previously high functioning, living alone in her own home. One morning upon getting out of bed, she fell forward when bending for her slippers, falling

L. J. Kinsella, MD (✉)
Department of Neurology, SSM Neuroscience Institute, St. Louis, MO, USA

Department of Neurology, St. Louis University School of Medicine, St. Louis, MO, USA
e-mail: Laurence.Kinsella@ssmhealth.com

© Springer International Publishing AG, part of Springer Nature 2018 181
G. T. Grossberg, L. J. Kinsella (eds.), *Clinical Psychopharmacology for Neurologists*, https://doi.org/10.1007/978-3-319-74604-3_10

to the floor without injury. She denied vertigo or loss of consciousness but felt "top heavy." Two weeks later, she had a second event while on the commode, felt suddenly unwell, and then fell off the commode, fracturing the left ankle. In the hospital, a carotid US showed a 90% stenosis of the left internal carotid artery. She underwent urgent endarterectomy and was discharged to short-term rehab. While there, she had a third event of dizziness, light-headedness, and loss of consciousness while on the commode, falling to the floor with confusion and slurred speech, lasting several minutes.

In the hospital, she had no orthostatic hypotension, and Dix-Hallpike testing was normal. She was found to have hypokalemia, hypocalcemia, and hypomagnesemia.

It was noted on her medication that she takes metoprolol. When asked, she admitted to taking nightly acetaminophen with diphenhydramine (Tylenol PM) for sleep.

Diphenhydramine, an antihistamine, is a common over-the-counter sleep aid. It is a substrate and an inhibitor of the P450 enzyme 2D6, which metabolizes 25% of all commercially available medications [1]. Metoprolol is also a substrate of 2D6. Coadministration of a substrate (metoprolol) and an inhibitor (diphenhydramine) of the same enzyme may increase serum concentrations of the substrate. In the case of metoprolol, an already active parent compound, this may lead to toxicity, resulting in bradycardia and hypotension [2]. It is suspected that the patient may have had syncope due to the interaction of diphenhydramine with metoprolol [3].

The converse is true in the case of a prodrug such as hydrocodone, which must be converted to its active metabolite, hydromorphone. When codeine cannot be converted to morphine due to P450 enzyme inhibition, the patient may have inadequate analgesia [4].

Pharmacogenomic differences may also contribute to drug-drug interactions. Five to 10% of Caucasians are poor metabolizers of CYP2D6, meaning they have fewer than two copies of the gene for the enzyme [5]. Metabolically active parent compounds like diphenhydramine and metoprolol will have higher concentrations in poor metabolizers, increasing the risk of toxicity [1]. Prodrugs such as hydrocodone and clopidogrel, metabolized by 2D6 and 2C19, respectively, lose efficacy in poor metabolizers, due to an inability to convert to the active metabolite [4].

The Impact of Libby Zion on Resident Education

In 1984, an 18-year-old college freshman died in New York Hospital. Few events have had as great an impact on medical resident education [6]. Libby Zion was admitted for agitation, confusion, and muscular twitching. She had a history of depression and was taking phenelzine, an MAO inhibitor. The house officers assigned to her care prescribed meperidine and haloperidol for sedation and placed restraints to prevent self-harm. By the following morning, she had a fever of 107F and died from a cardiac arrest. Her father Sidney Zion, a prominent journalist, brought charges against the hospital and the physicians, indicting the medical training system for excessive work hours and poor supervision that, he argued, contributed to poor judgment and medical negligence [6, 7].

In 1995, the jury in the *Zion v. New York Hospital* trial returned a mixed verdict, finding that the doctors were partially responsible for Libby's death but that Libby was also responsible based on autopsy samples positive for cocaine metabolites. Later, the New York Supreme Court threw out the cocaine evidence. They upheld the damages against the doctors and found the hospital not guilty of negligent trainee supervision given the training standards of the time [6, 7].

As a result of Libby's death, and her father Sidney Zion's considerable influence, the Bell Commission was convened in New York to address the issue of residency work hours [8]. In 2003, the ACGME adopted most of the Bell Commission's recommendations, restricting residency work hours at all US training programs to 80 h per week [9].

But would the current work hour restrictions have saved Libby Zion? Would a well-rested resident have recognized the signs and symptoms of serotonin syndrome that Libby Zion exhibited, namely, confusion, agitation, and muscular hyperactivity? Would the doctor have known that meperidine is associated with significant drug interactions that might worsen serotonin syndrome? Libby Zion's death was more likely due to a knowledge deficit than a sleep deficit.

An important lesson from Libby Zion's death is that drug-drug interactions (DDIs) and adverse drug events (ADEs) are common and under-recognized. Prescribers are often unaware of the potential for harm in many commonly prescribed medications.

Scope of the Problem

Adverse drug events (ADEs) are common. In an ambulatory setting, the rate of ADEs is 50 per 1000 person-years, of which 28% are considered preventable. Cardiovascular medications were the most common cause, followed by diuretics, nonopioid analgesics, hypoglycemics, and anticoagulants [10].

Almost 6.5% of all hospitalized patients are admitted due to ADEs, with a fatality rate of 0.15% [12]. Fear of receiving the wrong medication while in hospital is a common concern of patients [12]. High rates of hospitalization have been confirmed in multiple studies, of which two thirds are considered preventable [11, 13, 14].

Drug-drug interactions (DDIs) are a fraction of all ADEs [15]. However, most potential drug-drug interactions do not actually occur [16]. Despite the frequency of theoretically dangerous medication combinations, actual harm is relatively infrequent. Using a computerized interaction tool, Marino found 12,578 potential drug-drug interactions among 3473 emergency department patients, with 9% actually having the expected interaction [17].

Electronic medical records frequently flag potential drug interactions, but the relative infrequency of DDI may cause busy clinicians to ignore repetitive notifications when ordering medications, something known as alert fatigue [18].

Table 10.1 High Risk medications for side effects and interactions [22]

Amiodarone	Clonidine	Meprobamate
Amphetamine	Desmopressin	Metoclopramide
Anorexiants	Desiccated thyroid	Methyldopa
Anticholinergics	Disopyridine	Muscle relaxants
Antihistamines	Fluoxetine	Nifedipine
Antispasmodics	Indomethacin	Nitrofurantoin
Barbiturates	Ketoralac	Proton pump inhibitor
Benzodiazepines	Linezolid	Tricyclic antidepressants
Bisacodyl	Long-acting NSAIDs	Theophylline
Sulfonylureas	Meperidine	Typical antipsychotics

Despite the emphasis on detection and prevention of DDIs, the advent of computerized order entry has not substantially reduced the frequency of these events [19].

The adverse drug events reporting system of the FDA estimate roughly 15,000 deaths per year can be attributed to medication effects [20]. ADEs account for up to 6.5% of hospital admissions [11]. In 2011, there were an estimated 100,000 emergency visits for ADEs, 48% occurring over age 80 and two thirds due to unintentional overdose [21]. The most common medications were warfarin, insulin, antiplatelets, and oral hypoglycemic agents. Only 1.2% were due to a high-risk medication as listed in Beers list [22] (Table 10.1).

One third of all ED visits for ADRs involved just three medications: warfarin (17.3%), insulin (13.0%), and digoxin (3.2%) [21, 23].

It is no wonder that ADEs are so common. In 2006, the Slone Survey reported 82% of adults and 56% of children in the USA take at least one prescription or nonprescription medication or dietary supplement. Over age 65, 17% take ten or more medications in a given week [24].

Risk factors for ADEs and DDIs include age greater than 65, multiple medications and OTCs, genetic variability in drug metabolism, and medical comorbidity [13, 15]. Drug-drug interactions represented 3–5% of all in-hospital medication errors [16]. A lack of awareness of drug interactions by physicians also contributes to the problem [25].

Adverse drug reactions may occur by a variety of mechanisms as listed in Table 10.2 [26].

Clinical Syndromes of Drug Toxicity

There are many clinical syndromes relevant to neurologic practice that result from drug toxicity (Table 10.3).

Several are associated with acute confusional states, a common reason for neurologic consultation. Many of these agents are present on the Beers list of potentially inappropriate medications (Table 10.1).

Table 10.2 Types of adverse drug events

Type A – predictable based on drug concentration
Pt receives too much (benzos and confusion)
Pt metabolizes slowly, causing toxicity
Genetic variation (2D6 deficiency and venlafaxine)
Pharmacokinetic drug-drug interaction (fluvoxamine and clozapine- encephalopathy)
Pt metabolizes slowly, inactivating prodrug
Genetic variation (2D6 deficiency and codeine)
Pt has side effects at therapeutic levels (constipation w/ opioids)
Type B – aberrant reaction, not predictable
Drug allergy – rash with phenytoin
Idiosyncratic –Stevens-Johnson w/ carbamazepine

Table 10.3 Clinical syndromes related to medication toxicity

Clinical syndrome	Medication examples
Serotonin syndrome	SSRI, meperidine, MAOI, linezolid [27]
Neuroleptic malignant syndrome	Haloperidol, chlorpromazine [28]
Extrapyramidal syndromes	Metoclopramide, neuroleptics [29]
Myoclonus, falls, asterixis	Gabapentin [30]
Anticholinergic syndrome	TCA, trihexiphenadyl, atropine [31]
Stevens-Johnson syndrome	Carbamazepine, lamotrigine [32]
Drug-induced seizure	Bupropion, diphenhydramine, TCA [33]
Syncope from prolonged QT	Many SSRIs, TCAs, Haldol [34]
Reversible cerebral vasoconstriction syndrome (RCVS)	Sympathomimetic amines, marijuana, cocaine, fingolimod [35]
Posterior reversible encephalopathy syndrome (PRES)	Phentermine [36]

A number of commonly prescribed medications may induce neurotoxicity including confusion, myoclonus, asterixis, and increased risk of falls in patients with low creatinine clearance (<60 ml/min). The most common is gabapentin but also duloxetine, levetiracetam, pregabalin, and tramadol [22]. Gabapentin is a common cause of neurotoxicity in patients with low creatinine clearance [37, 38]. Patients may develop confusion, myoclonus, asterixis, and obtundation [30, 39]. They may present as recurrent falls due to asterixis of the legs, inducing unexpected knee buckling [40, 41].

The term serotonin syndrome was first coined by Sternbach in 1991 [42]. It is a potential complication of serotonergic drugs, especially when used in combination [43, 44].The incidence is unclear, since most cases are probably unrecognized. On occasion, cases are overestimated. An FDA alert warning of the risk of serotonin syndrome with the combination of SSRI and triptans was likely unwarranted based on poor documentation [45]. Toxicity occurs in 27% and deaths in 0.3% of patients overdosing on SSRIs [46]. For nefazodone, the incidence is 0.4 cases per 1000 patient-months [47].

Table 10.4 Clinical features of serotonin syndrome [48]

Cognitive dysfunction	Autonomic instability	Motor manifestations
Confusion	Tachycardia	Shivering
Disorientation	Hyperthermia	Multifocal myoclonus
Agitation	Diaphoresis	Tremor
Irritability	Hypertension	Asterixis
Euphoria	Mydriasis	Muscular rigidity
Hypomania	Hypotension	Hyperreflexia
Hallucinations	Pupillary dilatation	Ataxia
Coma	Diarrhea	Seizures
	Abdominal cramping	Clonus
		Nystagmus

Patients present with a clinical triad of mental status changes, autonomic instability, and motor hyperexcitability, usually within 24 h of a change in medication [43]. Most patients recover within 1–2 days after drug withdrawal; however some may develop respiratory failure, seizures, rhabdomyolysis, and cardiac arrest (Table 10.4). Mortality from serotonin syndrome was associated with use of MAO inhibitors but now is quite rare in recent series [27].

Some overlap of symptoms and signs exist for serotonin syndrome, neuroleptic malignant syndrome, and anticholinergic toxicity. They can generally be distinguished by the motor hyperexcitability, rapidity of onset, and recent addition or increase of a serotonergic medication [43].

Serotonergic drugs may act by increasing serotonin synthesis (tryptophan), decreasing serotonin metabolism (phenelzine, selegiline), increasing serotonin release (amphetamines, cocaine), and inhibiting reuptake (SSRIs, SNRIs, TCAs, meperidine, dextromethorphan). Some act directly on serotonin receptors (buspirone, triptans).

The treatment of serotonin syndrome is supportive care, with no randomized trials of any specific therapy. Most respond to withdrawal of the offending agent, intravenous fluids, benzodiazepines for agitation and myoclonus, anticonvulsants for seizures, critical care monitoring for autonomic instability, and airway protection. Cyproheptadine, a nonspecific serotonin receptor blocker, may be used in doses of 4–24 mg/day administered by nasogastric tube. Other agents have been tried anecdotally including dantrolene, propranolol, mirtazapine, and atypical antipsychotics. Bromocriptine, an agent commonly used for neuroleptic malignant syndrome, may exacerbate serotonin syndrome due to its indirect effect on serotonin metabolism and should be avoided [43].

P450 Metabolism

Over 95% of commercially available drugs are metabolized by the P450 system. Most are metabolized by just five enzymes: CYP1A2, CYP2C9, CYP2C19, CYP2D6, and CYP3A4.

The p450 enzyme system is an important determinant of drug interactions. With the exception of renal failure, alterations in protein binding are less clinically relevant than the P450 system [49, 50]. Even highly protein-bound drugs such as phenytoin and warfarin quickly alter binding ratios when coadministered and achieve a new steady state. Less well appreciated by practicing physicians is that medications may compete with, inhibit, or induce the metabolism of other drugs. Further, some of these enzymes are subject to genetic variation, making affected patients susceptible to toxicity at lower than expected doses [5, 51].

Drugs undergo phase I, II, and III metabolism. Phase I is carried out by the P450 system, primarily in the liver, and includes oxidation, hydroxylation, acetylation, and methylation [52].

Monamine oxidation, also phase I, is not part of the P450 system.

Phase II prepares the drug for elimination. Glucuronidation and sulfation increase water solubility, enhancing elimination in the urine or stool. Important drug interactions occur during phase II metabolism, such as the interaction of lamotrigine with valproate leading to Stevens-Johnson syndrome [53]. Further discussion of phase II metabolism may be found in Sirot et al. [26].

Phase III refers to the action of P-glycoprotein and other intracellular transporters. They account for the blood-brain barrier. Inhibitors of P-glycoprotein increase the permeability of the blood-brain barrier, allowing certain compounds to penetrate the CNS. An example is the combination of quinidine, a P-glycoprotein inhibitor, with loperamide, a peripherally acting opioid used for diarrhea. Patients on both may experience a central narcotic effect of loperamide in the presence of quinidine [54, 55].

P450 Enzyme System (Fig. 10.1)

These enzymes are located primarily in the liver, kidney, intestine, lungs, and brain. Six enzymes metabolize over 80% of all medications [2, 52]. They are CYP1A2, 2B6, 2C9, 2C19, 2D6, and 3A4.

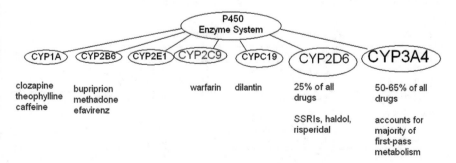

Fig. 10.1 P450 enzymes and some examples of representative drugs

CYP2D6, 2C19, and 2C9 are especially prone to genetic variability. Depending upon the number of gene copies of a particular allele, patients may be poor metabolizers (no functioning alleles), intermediate metabolizers (1 copy), extensive metabolizers (2 copies – the normal state), or ultrametabolizers (3–13 copies).

Substrates/Inducers/Inhibitors

Drugs may be substrates (requiring the enzyme for its metabolism/activation), inhibitors (preventing the metabolism of other substrates of the enzyme), or inducers of enzymatic activity, leading to accelerated metabolism/activation of another drug. Some drugs such as fluoxetine may be both a substrate of 2D6 at low concentrations and an inhibitor at higher concentrations [2]. The pharmacokinetic mechanism of drug interactions may be enzyme competition from two substrates [4], enzyme inhibition of a substrate by an inhibitor [4, 56], or enzyme hyper- or hypo-metabolism of a substrate medication due to pharmacogenetic variants of P450 enzymes [5, 57, 58].

Genetic Variants and Pharmacogenomics

Pharmacogenomics is the study of the variability in drug metabolism in individuals. Most P450 enzymes have two gene copies. However, an individual may have none, one, or more than two copies, thus increasing or reducing the rate of metabolism of the substrate medication. The multiple variants of the enzymes are termed polymorphisms. Screening tests are available from commercial laboratories that assess the likelihood of genetic susceptibility to drug interaction. Phillips reviewed 18 studies of ADEs related to genetic variations of CYP enzymes. Two thirds of the 27 drugs most commonly identified are metabolized by an enzyme with genetic variants [59].

Although 2D6 polymorphisms are present in 7% of the population, 14% of hospitalized psychiatric patients have 2D6 variants, suggesting a far greater risk of adverse drug events requiring hospitalization [60] (Table 10.5).

Table 10.5 Genetic polymorphisms and clinical relevance [26]

Polymorphism	Frequency	Drugs affected
CYP2C9 poor metabolizer	6–10% Caucasian	Phenytoin, warfarin, tolbutamide or glipizide
CYP2C19 poor metabolizer	13–23% Asian	Barbiturate, benzodiazepine
CYP2D6 poor metabolizer	1–10% Caucasians 1–4% African	Toxicity with TCAs, typical antipsychotics
CYP2D6 ultra metabolizer	25% Ethiopians 5–20% Turks, Southern European, Saudi Arabia	Opioid intoxication with codeine

Prodrugs

Some agents like hydrocodone and clopidogrel are prodrugs. They must be converted by 2D6 or 2C19, respectively, to the active compound. Other agents like metoprolol are metabolically active prior to 2D6 metabolism. Therefore coadministration of codeine and an inhibitor of 2D6 such as diphenhydramine or paroxetine may lead to inadequate analgesia due to lack of conversion of codeine to its active metabolite, morphine. Conversely, coadministration of metoprolol with an inhibitor of 2D6 such as amiodarone may lead to metoprolol toxicity with hypotension and bradycardia [4, 56].

P450 Enzyme Subtypes

CYP1A2 metabolizes 15% of all drugs, including caffeine, benzodiazepines, SSRIs, haloperidol, and clozapine [61]. Activity of metabolism is induced by tobacco [62] and inhibited by fluvoxamine, quinolones, and cimetidine. There is mild genetic variability.

CYP2C9 metabolizes 20% of the most commonly prescribed drugs, most importantly warfarin. Other "substrates" include phenytoin, tolbutamide, glipizide, losartan, fluvastatin, and NSAIDs. It is inhibited by fluconazole and induced by phenobarbital and rifampin. Up to 10% of Caucasians may be 2C9 deficient and may develop bleeding on usual doses of warfarin due to an inability to metabolize the drug. An FDA alert encourages physicians to consider genetic screening in patients whose anticoagulation is difficult to manage [63].

CYP2C19 metabolizes citalopram, diazepam, and omeprazole. It is inhibited by fluoxetine, fluvoxamine, omeprazole, and certain HIV drugs. It is induced by phenobarbital and rifampin. Up to 20% of Asians may be 2C19 poor metabolizers and are susceptible to toxicity on standard doses of diazepam [52, 63].

CYP2D6 is responsible for 25% of P450 drug metabolism, particularly the SSRIs, TCAs, phenothiazines, risperidone, and codeine. It is inhibited by amiodarone, fluoxetine, paroxetine, cimetidine, and quinidine. It may be induced by dexamethasone. 2D6 has significant polymorphisms. One in 10–14 Caucasians and 4% of African Americans are poor metabolizers. Because codeine must be converted to morphine to have an analgesic effect, these patients experience no analgesia with codeine. A small percentage are ultrametabolizers (1–7% of Caucasians, 25% of Ethiopians), leading to excessive narcosis on standard doses of codeine [51]. Conversely, patients deficient in 2D6 may develop toxicity on standard doses of active compounds such as haloperidol, due to inability to convert to inactive metabolites [64, 65].

CYP3A4 metabolizes 60% of currently available medications, including calcium channel blockers, HIV drugs, statins, cyclosporin, antihistamines, and cisapride. It is present in the intestinal mucosa and liver and accounts for the majority of first-pass metabolism. The enzyme lining the intestine is strongly inhibited by grapefruit juice [66]. The furanocoumarins in the fruit inactivate the enzyme in the gut, reducing first-pass metabolism, and allows for higher concentrations of drug leading to toxicity [52]. Other inhibitors include ketoconazole, metronidazole, AZT, omeprazole, erythromycin, and verapamil. The enzyme is induced by *Hypericum* (St John's-wort), carbamazepine, phenobarbital, and phenytoin [67].

Substrates/Inducers/Inhibitors

The majority of clinically useful medications are P450 substrates, meaning that they are metabolized by one or more P450 enzymes [52]. Medications may also be inhibitors or inducers (activators) of enzyme metabolism. Inducers are medications that increase the activity of enzyme. Inhibitors reduce enzyme activity. An agent may be both a substrate at low concentrations, and an inhibitor at higher levels, thus providing a potential check on toxicity. Some medications may be metabolized preferentially by one P450 enzyme at lower concentrations and by one or more others enzymes at higher concentrations. An example is codeine, a prodrug, which is a substrate of 2D6 but also 3A4 [51] (Table 10.6).

Prodrugs

Tamoxifen, a common antihormonal agent for the treatment of breast cancer, is a substrate of both 3A4 and 2D6. If taken with potent inhibitors of 2D6 metabolism such as fluoxetine, duloxetine, or diphenhydramine, tamoxifen is unable to be converted to its active form endoxifen, rendering it ineffective (Table 10.7).

Table 10.6 Significant P450 enzymes and clinically relevant drug-drug interactions [2]

Drug 1	Enzyme inhibitor or inducer	Drug 2	Metabolizing enzyme	Clinical effects
Fluoxetine, paroxetine	CYP2D6 inhibitor	Risperidone, tramadol	CYP2D6	Risperidone toxicity, inadequate pain relief
Grapefruit juice	CYP3A4 inhibitor	Buspirone	CYP3A4	Toxicity, serotonin syndrome
Diphenhydramine	CYP2D6 inhibitor	Amitriptyline	CYP2D6	Dry mouth, cardiac arrhythmia [68]

Table 10.7 Common prodrugs

Common prodrugs in clinical practice
Hydrocodone
Tramadol
Clopidogrel
Tamoxifen
Midodrine
Losartan
Azathioprine

Table 10.8 A top ten list of potential DDIs

Substrate	Inhibitor or inducer	Toxicity
Risperidone	Fluoxetine, paroxetine	Inhibits 2D6, leading to risperidone excess, sedation
Buspirone	Grapefruit juice	Increased absorption of buspirone due to 3A4 inhibition in the gut, leading to somnolence
Hydrocodone	Amiodarone, SSRIs	Lack of pain relief due to 2D6 inhibition
Metoprolol	Diphenhydramine	2D6 inhibition leading to bradycardia, hypotension
Meperidine	SSRIs, MAOIs	Serotonin syndrome
Oral contraceptives	Carbamazepine, phenytoin	3A4 induction, possible pregnancy
Clopidogrel	Omeprazole	2C19 inhibition, loss of prodrug clopidogrel efficacy
Amitriptyline	Fluvoxamine	2D6 inhibition
Theophylline	Fluoroquinolone	Seizures related to 1A2 inhibition
Marijuana	Fluvoxamine	Increased marijuana levels due to 2C9 inhibition

A Top Ten List of DDIs: Table 10.8

A Top Ten list would include commonly prescribed medications in combination with known P450 enzyme inhibitors or inducers or enzymes with marked pharmacogenomic variation. That list might include combinations of diphenhydramine, metoprolol, fluoxetine, SSRIs, first-generation anticonvulsants, oral contraceptives, meperidine and other opioids, amiodarone, fluoroquinolone, omeprazole, theophylline, antifungals, and clopidogrel.

Combining risperidone with carbamazepine, commonly used as a mood stabilizer, may lead to reduced therapeutic levels of risperidone due to enzyme induction [69].

Prevention/Recognition (Table 10.9)

Prevention of DDIs begins with a careful assessment of the patients medications and dietary supplements. A mnemonic such as AVOID MISTAKES serves as a helpful reminder of risk factors for drug interactions.

Table 10.9 A stepwise approach to drug-drug interactions

1. Take a medication history
Mnemonic – **Avoid m**istakes
Allergies?
Vitamins and dietary supplements
That is, grapefruit juice, St John's-wort (*Hypericum*)
Old drugs and **OTC**?
Interactions risk?
Dependence?
Mendel: any family history of drug sensitivity
2. Identify high-risk patients
>3 medications
Red flag drugs – anticonvulsants, antibiotics, digoxin, warfarin, amiodarone
3. Check pocket reference card
4. Consult pharmacist/drug specialist
5. Check computer programs
www.epocrates.com
Medical letter drug interaction program

www.fda.gov/cder-archived lecture

DDI Card

Patients frequently want to know whether the medication we are about to prescribe is likely to interact with others on their list. The tables listed below may be reprinted for use in the patient exam rooms and serve as a guide when counselling on potential drug interactions.

The most common mechanism of DDI is the coadministration of a substrate with an inhibitor or inducer of the same P450 enzyme. The tables below list common and clinically relevant drugs likely to interact.

First, determine whether there are any inhibitors on the patient's medication list. Next, identify any substrates of the inhibited or induced enzyme in question. Finally, discuss the symptoms and warning signs of possible interactions and whether the drug should be abruptly discontinued or weaned in the event of an interaction.

Cytochrome P450 drug interactions

CYP1A2

Substrates

Acetaminophen	Frovatriptan	Quinine
Amitriptyline	**Haloperidol**	Ranitidine
Bupropion	**Imipramine**	**Rasagiline**
Caffeine	Melatonin	
Clomipramine	Metoclopramide	**Theophylline**
Clozapine	**Mexiletine**	**Tizanidine**
	Mirtazapine	**R-warfarin**
Cyclobenzaprine	Naproxen	
Doxepin	**Olanzapine**	Zolmitriptan
Duloxetine		
	Propranolol	
Fluvoxamine		

Inhibitors

Amiodarone	Fluphenazine	Paroxetine
Amlodipine	Fluoxetine	Perphenazine
Caffeine	**Fluvoxamine**	**Refecoxib**
Cimetidine	**Levofloxacin**	Sertraline
	Lidocaine	
	Mexiletine	**Verapamil**
Ciprofloxacin	Nifedipine	
Diclofenac	Norfloxacin	**Herbal tea**
Duloxetine		Peppermint, Chamomile Teas
	Olanzapine	
	Oral contraceptives	

Inducers

Brussels sprouts	Phenobarbital	
Cruciferous veggies	Rifampin	
Carbamazepine	**Tobacco smoke**	Marijuana
Char-grilled meats	**St. John's Wort**	
	Paclitaxol	

Key- **bold**= common drug interactions, or dominant pathway

MAO, Phase II and Phase III (P-glycoprotein) drug interactions are not included

Important Prodrugs*

Codeine		**Tramadol**
Clopidogrel	**Tamoxifen**	**Azathioprine**
Midodrine		**Mycophenolate**

CYP3A4

Substrates			
Alprazolam	Doxepin	Methadone	**Quetiapine**
Amiodarone		**Midazolam**	Quinidine
Amlodipine	Erythromycin	Mirtazapine	
	Esomeprazole	Marijuana	**Sildenafil**
Atorvastatin		Modafinil	**Simvastatin**
Bromocriptine	Ethosuximide	Nefazodone	**Tacrolimus**
Bupropion	Felbamate	**Nicardipine**	**Tamoxifen**
Buspirone	Felodipine		
Caffeine		Omeprazole	Tiagabine
Carbamazepine	Fentanyl	Ondansetron	
	Fluconazole	**Oral contraceptives**	Ttramadol
Clarithromycin	Fluvoxamine	Oxcarbazepine	
Cocaine	**Haloperidol**		Trazodone
Cyclophosphamide			Venlafaxine
Cyclosporine	Hydrocortisone	Pravastatin	**Verapamil**
	Ketoconazole		
Dexamethasone	**Lansoprazole**	**Prednisone**	Warfarin
Diazepam	Lidocaine	**Progesterone**	
Diltiazem	Losartan		Zolpidem
	Lovastatin		
Inhibitors			
Amiodarone	Fentanyl	**Ketoconazole**	
Atorvastatin	**Fluconazole**	Lovastatin	**Saquinavir**
Cimetidine	Fluoxetine	Nicardipine	Simvastatin
Ciprofloxacin	Fluvoxamine		
Clarithromycin		Nifedipine	Sertraline
Cyclosporine	**Grapefruit juice (functional inducer)**	**Nefazodone**	Tacrolimus
Diltiazem			
Erythromycin		Omeprazole	Valproic acid
	Isoniazid		
		Paroxetine	Verapamil
		Quinidine	**Voriconazole**
Inducers			
Carbamazepine	Oxcarbazepine	**Prednisone**	**St. John's Wort**
Dexamethasone	**Phenobarbital**	**Primidone**	**Topiramate (>200 mg)**
Modafinil	**Phenytoin**	**Rifampin**	

Important notice: These tables are not all-inclusive. New information is continually identified

CYP2D6

Substrates

Poor metabolizers- 7–10% of Caucasians, 4% African Americans

Ultrarapid metabolizers- 1–7% Caucasians, 25% of Ethiopians

Amitriptyline	Duloxetine	Nortriptyline
Bupropion	**Fluoxetine**	**Oxycodone**
Carvedilol	Fluphenazine	Paroxetine
Codeine*	Fluvoxamine	Propafenone
Desipramine	Haloperidol	**Propranolol**
Dextromethorphan	Hydrocodone	**Risperidone**
Donepezil	Imipramine	Sertraline
Doxepin	Lidocaine	**Tamoxifen***
Doxorubicin	Methadone	Thioridazine
	Metoclopramide	**Timolol**
	Metoprolol	**Tramadol***
	Mexiletine	Venlafaxine
	Mirtazapine	

Inhibitors

Amiodarone	**Duloxetine**	Nortriptyline
Amitriptyline	**Fluoxetine**	**Paroxetine**
Atorvastatin	Fluvoxamine	**Pimozide**
Bupropion	**Haloperidol**	Pioglitazone
Celecoxib	Isoniazid	**Quinidine**
Clozapine	Lansoprazole	Risperidone
Cocaine	Methadone	**Ritonavir**
Desipramine		Sertraline
Diclofenac		Thioridazine
Diphenhydramine		Trazodone
		Venlafaxine

Inducers

Probably none

CYP2C9

Substrates

2C9 Impaired in 1–10% Caucasians

Bupropion	**Glipizide**	**Naproxen**	Valproic acid
Carvedilol	**Ibuprofen**	Phenobarbital	Voriconazole
Celecoxib	**Indomethacin**	Phenytoin	**S-warfarin**
Cyclophosphamide	**Irbesartan**	**Piroxicam**	Marijuana
Dapsone	**Losartan***	Sildenafil	
Diclofenac	**Meloxicam**	SMX/TMP	
Fluoxetine	Methadone	Tamoxifen	

Inhibitors

Amiodarone	**Fluvoxamine**	**Metronidazole** nicardipine	Sertraline
Cimetidine	**Ginkgo Biloba**	Pantoprazole	Simvastatin
Fluconazole	Ibuprofen	**Paroxetine**	**Valproic acid**
Fluoxetine	Indomethacin	Piroxicam	**Zafirlukast**
Fluvastatin	**Ketoconazole**	Quinine	
	Losartan	Ritonavir	

Inducers

Carbamazepine	**Phenobarbital**	Primidone	Ritonavir
Dexamethasone	**Phenytoin**	**Rifampin**	**St. John's Wort**
Oxcarbazepine			

CYP2C19

Substrates

2C19 impaired in 15–30% of Asians

Amitriptyline	**Diazepam**	**Omeprazole**	Progesterone
Carisoprodol	**Esomeprazole**	Pantoprazole	Sertraline
Clomipramine	**Fluoxetine**	Phenobarbital	Voriconazole
Citalopram	**Imipramine**	**Phenytoin**	Warfarin
Clopidogrel*	Indomethacin		
Cyclophosphamide	**Lansoprazole**		
Dapsone	Methadone		

Inhibitors

Amiodarone	**Fluoxetine**	**Isoniazid**	**Oral contraceptive** paroxetine
Amitriptyline	**Fluvoxamine**	Ketoconazole	Sertraline
Cimetidine	Imipramine	**Lansoprazole**	**Topiramate**
Felbamate	Indomethacin	Modafinil	**Valproic acid**
Fluconazole		Nicardipine	
		Omeprazole	

Inducers

Carbamazepine	Pentobarbital	**Rifampin**	**St. John's Wort**
Oxcarbazepine	Phenytoin		**Glucocorticoids**

Prevention/Recognition

An effective means of preventing adverse drug reactions and drug-drug interactions is rounding with a hospital-based clinical pharmacist. Rivkin found that rounding with a pharmacist who screened ICU patients for potential drug interactions reduced ADEs by 65% and reduced length of stay and mortality [70]

DDI Websites

http://medicine.iupui.edu/CLINPHARM/DDIS
https://www.drugs.com/drug_interactions.html
www.themedicalletter.com [17]
www.druginteractioninfo.org
www.pharmvar.org
www.fda.gov/drugs/developmentapprovalprocess/developmentresources/drugin-teractionslabeling/ucm080499.htm

References

1. Samer CF, Lorenzini KI, Rollason V, Daali Y, Desmeules JA. Applications of CYP450 testing in the clinical setting. Mol Diag Ther. 2013;17(3):165–84. https://doi.org/10.1007/s40291-013-0028-5.
2. Lynch T, Price A. The effect of cytochrome P450 metabolism on drug response, interactions, and adverse effects. Am Fam Physician. 2007;76:391–9.
3. Sharma A, Pibarot P, Pilote S, et al. Toward optimal treatment in women: the effect of sex on metoprolol-diphenhydramine interaction. J Clin Pharmacol. 2010;50(2):214–25. https://doi.org/10.1177/0091270009340417.
4. Monte AA, Heard KJ, Campbell J, Hamamura D, Weinshilboum RM, Vasiliou V. The effect of CYP2D6 drug-drug interactions on hydrocodone effectiveness. Acad Emerg Med. 2014;21(8):879–85. https://doi.org/10.1111/acem.12431.
5. Chang K-L, Weitzel K, Schmidt S. Pharmacogenetics: using genetic information to guide drug therapy. Am Fam Physician. 2015;92(7):588–94.
6. Lerner B. A case that shook medicine. Washington Post. http://www.washingtonpost.com/wp-dyn/content/article/2006/11/24/AR2006112400985.html. Published November 28, 2006.
7. Hoffman J. Judge sets aside use of cocaine as part of verdict in zion case. New York Times. http://query.nytimes.com/gst/fullpage.html?res=990CE6DE1F38F931A35756C0A963958260&sec=&spon=&pagewanted=2. Published 1995.
8. Asch DA, Parker RM. The libby zion case. N Engl J Med 1988;318:771–75.
9. Nasca TJ, Day SH, Amis ESJ. The new recommendations on duty hours from the ACGME Task Force. N Engl J Med. 2010;363(2):e3. https://doi.org/10.1056/NEJMsb1005800.
10. Gurwitz JH, Field TS, Harrold LR, et al. Incidence and preventability of adverse drug events among older persons in the ambulatory setting. JAMA. 2003;289(9):1107–16. https://doi.org/10.1001/jama.289.9.1107.
11. Pirmohamed M, James S, Meakin S, et al. Adverse drug reactions as cause of admission to hospital: prospective analysis of 18 820 patients. BMJ. 2004;329(7456):15–9. https://doi.org/10.1136/bmj.329.7456.15.

12. Burroughs TE, Waterman AD, Gallagher TH, et al. Patient concerns about medical errors in emergency departments. Acad Emerg Med. 2005;12(1):57–64. https://doi.org/10.1111/j.1553-2712.2005.tb01480.x.

13. McDonnell PJ, Jacobs MR. Hospital admissions resulting from preventable adverse drug reactions. Ann Pharmacother. 2016;36(9):1331–6. https://doi.org/10.1345/aph.1A333.

14. Franceschi M, Scarcelli C, Niro V, et al. Prevalence, clinical features and avoidability of adverse drug reactions as cause of admission to a geriatric unit. Drug Saf. 2008;31(6):545–56. https://doi.org/10.2165/00002018-200831060-00009.

15. Becker ML, Kallewaard M, Caspers PW, Visser LE, Leufkens HG, Stricker BH. Hospitalisations and emergency department visits due to drug–drug interactions: a literature review. Pharmacoepidemiol Drug Saf. 2007;16(6):641–51. https://doi.org/10.1002/pds.1351.

16. Leape LL, Bates DW, Cullen DJ, et al. Systems analysis of adverse drug events. JAMA. 1995;274(1):35–43. https://doi.org/10.1001/jama.1995.03530010049034.

17. Marino A, Capogrosso-Sansone A, Tuccori M, et al. Expected and actual adverse drug-drug interactions in elderly patients accessing the emergency department: data from the ANCESTRAL-ED study. Expert Opin Drug Saf. 2016;15(sup2):45–50. https://doi.org/10.1080/14740338.2016.1221400.

18. Phansalkar S, van der Sijs H, Tucker AD, et al. Drug–drug interactions that should be non-interruptive in order to reduce alert fatigue in electronic health records. J Am Med Inform Assoc. 2013;20(3):489–93. https://doi.org/10.1136/amiajnl-2012-001089.

19. Nebeker JR, Hoffman JM, Weir CR, Bennett CL, Hurdle JF. High rates of adverse drug events in a highly computerized hospital. Arch Intern Med. 2005;165(10):1111–6. https://doi.org/10.1001/archinte.165.10.1111.

20. Moore TJ, Cohen MR, Furberg CD. Serious adverse drug events reported to the Food and Drug Administration, 1998-2005. Arch Intern Med. 2007;167(16):1752–9. https://doi.org/10.1001/archinte.167.16.1752.

21. Budnitz DS, Lovegrove MC, Shehab N, Richards CL. Emergency hospitalizations for adverse drug events in older Americans. N Engl J Med. 2011;365(21):2002–12. https://doi.org/10.1056/NEJMsa1103053.

22. By the American Geriatrics Society 2015 Beers Criteria Update Expert Panel. American Geriatrics Society 2015 updated beers criteria for potentially inappropriate medication use in older adults. J Am Geriatr Soc. 2015;63(11):2227–46. https://doi.org/10.1111/jgs.13702.

23. Budnitz DS, Shehab N, Kegler SR, Richards CL. Medication use leading to emergency department visits for adverse drug events in older adults. Ann Intern Med. 2007;147(11):755–65. https://doi.org/10.7326/0003-4819-147-11-200712040-00006.

24. Patterns of medication use in the United States. http://www.bu.edu/slone/files/2012/11/SloneSurveyReport2006.pdf. Published 2006. Accessed 4 Sept 2017.

25. Leone R, Magro L, Moretti U, et al. Identifying adverse drug reactions associated with drug-drug interactions. Drug Saf. 2010;33(8):667–75. https://doi.org/10.2165/11534400-000000000-00000.

26. Sirot EJ, van der Velden JW, Rentsch K, Eap CB, Baumann P. Therapeutic drug monitoring and pharmacogenetic tests as tools in pharmacovigilance. Drug Saf. 2006;29(9):735–68. https://doi.org/10.2165/00002018-200629090-00001.

27. Pedavally S, Fugate JE, Rabinstein AA. Serotonin syndrome in the intensive care unit: clinical presentations and precipitating medications. Neurocrit Care. 2014;21(1):108–13. https://doi.org/10.1007/s12028-013-9914-2.

28. Jeffrey R, Strawn MD, Paul E, Keck MD Jr, Stanley N, Caroff MD. Neuroleptic malignant syndrome. Am J Psychiatr. 2007. https://doi.org/10.1176/ajp.2007.164.issue-6;page:string:Article/Chapter.

29. Christodoulou C, Kalaitzi C. Antipsychotic drug-induced acute laryngeal dystonia: two case reports and a mini review. J Psychopharmacol (Oxford). 2005;19(3):307–11. https://doi.org/10.1177/0269881105051543.

30. Bookwalter T, Gitlin M. Gabapentin-induced neurologic toxicities. Pharmacother J Hum Pharmacol Drug Ther. 2005;25(12):1817–9. https://doi.org/10.1592/phco.2005.25.12.1817.

31. Lee C-P, Chen P-J, Chang C-M. Heat stroke during treatment with olanzapine, trihexypheni-dyl, and trazodone in a patient with schizophrenia. Acta Neuropsychiatr. 2015;27(6):380–5. https://doi.org/10.1017/neu.2015.29.

32. Locharernkul C, Loplumlert J, Limotai C, et al. Carbamazepine and phenytoin induced Stevens-Johnson syndrome is associated with HLA-B*1502 allele in Thai population. Epilepsia. 2008;49(12):2087–91. https://doi.org/10.1111/j.1528-1167.2008.01719.x.

33. Thundiyil JG, Kearney TE, Olson KR. Evolving epidemiology of drug-induced seizures reported to a poison control center system. J Med Toxicol. 2007;3(1):15–9. https://doi.org/10.1007/BF03161033.

34. Gupta A, Lawrence AT, Krishnan K, Kavinsky CJ, Trohman RG. Current concepts in the mechanisms and management of drug-induced QT prolongation and torsade de pointes. Am Heart J. 2007;153(6):891–9. https://doi.org/10.1016/j.ahj.2007.01.040.

35. Sheikh HU, Mathew PG. Reversible cerebral vasoconstriction syndrome: updates and new perspectives. Curr Pain Headache Rep. 2014;18(5):414. https://doi.org/10.1007/s11916-014-0414-7.

36. Wong VSS, Singh H, Verro P. Posterior reversible encephalopathy syndrome in the context of phentermine use resulting in intracranial hemorrhage. Neurologist. 2011;17(2):111–3. https://doi.org/10.1097/NRL.0b013e31820a9ddc.

37. Hung T-Y, Seow V-K, Chong C-F, Wang T-L, Chen C-C. Gabapentin toxicity: an important cause of altered consciousness in patients with uraemia. Emerg Med J. 2008;25(3):178–9. https://doi.org/10.1136/emj.2007.053470.

38. Zand L, McKian KP, Qian Q. Gabapentin toxicity in patients with chronic kidney disease: a preventable cause of morbidity. Am J Med. 2010;123(4):367–73. https://doi.org/10.1016/j.amjmed.2009.09.030.

39. Chau V, Prasad S, Stewart D, Heckman G. Creutzfeldt–Jakob disease-like syndrome induced by gabapentin toxicity. Age Res. 2010;1(1):3. https://doi.org/10.4081/ar.2010.e3.

40. Babiy M, Stubblefield MD, Herklotz M, Hand M. Asterixis related to gabapentin as a cause of falls. Am J Phys Med Rehabil. 2005;84(2):136–40. https://doi.org/10.1097/01.PHM.0000151943.06257.64.

41. Clark SL, Rabinstein AA, Hocker SE. Disabling asterixis induced by gabapentin. J Med Case. 2015;6(7):285–6. https://doi.org/10.14740/jmc.v6i7.2143.

42. Sternbach H. The serotonin syndrome. Am J Psychiatr. 1991;148:705–16.

43. Boyer EW, Shannon M. The serotonin syndrome. N Engl J Med. 2009;352(11):1112–20. https://doi.org/10.1056/NEJMra041867.

44. Bodner RA, Lynch T, Lewis L, Kahn D. Serotonin syndrome. Neurology. 1995;45(2):219–23. https://doi.org/10.1212/WNL.45.2.219.

45. Evans RW, Tepper SJ, Shapiro RE, Sun Edelstein C, Tietjen GE. The FDA alert on sero-tonin syndrome with use of triptans combined with selective serotonin reuptake inhibi-tors or selective serotonin-norepinephrine reuptake inhibitors: American Headache Society position paper. Headache J Head Face Pain. 2010;50(6):1089–99. https://doi.org/10.1111/j.1526-4610.2010.01691.x.

46. Watson WA, Litovitz TL, Rodgers GC, Klein-Schwartz W, Youniss J, Rose SR, Borys D, May ME. 2002 annual report of the American Association of poison control centers toxic exposure surveillance system. Am J Emerg Med. 2003;21(5):353–421.

47. Mackay FJ, Dunn NR, Mann RD. Antidepressants and the serotonin syndrome in general practice. Br J Gen Pract. 1999;49(448):871–4.

48. Dunkley EJ, Isbister GK, Sibbritt D, Dawson AH, Whyte IM. The hunter serotonin toxicity criteria: simple and accurate diagnostic decision rules for serotonin toxicity. QJM. 2003 Sep 1;96(9):635–42.

49. Roberts JA, Pea F, Lipman J. The clinical relevance of plasma protein binding changes. Clin Pharmacokinet. 2013;52(1):1–8. https://doi.org/10.1007/s40262-012-0018-5.

50. Benet LZ, Hoener BA. Changes in plasma protein binding have little clinical relevance. Clin Pharmacol Therap. 2002;71(3):115–21. https://doi.org/10.1067/mcp.2002.121829.

51. Gasche Y, Daali Y, Fathi M, et al. Codeine intoxication associated with ultrarapid CYP2D6 metabolism. N Engl J Med. 2009;351(27):2827–31. https://doi.org/10.1056/NEJMoa041888.

52. Wilkinson GR. Drug metabolism and variability among patients in drug response. N Engl J Med. 2005;352(21):2211–21. https://doi.org/10.1056/NEJMra032424.
53. Patsalos PN, Perucca E. Clinically important drug interactions in epilepsy: general features and interactions between antiepileptic drugs. Lancet Neurol. 2003;2(6):347–56. https://doi.org/10.1016/S1474-4422(03)00409-5.
54. Xu C, Li CY-T, Kong A-NT. Induction of phase I, II and III drug metabolism/transport by xenobiotics. Arch Pharm Res. 2005;28(3):249–68. https://doi.org/10.1007/BF02977789.
55. Marchetti S, Mazzanti R, Beijnen JH, Schellens JHM. Concise review: clinical relevance of drug drug and herb drug interactions mediated by the ABC transporter ABCB1 (MDR1, P-glycoprotein). Oncologist. 2007;12(8):927–41. https://doi.org/10.1634/theoncologist.12-8-927.
56. Werner D, Wuttke H, Fromm MF, et al. Effect of amiodarone on the plasma levels of metoprolol. Am J Cardiol. 2004;94(10):1319–21. https://doi.org/10.1016/j.amjcard.2004.07.125.
57. Wuttke H, Rau T, Heide R, et al. Increased frequency of cytochrome P450 2D6 poor metabolizers among patients with metoprolol-associated adverse effects. Clin Pharmacol Therap. 2002;72(4):429–37. https://doi.org/10.1067/mcp.2002.127111.
58. Weinshilboum R. Inheritance and drug response. N Engl J Med. 2009;348(6):529–37. https://doi.org/10.1056/NEJMra020021.
59. Phillips KA, Veenstra DL, Oren E, Lee JK, Sadee W. Potential role of pharmacogenomics in reducing adverse drug reactions: a systematic review. JAMA. 2001;286(18):2270–9. https://doi.org/10.1001/jama.286.18.2270.
60. de Leon J, Susce MT, Pan RM, Fairchild M, Koch WH, Wedlund PJ. The CYP2D6 poor metabolizer phenotype may be associated with risperidone adverse drug reactions and discontinuation. J Clin Psychiatry. 2005;66(1):15–27.
61. Raaska K, Neuvonen PJ. Ciprofloxacin increases serum clozapine and N-desmethylclozapine: a study in patients with schizophrenia. Eur J Clin Pharmacol. 2000;56(8):585–9.
62. Zevin S, Benowitz NL. Drug interactions with tobacco smoking. Clin Pharmacokinet. 1999;36(6):425–38. https://doi.org/10.2165/00003088-199936060-00004.
63. Huang SM, Temple R. Is this the drug or dose for you?: impact and consideration of ethnic factors in global drug development, regulatory review, and clinical practice. Clin Pharmacol Ther. 2008;84(3):287–94. https://doi.org/10.1038/clpt.2008.144.
64. Hartmann AM, Giegling I, Genius J, Schäfer M, Bondy B, Möller HJ, Rujescu D. A study on pharmacogenetics of haloperidol treatment. Pharmacopsychiatry. 2007 Sep;40(05):A078.
65. Šimić I, Potočnjak I, Kraljičković I, et al. CYP2D6 *6/*6 genotype and drug interactions as cause of haloperidol-induced extrapyramidal symptoms. 2016 Pharmacogenomics;17(13):1385–1389. doi:https://doi.org/10.2217/pgs-2016-0069. http://dxdoiorgezpsluedu/102217/pgs-2016-0069
66. Bressler R. Grapefruit juice and prescription drug interactions. Geriatrics. 2006;61:12–18.
67. Gurley BJ, Gardner SF, Hubbard MA, et al. In vivo effects of goldenseal, kava kava, black cohosh, and valerian on human cytochrome P450 1A2, 2D6, 2E1, and 3A4/5 phenotypes. Clin Pharmacol Therap. 2005;77(5):415–26. https://doi.org/10.1016/j.clpt.2005.01.009.
68. Fosnight SM, Holder CM, Allen KR, Hazelett S. A strategy to decrease the use of risky drugs in the elderly. Cleve Clin J Med. 2004;71(7):561–8.
69. Schoretsanitis G, Haen E, Gründer G, et al. Pharmacokinetic drug-drug interactions of mood stabilizers and risperidone in patients under combined treatment. J Clin Psychopharmacol. 2016;36(6):554–61. https://doi.org/10.1097/JCP.0000000000000601.
70. Rivkin A, Yin H. Evaluation of the role of the critical care pharmacist in identifying and avoiding or minimizing significant drug-drug interactions in medical intensive care patients. J Crit Care. 2011;26(1):104.e1–6. https://doi.org/10.1016/j.jcrc.2010.04.014.

Chapter 11
Mood Stabilizers, Anticonvulsants, and Anti-agitants

William J. Newman

This chapter addresses the use of mood stabilizers, including various anticonvulsants, for both FDA-approved and off-label uses in treating psychiatric disorders. Additionally, this chapter provides a focused overview of the management of adults with aggressive behaviors related to major psychiatric disorders, with an emphasis on conditions most likely to be encountered by neurologists. The classifications of the disorders in this chapter are consistent with diagnostic criteria in the *Diagnostic and Statistical Manual of Mental Disorders*, Fifth Edition [1].

There are no currently FDA-approved pharmacological treatments of aggression, regardless of the diagnosis or the origin of the behaviors. The treatments used to target aggression (beyond primary treatment of psychiatric disorders) are therefore off-label interventions and should be carefully considered after reviewing the available evidence. This chapter presents some of the relevant evidence supporting off-label pharmacological treatments targeting aggression related to specific diagnoses. Other sources provide more detailed overviews of the assessment and management of aggression.

Bipolar and Related Disorders

Diagnostic Clarity

Mood stabilizers are most commonly used in psychiatry to treat bipolar disorder, a diagnosis that is commonly misunderstood (even among mental health professionals). It is therefore important to first develop a clear understanding of what bipolar disorder is and what it is not. There are two types of bipolar disorder described in the DSM-5. One or more manic episodes are required to establish a diagnosis of bipolar I disorder. The presence of one or more hypomanic episodes, in addition to

W. J. Newman, MD (✉)
Department of Psychiatry and Behavioral Neuroscience, Saint Louis University
School of Medicine, St. Louis, MO, USA
e-mail: newmanwj@slu.edu

© Springer International Publishing AG, part of Springer Nature 2018　　　　201
G. T. Grossberg, L. J. Kinsella (eds.), *Clinical Psychopharmacology for Neurologists*, https://doi.org/10.1007/978-3-319-74604-3_11

Table 11.1 Differentiating bipolar I disorder, bipolar II disorder, and borderline personality disorder

	Bipolar I disorder	Bipolar II disorder	Borderline PD
Mood episodes	Manic episodes, major depressive episodes	Hypomanic episodes, major depressive episodes	Not episodic
Irritability	Episodic, during manic episodes	Episodic, during hypomanic episodes	Chronic and situational
Female-male ratio	Nearly equal	Nearly equal	3:1
Psychosis possible	Yes	Not as part of primary diagnosis	Not as part of primary diagnosis

one or more major depressive episodes, is required to establish a diagnosis of bipolar II disorder. Table 11.1 differentiates bipolar I disorder, bipolar II disorder, and borderline personality disorder (which is frequently confused with bipolar spectrum disorders).

Many individuals report having bipolar disorder despite not actually having an overall history consistent with the diagnosis. There are several potential contributing factors to misdiagnosis. One common factor, particularly for providers not typically accustomed to providing mental health treatment, is a limited understanding of the core criteria and common course of manic and hypomanic episodes. Another common factor is individuals sometimes having a preference of being diagnosed with a mood disorder (such as bipolar disorder), as opposed to being diagnosed with a personality disorder that better explains their chronic interpersonal problems, mood lability, and poor decision making. For instance, a longtime perpetrator of intimate partner violence may explain his behavior by stating, "I can't control myself because of my bipolar disorder." However, his history of interpersonal violence may be persistent and not better accounted for by a mood disorder.

One important point to remember about bipolar disorder is that it is an episodic illness. Individuals with persistent characterological traits must therefore be differentiated from individuals with behaviors that occur solely in the context of manic or hypomanic episodes. The former may exhibit compulsive gambling and disrupt their family's finances by taking every paycheck to the local casino hoping to strike it big. In contrast, a manic individual may blow a large amount of money at the casino during a manic episode, gambling and purchasing drinks for large numbers of newfound friends.

Treatment of Bipolar Disorder

Typical treatment involves the daily use of a mood stabilizer, such as lithium or valproate, with the potential addition of an antipsychotic when there are concurrent psychotic symptoms in patients with bipolar I disorder. Regarding combination treatment for individuals with mania and psychosis, the American Psychiatric

Table 11.2 Mood stabilizers with FDA indications for psychiatric illness

Generic name	Common brand name(s)	FDA-approved indication(s) for psychiatric illnesses
lithium	Eskalith, Eskalith CR, Lithobid, lithium citrate (liquid)	Bipolar disorder (manic episodes and maintenance treatment)
valproate	Depakote, Depakote ER, Depakene (liquid)	Bipolar disorder (acute manic and mixed episodes)
lamotrigine	Lamictal	Bipolar disorder (maintenance treatment)
carbamazepine	Tegretol, Tegretol XR	Bipolar disorder (acute manic and mixed episodes)[a]
oxcarbazepine	Trileptal	None
topiramate	Topamax	None
levetiracetam	Keppra	None
gabapentin	Neurontin	None

[a]Only the extended-release formulation has been FDA approved for the treatment of bipolar disorder, though the immediate-release formulation is also commonly prescribed

Table 11.3 Initiating and monitoring lithium or valproate for bipolar disorder

	Check before prescribing	Potential birth defect	Target serum level
Lithium	Renal function, thyroid function, pregnancy test, EKG (for age 40+ or known cardiac history)	Ebstein's anomaly	0.7–1.2
Valproate	LFTs, pregnancy test, CBC	Neural tube defects, ovarian dysplasia	50–150

Association (APA) practice guidelines note, "The *combination* [emphasis included] of an antipsychotic with either lithium or valproate may be more effective than any of these agents alone. Thus, the first-line pharmacological treatment for patients with severe mania is the initiation of either lithium plus an antipsychotic or valproate plus an antipsychotic" [2].

There are several considerations that go into deciding which mood stabilizers to prescribe to patients with bipolar spectrum disorders. Table 11.2 summarizes mood stabilizers that are commonly used in the treatment of bipolar spectrum disorders, highlighting FDA-approved indications. Prescribers sometimes consider using levetiracetam as a mood stabilizer. However, levetiracetam is not an effective mood stabilizer and in fact may cause or exacerbate aggression or excessive motoric activity. Lithium and valproate are the first two mood stabilizers typically used to treat patients with bipolar disorder. Table 11.3 presents an overview of factors to consider when initiating and monitoring lithium or valproate for bipolar disorder. Women of childbearing age should be informed about the potential risks of birth defects when treated with either medication. For patients with bipolar II disorder who have prominent major depressive episodes, lithium and lamotrigine should generally be tried first. Patients with the rapid cycling subtype of bipolar disorder often respond well to valproate.

When patients do not improve as expected, clinicians should consider that the patient may not be taking the medications as prescribed. When clinically indicated, this issue can be addressed by obtaining serum levels that are easily tracked. Examples of medications with available serum levels include lithium, valproate, and carbamazepine. Serum levels allow the prescriber to at least have basic knowledge of the patient's recent adherence and to make an informed decision regarding the course of treatment. Obtaining a serum level that is markedly different from the anticipated level allows clinicians to consider potential causes for the discrepancy. Some patients are simply rapid metabolizers and need to be prescribed an increased dose. Other patients do not have a full understanding of their medication regimen and would benefit from additional education. Others consciously choose not to take their medications, in which case a frank discussion about why could be beneficial to both parties. Patients may choose not to take their mood stabilizers because they enjoy the experience of being manic or hypomanic and do not want the medications to bring them down. Alcohol and illicit drug use can also negatively impact treatment.

Managing Aggressive Behaviors in Bipolar Disorder

Aggressive behaviors by manic individuals are often impulsive and related to their elevated mood, grandiosity, or sense of invulnerability. The primary intervention is therefore treatment of the underlying mania. Aggressive behaviors are often the precipitating factors that lead to manic patients being hospitalized or arrested. Patients with bipolar disorder are at an overall increased risk of being arrested. In one study of individuals with bipolar disorder who had been arrested, the majority were manic (74.2%) and/or psychotic (59.0%) at the time of their arrest [3]. The presence of psychosis or comorbid substance use can further increase their risk of aggression [4].

Case Example

Mr. A is a 36-year-old man with a bipolar I disorder diagnosis dating back to age 21. He has been stable on lithium for 12 years. He is now also being prescribed levetiracetam for seizures that he began experiencing after a traumatic brain injury that he suffered during a motor vehicle accident when he was 35 years old. Over time, he has developed a significant tremor despite being in the therapeutic window for his lithium. His thyroid function has also been declining over the last few years, which is thought to likely be related to his lithium. Mr. A's psychiatrist and neurologist discuss potential treatment options and decide on valproate as a single agent that could be used to control both his bipolar disorder and his seizures. They coordinate to get him on a target dose of valproate 1000 mg bid, based on his weight of 200 lbs. After checking a serum valproate level 5 days later, his level is 84. They then discontinue his lithium and levetiracetam.

Schizophrenia Spectrum and Other Psychotic Disorders

The primary pharmacological treatment of schizophrenia involves management using typical or atypical antipsychotic medications, either as daily pills or long-acting injectable formulations. However, mood stabilizers can be used for adjunctive management of aggression in patients with schizophrenia who do not respond to antipsychotic medications alone [5]. There is some published evidence supporting augmentation with various mood stabilizers including valproate [6, 7], lithium [8], carbamazepine [9], and lamotrigine [10]. However, the use of mood stabilizers for this purpose is neither FDA approved nor based on large-scale, double-blind/controlled studies. The addition of a mood stabilizer is unlikely to significantly address aggressive behaviors related to residual psychotic symptoms. They are most likely to be beneficial in patients with schizophrenia who display impulsive acts of aggression.

Personality Disorders

Individuals with certain personality disorders are prone to displaying increased aggression related to their personality structure. Antisocial and borderline personality disorders are the two that are most frequently linked to aggression. The link is common enough that a pattern of aggressive behavior is a diagnostic criterion for both antisocial and borderline personality disorders based on the DSM-5 [1]. Substance misuse (including alcohol) is also particularly common in both populations, which can worsen the frequency and severity of aggressive behaviors.

There is published evidence regarding the pharmacological management of aggression in individuals with certain personality disorders. One double-blind, placebo-controlled study presented the benefits of using valproate to target impulsive aggression in patients with cluster B personality disorders. Cluster B personality disorders include the following: antisocial personality disorder, borderline personality disorder, histrionic personality disorder, and narcissistic personality disorder. The subjects received average daily doses of 1400 mg, with average serum valproate levels of 65.5 [11]. Another double-blind, placebo-controlled study presented the benefits of lithium to target impulsive aggression in incarcerated individuals with "nonpsychotic personality disorders," with serum lithium levels typically under 1.0 mEq/L [12].

No pharmacological intervention has consistently proven effective in the overall management of individuals with antisocial personality disorder. These individuals are often prone to display preconceived, predatory acts of aggression, for which there is not a helpful pharmacological intervention. Individuals with antisocial personality disorder may separately display impulsive acts of aggression. One case report described the benefits of targeting impulsive aggression in patients diagnosed with antisocial personality disorder using propranolol [13].

Multiple studies have also been published about pharmacological interventions targeting the impulsivity and anger that often contribute to acts of impulsive aggression by individuals with borderline personality disorder. Various articles have described decreased anger in patients with borderline personality disorder using mood stabilizers including lamotrigine, topiramate, and valproate [14–18]. Impulsivity is another common trait in borderline personality disorder that can contribute to aggressive behaviors. The same three mood stabilizers reported to improve anger in this population also improved impulsivity [14–19].

Neurocognitive Disorders

Neurocognitive Disorder Due to Traumatic Brain Injury (TBI), with Behavioral Disturbance

Agitation and aggression displayed by patients with major neurocognitive disorder are covered in a separate chapter. However, aggression is an issue frequently encountered by clinicians when managing patients with acquired brain injuries. In the DSM-5, the condition is termed neurocognitive disorder due to traumatic brain injury. The DSM-5 allows for further diagnostic specification regarding behavioral disturbances related to the TBI. Patients with a history of TBI do not necessarily need prophylactic treatment for behavioral disturbances. When the behavioral changes limit functioning, impact medical treatment, and/or put the patient or others at danger, treatment of the behavioral disturbance may be warranted.

Various medications have been used over the years to target aggression in this population. Beta blockers represent one effective strategy for specifically targeting aggression in patients with acquired brain injuries. The published research, though largely limited to small studies, is overall encouraging. One research group published multiple reports involving double-blind, placebo-controlled studies describing the benefits of beta blockers for individuals with acquired brain injuries [20–22].

Most published reports involving beta blockers to target the management of aggression have studied the use of propranolol and pindolol. Many of the doses utilized in these early studies were higher than are typically used for hypertension. At the higher doses, there were numerous reports of adverse events related to bradycardia and hypotension. Recent studies, however, have found similarly encouraging anti-aggressive effects using lower doses of beta blockers. For instance, Caspi et al. [23] published positive outcomes in a study using pindolol 5 mg tid.

Some researchers have specifically studied pindolol as opposed to other beta blockers due to it displaying intrinsic sympathomimetic activity (ISA), a partial agonism particularly apparent at higher doses. The ISA results in less problematic drops in heart rate and blood pressure than would typically happen with pro-pranolol. Pindolol comes in generic formulations and can also be easily titrated in patients whose vital signs and medical histories make them appropriate candidates.

Other pharmacological treatment options for patients with acquired brain injuries have also been described in the literature. Mood stabilizers are the other class that has shown significant benefits in this population. Multiple studies note the apparent benefits of valproate for curbing aggression in individuals with acquired brain injuries [24–26]. Another article addresses the benefits of carbamazepine in addressing aggression in individuals with severe closed-head injuries [27]. One case report alludes to the benefits of using lithium in a patient with an acquired brain injury who had not responded to other treatment options [28]. However, since individuals with acquired brain injuries may be more likely to experience side effects, lower total doses should be used [29]. Antipsychotics are frequently prescribed to address agitated/aggressive behaviors in this population. However, there is more data to support the use of mood stabilizers, including anticonvulsant medications, for this purpose [30].

Delirium

Patients with delirium can at times display both purposeful and purposeless (arm flailing, kicking, etc.) aggressive behaviors (Fig. 11.1). These actions are most commonly related to underlying disorientation and confusion. Low-dose typical and atypical antipsychotics are commonly used to address these behaviors [31]. The American Association for Emergency Psychiatry Project BETA Psychopharmacology Workgroup suggests prescribing low-dose haloperidol or atypical antipsychotics for agitation and related aggression [32].

If alcohol or benzodiazepine withdrawal is a potential cause of the delirium, appropriate doses of benzodiazepines should be administered immediately. Unless alcohol or benzodiazepine withdrawal is likely as a cause of the delirium, benzodiazepines should generally be avoided. Benzodiazepines can worsen levels of disorientation and aggravate delirium. This is particularly evident in cases of ICU delirium [33].

Antipsychotic medications should be viewed as a short-term intervention to target agitation while the cause of the delirium is being addressed. Delirium sometimes resolves naturally and antipsychotics may prevent further neurological injury during this period. Delirium is a potentially life-threatening condition and should be managed aggressively until the underlying cause has been discovered or the delirium resolves. Aggression is a secondary manifestation and will resolve along with the delirium. If the aggression persists after resolution of the delirium, other potential causes should be considered.

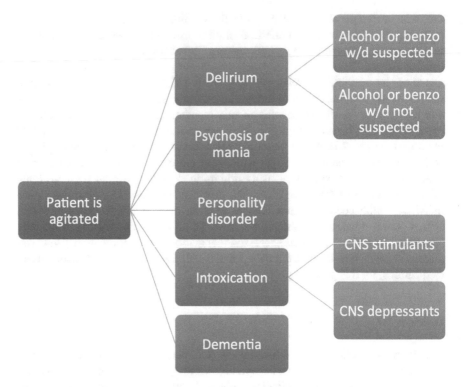

Fig. 11.1 Considering causes of agitation (Adapted from Wilson et al. [32])

Neurodevelopmental Disorders

Intellectual Disability

Individuals with intellectual disability (formerly mental retardation in earlier DSM versions) can display aggressive behaviors for a variety of reasons. They commonly have impaired impulse control, difficulty with long-term planning, and trouble handling stressful or emotional situations. Pharmacological treatments have shown some benefits in targeting aggression in this population. Although much of the published evidence uses the antiquated term "mental retardation," the term intellectual disability will be employed through the remainder of this section.

Treatment with lithium has been shown as beneficial for managing aggression in individuals with intellectual disability. The published reports have typically proposed suggested lithium levels ranging from 0.5 to 1.0 mEq/L [34–36]. Valproate has also been reported as beneficial in managing aggression in this population [37]. Antipsychotics can be helpful in managing aggressive behaviors in individuals with intellectual disability [38]. Risperidone has particularly been reported as having benefits in this population, at doses typically ranging from 0.5

to 4 mg/day [39]. Beta blockers also have reported benefits in curbing aggression in patients with intellectual disability [40].

Clinical Pearls

- Consider medications indicated for treating neurological conditions that could also be used to address comorbid psychiatric issue or aggression.
- There is not currently an FDA-approved pharmacological treatment specifically for managing aggression.
- Bipolar disorder, the condition most commonly treated using mood stabilizers, is commonly misdiagnosed for various reasons.
- Many individuals with antisocial and borderline personality disorders behave aggressively.
- Much of the existing evidence for addressing aggression using pharmacological interventions derives from case reports and small studies.

References

1. American Psychiatric Association. Diagnostic and statistical manual of mental disorders. 5th ed. Arlington: American Psychiatric Association; 2013.
2. American Psychiatric Association. Practice guidelines for the treatment of patients with bipolar disorder [Electronic Version]. 2002 Retrieved July 21, 2015 from http://psychiatryonline.org/pb/assets/raw/sitewide/practice_guidelines/guidelines/bipolar.pdf.
3. Quanbeck CD, Stone DC, Scott CL, et al. Clinical and legal correlates of inmates with bipolar disorder at time of criminal arrest. J Clin Psychiatry. 2004;65(2):198–203.
4. Asnis GM, Kaplan ML, Hundorfean G, et al. Violence and homicidal behaviors in psychiatric disorders. Psychiatr Clin North Am. 1997;20(2):405–25.
5. McEvoy JP, Scheifler PL, Frances A. Treatment of schizophrenia 1999. The expert consensus guideline series. J Clin Psychiatry. 1999;60:S3–80.
6. Wang Y, Xia J, Helfer B, Li C, Leucht S. Valproate for schizophrenia. Cochrane Database Syst Rev. 2016;11:CD004028.
7. Dose M, Hellweg R, Yassouridis A, Theison M, Emrich HM. Combined treatment of schizophrenic psychoses with haloperidol and valproate. Pharmacopsychiatry. 1998;31:122–5.
8. Bender S, Linka T, Wolstein J, Gehendges S, Paulus HJ, Schall U, Gastpar M. Safety and efficacy of combined clozapine-lithium pharmacotherapy. Int J Neuropsychopharmacol. 2004;7(1):59–63.
9. Okuma T, Yamashita I, Takahashi R, Itoh H, Otsuki S, Watanabe S, Sarai K, Hazama H, Inanaga K. A double-blind study of adjunctive carbamazepine versus placebo on excited states of schizophrenic and schizoaffective disorders. Acta Psychiatr Scand. 1989;80:250–9.
10. Pavlovic ZM. Augmentation of clozapine's antiaggressive properties with lamotrigine in a patient with chronic disorganized schizophrenia. J Clin Psychopharmacol. 2008;28(1):119–20.
11. Hollander E, Tracy KA, Swann AC, Coccaro EF, McElroy SL, Wozniak P, Sommerville KW, Nemeroff CB. Divalproex in the treatment of impulsive aggression: efficacy in cluster B personality disorders. Neuropsychopharmacology. 2003;28(6):1186–97.

12. Sheard MH, Marini JL, Bridges CI, Wagner E. The effect of lithium on impulsive aggressive behavior in man. Am J Psychiatry. 1976;133:1409–13.
13. Newman WJ, McDermott BE. Beta blockers for violence prophylaxis – case reports. J Clin Psychopharmacol. 2011;31(6):785–7.
14. Hollander E, Allen A, Lopez RP, Bienstock CA, Grossman R, Siever LJ, Merkatz L, Stein DJ. A preliminary double-blind, placebo-controlled trial of divalproex sodium in borderline personality disorder. J Clin Psychiatry. 2001;62(3):199–203.
15. Loew TH, Nickel MK, Muehlbacher M, Kaplan P, Nickel C, Kettler C, Fartacek R, Lahmann C, Buschmann W, Tritt K, Bachler E, Mitterlehner F, Pedrosa Gil F, Leiberich P, Rother WK, Egger C. Topiramate treatment for women with borderline personality disorder: a double-blind, placebo-controlled study. J Clin Psychopharmacol. 2006;26(1):61–6.
16. Nickel MK, Nickel C, Mitterlehner FO, Tritt K, Lahmann C, Leiberich PK, Rother WK, Loew TH. Topiramate treatment of aggression in female borderline personality disorder patients: a double-blind, placebo-controlled study. J Clin Psychiatry. 2004;65(11):1515–9.
17. Stoffers J, Völlm BA, Rücker G, Timmer A, Huband N, Lieb K. Pharmacological interventions for borderline personality disorder. Cochrane Database Syst Rev. 2010;6:CD005653.
18. Tritt K, Nickel C, Lahmann C, Leiberich PK, Rother WK, Loew TH, Nickel MK. Lamotrigine treatment of aggression in female borderline patients: a randomized, double-blind, placebo-controlled study. J Clin Psychopharmacol. 2005;9(3):287–91.
19. Reich DB, Zanarini MC, Bieri KA. A preliminary study of lamotrigine in the treatment of affective instability in borderline personality disorder. Int Clin Psychopharmacol. 2009;24(5):270–5.
20. Greendyke RM, Kanter DR. Therapeutic effects of pindolol on behavioral disturbances associated with organic brain disease: a double-blind study. J Clin Psychiatry. 1986;47:423–6.
21. Greendyke RM, Kanter DR, Schuster DB, Verstreate S, Wootton J. Propranolol treatment of assaultive patients with organic brain disease. J Nerv Ment Dis. 1986;174:290–4.
22. Greendyke RM, Berkner JP, Webster JC, Gulya A. Treatment of behavioral problems with pindolol. Psychosomatics. 1989;30(2):161–5.
23. Caspi N, Modai I, Barak P, Waisbourd A, Zbarsky H, Hirschmann H, Ritsner M. Pindolol augmentation in aggressive schizophrenic patients: a double-blind crossover randomized study. Int Clin Psychopharmacol. 2001;16(2):111–5.
24. Geracioti TD. Valproic acid treatment of episodic explosiveness related to brain injury. J Clin Psychiatry. 1994;55:416–7.
25. Horne M, Lindley SE. Divalproex sodium in the treatment of aggressive behavior and dysphoria in patients with organic brain syndromes. J Clin Psychiatry. 1995;56:430–1.
26. Wroblewski BA, Joseph AB, Kupfer J, Kalliel K. Effectiveness of valproic acid on destructive and aggressive behaviors in patients with acquired brain injury. Brain Inj. 1997;11:37–47.
27. Azouvi P, Jokic C, Attal N, Denys P, Markabi S, Bussel B. Carbamazepine in agitation and aggressive behavior following severe closed-head injury: results of an open trial. Brain Inj. 1999;13:797–804.
28. Haas JF, Cope DN. Neuropharmacologic management of behavior sequelae in head injury: a case report. Arch Phys Med Rehabil. 1985;66:472–4.
29. Hornstein A, Seliger G. Cognitive side effects of lithium in closed head injury. J Neuropsychiatr Clin Neurosci. 1989;1:446–7.
30. Deb S, Crownshaw T. The role of pharmacotherapy in the management of behaviour disorders in traumatic brain injury patients. Brain Inj. 2004;18:1–31.
31. Lonergan E, Britton AM, Luxenberg J. Antipsychotics for delirium. Cochrane Database Syst Rev. 2007;2:CD005594.
32. Wilson MP, Pepper D, Currier GW, Holloam GH, Feifel D. The psychopharmacology of agitation: consensus statement of the American Association for Emergency Psychiatry Project BETA Psychopharmacology Workgroup. West J Emerg Med. 2012;13:26–34.
33. Pun BT, Ely EW. The importance of diagnosing and managing ICU delirium. Chest. 2007;132:624–36.

34. Craft M, Ismail IA, Krishnamurti D, Mathews J, Regan A, Seth RV, North PM. Lithium in the treatment of aggression in mentally handicapped patients. A double-blind trial. Br J Psychiatry. 1987;150:685–9.
35. Spreat S, Behar D, Reneski B, Miazzo P. Lithium carbonate for aggression in mentally retarded persons. Compr Psychiatry. 1989;30:505–11.
36. Tyrer SP, Walsh A, Edwards DE, Berney TP, Stephens DA. Factors associated with a good response to lithium in aggressive mentally handicapped subjects. Prog Neuro-Psychopharmacol Biol Psychiatry. 1984;8:751–5.
37. Mattes JA. Valproic acid for nonaffective aggression in the mentally retarded. J Nerv Ment Dis. 1992;180:601–2.
38. Amore M, Bertelli M, Villani D, Tamborini S, Rossi M. Olanzapine vs. risperidone in treating aggressive behaviors in adults with intellectual disability: a single blind study. J Intellect Disabil Res. 2011;55(2):210–8.
39. Hassler F, Reis O. Pharmacotherapy of disruptive behavior in mentally retarded subjects: a review of the current literature. Dev Disabil Res Rev. 2010;16(3):265–72.
40. Ruedrich SL, Grush L, Wilson J. Beta adrenergic blocking medications for aggressive or self-injurious mentally retarded persons. Am J Ment Retard. 1990;95(1):110–9.

Chapter 12
Drug-Dietary Interactions: Over-the-Counter Medications, Herbs, and Dietary Supplements

Laurence J. Kinsella, George T. Grossberg, and Neha Prakash

Case Vignette

A 35-year-old man presents with sudden onset of severe throbbing headache, nausea, and light sensitivity. He has no prior history of headaches and migraine. In the emergency department, his examination is normal except for mild neck stiffness and photophobia. Computed tomography (CT) of the brain was unrevealing, and lumbar puncture showed no evidence of subarachnoid hemorrhage. Magnetic resonance imaging (MRI) was performed demonstrating multiple small white matter lesions on FLAIR sequences with normal diffusion-weighted imaging. An MR angiogram demonstrated multiple segmental arterial narrowing in the branches of the middle cerebral arteries. When questioned further, he admitted to using Hydroxycut for weight loss in the last 15 days. Symptoms resolved when the supplement was stopped [1].

L. J. Kinsella, MD (✉)
Department of Neurology, SSM Neuroscience Institute, St. Louis, MO, USA

Department of Neurology, St. Louis University School of Medicine, St. Louis, MO, USA
e-mail: Laurence.Kinsella@ssmhealth.com

G. T. Grossberg, MD
Division of Geriatric Psychiatry, Department of Psychiatry & Behavioral Neuroscience,
St. Louis University School of Medicine, St. Louis, MO, USA

N. Prakash, MD
Department of Neurology, Northwestern University Feinberg School of Medicine,
Chicago, IL, USA

© Springer International Publishing AG, part of Springer Nature 2018   213
G. T. Grossberg, L. J. Kinsella (eds.), *Clinical Psychopharmacology for Neurologists*, https://doi.org/10.1007/978-3-319-74604-3_12

Introduction

Herbal medications have been used throughout human history. Since the DHEAS Act of 1994, there has been an explosion of new products marketed to a welcoming public. Dietary supplements are far less rigorously regulated than drugs by the Federal Drug Administration (FDA). The FDA defines dietary supplement as "a product intended for ingestion that contains a 'dietary ingredient' intended to further nutritional value to supplement the diet. A 'dietary ingredient' may be one, or any combination, of the following substances: a vitamin, a mineral, an herb or other botanical" [2]. There are over 50,000 dietary supplements registered with the Office of Dietary Supplements, a division of the National Institutes of Health. The most popular include vitamin and minerals (43%), specialty supplements for weight loss and sexual health (20%), botanicals (20%), and sports (16%) [3]. Over half of American adults take dietary supplements, and about a third of older adults take over the counter medications (OTCs) [4].

Dietary supplements of interest to neurologists include the migraine remedies feverfew, riboflavin, magnesium and butterbur extract. Galantamine, a plant extract, is used in the treatment of Alzheimer's disease [3].

Without claiming to treat a disease, the dietary supplement industry may promote health and wellness benefits without the requirement of randomized controlled trials, although a number do exist [3].

Herbs may be complicated mixtures of organic and inorganic compounds, some with potentially toxic ingredients [5]. The strength and quantity of the active ingredient may differ among manufacturers. There are efforts to standardize supplement ingredients for consistency and safety [6]. As the use of herbs and over-the-counter (OTC) medications increases, so too the risk of interactions with prescribed medications. This review highlights potential side effects and drug interactions possible with OTCs, herbal medicines, and dietary supplements without undermining the potential, though often unproven, benefits when used appropriately.

In one study, 43% of patients in an outpatient practice were taking both a dietary supplement with prescribed medication. The most common products included vitamins and minerals, garlic, *Ginkgo biloba*, saw palmetto, and ginseng.

About 6% had potentially serious drug-OTC interactions [7]. This included patients taking both calcium and ciprofloxacin (reduced absorption of fluoroquinolones), potassium plus lisinopril (risk for hyperkalemia), and St John's wort plus paroxetine (increased risk of serotonin syndrome) [8].

Clinical Syndromes of Drug-Diet-OTC Toxicity

The presentation of herbal and OTC medication toxicity has a wide spectrum (Table 12.1). The use of excessive diphenhydramine as a sleep aid may induce somnolence and confusion, especially when combined with a beta blocker or other

Table 12.1 Some neurologic syndromes associated with dietary supplements

Neurologic syndrome	Medication examples
Reversible cerebral vasoconstriction syndrome	Sympathomimetic amines (khat, ephedra, ma huang, pseudoephedrine), caffeine, marijuana [9]
Drug-induced seizure	Khat, HCA, caffeine, diphenhydramine [10]
	Gingko [11]
Serotonin syndrome	Tryptophan [12]
Large fiber neuropathy	Pyridoxine (B6) [13, 14]
Rhabdomyolysis	Hydroxycut [15]
Acute renal failure	Orlistat [16]
Syncope from prolonged QT	Energy drinks, guarana, caffeine [17] diphenhydramine [18]
Intracerebral hemorrhage	Ginseng, garlic, gingko [19–21]
Delirium	Dextromethorphan, diphenhydramine [22]

Table 12.2 Dietary supplement toxicity

Agent	Mechanism of injury	Toxicity symptoms
Pyridoxine (vitamin B6)	Enzyme inhibition [27]	Large fiber neuropathy, sensory ataxia [13, 14, 28]
Chinese herbal remedies	Heavy metal intoxication [29]	Neuropathy, encephalopathy [5, 29]
Metabolife	Excitotoxicity (yohimbine, guarana)	QTc prolongation, arrhythmia [30]
Caffeine	Excitotoxicity	Cardiac arrhythmia [30]

inhibitor of P450 2D6. Vasoactive compounds such as pseudoephedrine (also known as ephedra and ma huang) in cough and weight loss remedies may induce stroke, seizures, or thunderclap headache. Since 2004, the FDA has banned the use of ephedra-containing compounds in dietary supplements [23].

One striking presentation of toxicity is reversible cerebral vasoconstriction syndrome (RCVS). It often presents as a thunderclap headache with or without neurological deficits. Angiography may show multifocal cerebral artery vasospasm [1, 9, 24]. RCVS has been reported secondary to vasoactive substances such as pseudoephedrine, caffeine, energy drinks, marijuana, and other naturally occurring stimulants. Another example is *khat*, a plant (*Catha edulis*) chewed in countries like Yemen. Its active ingredient is an amphetamine-like agent that may trigger cerebral vasospasm, stroke, and seizure [25, 26].

Dietary Supplement Toxicity

Toxicity may be direct or secondary to an interaction with a prescribed or OTC medication. Some examples of toxicity from dietary supplements are seen Table 12.2. Pyridoxine in doses >200 mg per day for several months or >1000 mg per day for several days may induce a severe peripheral neuropathy [13, 14, 31]. Chinese herbal remedies may be laced with heavy metals [5].

Mechanism of the Drug-Diet Interaction

Over-the-Counter Medications

Increasing over-the-counter (OTC) medication use has been associated with increasing reports of toxicity and abuse (Tables 12.3 and 12.4) [40]. OTCs can be categorized as:

1. Medications for common ailments (cough syrup, analgesics, antiseptics, antifungal/antibacterials, motion sickness medications, etc.)
2. Herbal and dietary supplements
3. Weight loss supplements

Finkelstein found that one-fourth of all poisoning cases in the pediatric population seen in an ER involve improper use of OTCs [22]. Abuse and misuse of OTCs has been associated with depression [41].

Dextromethorphan is a commonly consumed cough remedy. Side effects are dose dependent and vary from mild sedation at low doses to hallucinations and

Table 12.3 Ten examples of potential drug-OTC interactions

OTC	Rx drug	Interaction
Diphenhydramine	Metoprolol	Bradycardia
	SSRI/SNRI	Serotonin syndrome
Pseudoephedrine	SSRI/SNRI	Serotonin syndrome
Acetaminophen	Alcohol	Increased toxic acetaminophen metabolites, increased alcohol levels [32]
Caffeine	Alcohol	Inhibitor of CYP1A2, raising caffeine levels [30]
Aspirin	Valproate	Displaces VPA, raising levels [33]
Omeprazole	Ciprofloxacin	Reduced Cipro levels, CYP1A2 vs malabsorption [34]
Fexofenadine	Ketoconazole	Increased fexofenadine levels [35]
Dextromethorphan	Quinidine	Increased serum concentrations due to 2D6 inhibition, now FDA approved for pseudobulbar affect (NUEDEXTA) [36]
Loperamide	Quinidine	CNS depression due to PGP inhibition within blood-brain barrier [37]

Table 12.4 Mechanisms of drug-diet interactions

Example	Adverse event	Mechanism
Diphenhydramine and alcohol	Additive sedative properties	Pharmacodynamic interaction
Fluvoxamine and caffeine	Increased caffeine levels [38]	P450 1A2 enzyme inhibition [30]
Amitriptyline and St John's wort	Low amitriptyline levels [39]	P450 3A4 enzyme induction
Statins and grapefruit juice	Myalgias, statin myopathy	Inhibits first-pass metabolism of 3A4 enzyme
Warfarin and spinach	Reduced INR, increase thrombotic risk	Incomplete vitamin K inhibition

ataxia and coma at higher doses. In a review of adolescent overdose, 25% are OTC medications, and half were due to dextromethorphan [22]. Other common agents of overdose include diphenhydramine [42], aspirin, acetaminophen, motion sickness agents such as dramamine, and pseudoephedrine.

Weight Loss Supplements

Weight loss supplements are popular and are a dominant player in the dietary supplement industry. A quick review of Amazon shows hundreds of products marketed to the public [43]. Some of the most widely used supplements and their ingredients are listed in Table 12.5. Hydroxycut is among the most popular weight loss supplements. Prior to 2004, it contained both ephedra and caffeine. It has had several reformulations due to reports of toxicity and was pulled off the market in 2009 following an FDA warning [55]. Current versions contain up to 400 mg of caffeine. Hydroxycut has been linked with liver toxicity [44, 45], seizures [46], RCVS [1], mania [47], and rhabdomyolysis [48].

Hydroxycitric acid (HCA) is the active ingredient of *Garcinia cambogia extract (MOA)*, a fruit rind of *Garcinia gummi-gutta*, and is most commonly used in weight loss supplements. It is purported to regulate serotonin levels, promote lipid oxidation, and inhibit lipid synthesis [56]. Although HCA has potential beneficial effects, drug interactions and adverse effects do occur. Serotonin syndrome has been

Table 12.5 Weight loss supplements and toxicity

Weight loss supplement brand	Ingredients	Active ingredient known	Toxicity reported
Pure *Garcinia cambogia* extract 95% HCA	*Garcinia cambogia* extract (HCA), potassium, calcium, chromium	Hydroxycitric acid (HCA)	Liver toxicity [44, 45], seizures [46], RCVS [1], mania [47], and rhabdomyolysis [48]
Hydroxycut	230–340 mg caffeine, green coffee extract, yohimbe, L-theanine, *Coleus forskohlii*	Green coffee bean extract	Manic episodes [49]
			Serotonin syndrome with escitalopram [50]
			QTc prolongation with yohimbine [30]
Alli orlistat FDA approved	Orlistat (60 Mg). Inactive ingredients: FD&C Blue No. 2, edible ink, gelatin, iron oxide, microcrystalline cellulose, povidone, sodium lauryl sulfate, sodium starch glycolate, talc, titanium dioxide	Orlistat	Hepatotoxic [51] and nephrotoxic [16]
			Deficiency of fat-soluble vitamins [52]
			Inhibits absorption of some medications [53]
NatureWise CLA 1250	Safflower oil: 80% conjugated linoleic acid (CLA)	Conjugated linoleic acid (CLA)	Hepatic steatosis in animal studies [54]

reported in a woman on escitalopram and *Garcinia* for weight loss [50]. *Garcinia* has also been associated with manic episodes [49].

Another weight loss supplement, *orlistat*, is an over-the-counter, semisynthetic lipase inhibitor. It blocks gastric and pancreatic lipase, leading to a 30% reduction in absorption of dietary triglycerides [57]. Orlistat may reduce levels of cyclosporine [53], leading to loss of immunosuppression. It may cause hepatotoxic [51] and nephrotoxic [16] effects. Because of its mechanism of action, it has the potential to cause deficiency of fat-soluble vitamins [52]. Conjugated linoleic acid has been associated with hepatic steatosis in animal studies [54].

Other Herbal and Dietary Supplements

What follows is a list of dietary supplements that have been associated with direct toxicity or drug-diet interactions. The supporting literature is often weak and based upon case reports (Tables 12.6 and 12.7). More rigorous clinical studies of some previously suspect dietary supplements such as garlic, gingko, ginger, and cranberry show no significant interactions at recommended doses; however, megadosing may be associated with greater toxicity. The most important dietary supplement to cause clinically relevant interactions with prescription drugs is St John's wort [58, 59].

St John's wort has been used successfully for mild to moderate depression [66]. When taken together with an SSRI or SNRI, it may increase the risk of serotonin syndrome due to additive serotonergic effects [8]. It may lower the efficacy of various medications by its action as an inducer of P450 enzymes, especially CYP3A4, leading to lowered plasma levels (Table 12.7). Drug interactions have been seen with alprazolam, amitriptyline, cyclosporine, fexofenadine, indinavir, methadone, simvastatin, tacrolimus, warfarin, and oral contraceptives [59, 64]. St John's wort does not appear to interact with carbamazepine, dextromethorphan, mycophenolic acid, or pravastatin [8].

Hypoglycemia is more likely when St John's wort is used with oral hypoglycemic agents such as glipizide and rosiglitazone. It may induce delirium with loperamide, possibly due to its effects on P-glycoprotein [67]. St John's wort has been reported to trigger mania in bipolar patients [68] and psychosis in schizophrenia [69].

Garlic is commonly utilized for its purported cardiovascular benefits and antiplatelet and antineoplastic activities [70]. It may have modest antihypertensive effects [71]; however, caution is advised when using along with other antihypertensives as it may further lower blood pressure. Garlic has been reported to inhibit platelet aggregation [19], and concurrent use with ASA and clopidogrel has been associated with an increased bleeding tendency [20, 72] although this effect is contested [59].

Gingko biloba is a commonly used medicinal plant for memory enhancement, claudication, tinnitus, and vertigo. Like other herbs, there are case reports of increased risk of bleeding when used along with anticoagulant or antiplatelet therapies [73]. However, more rigorous studies have not confirmed a clinically important interaction [59, 39, 74].

Table 12.6 Case reports of drug-dietary supplement interactions

Dietary supplement	Purported mechanism of action/indication	Toxicity/interaction
Black cohosh	Menopausal symptoms	Case reports of hypotension with HCTZ, lisinopril, diltiazem not confirmed in clinical trials, likely safe [58]
Cranberry juice	Acidifies urine, reduce bacterial adherence	Case reports of warfarin and antiplatelet interaction not confirmed by controlled trials [59]
Garlic	HTN, atherosclerosis	Case reports of warfarin and antiplatelet interaction not confirmed by controlled trials [59]
Ginkgo biloba	Increase blood flow; memory promotor	Case reports of warfarin and antiplatelet interaction not confirmed by controlled trials [59]
Ginseng	Memory promotor	Possible bleeding risk with antiplatelet agents [60]
Goldenseal	Anticancer properties	May inhibit action of drugs metabolized by CYP2D6 and 3A4 [61]
Saw palmetto	Reduce Sx of prostatic hypertrophy	Single case report of warfarin interaction, likely safe [59, 62]
Soy	Relief of menopausal symptoms	Possible promotor of estrogen-sensitive tumor growth [63]
St John's wort	Depression, anxiety	Potent CYP3A4 inducer
		Reduces BCP, simvastatin, warfarin, alprazolam. Delirium with loperamide
		Serotonin syndrome with SSRI, buspirone [8, 64]

Table 12.7 Other drug-diet interactions

Dietary product	Rx drug	Interaction
Grapefruit juice	Statins	Myalgias, rhabdomyolysis
	Ca channel blocker	Hypotension, bradycardia
	Chemotherapy	Reduced efficacy
	Fexofenadine	Reduce efficacy (OATP inhibition) [65]
Caffeine	SSRI	Irritability, tremor
Hard cheese	MAOIs, selegiline	Serotonin syndrome
St John's wort	Cyclosporine	Lowers plasma levels by PGP and 3A4 induction [35]
St John's wort	Indinavir	Lowers plasma levels by PGP and 3A4 induction [35]
St John's wort	Cyclosporine	Lowers plasma levels by PGP and 3A4 induction [35]

The significance of herb-drug interactions in elderly patients receiving warfarin or in patients taking higher than recommended doses or combinations of herbal medicines is not yet established. Various case reports have shown seizure inducing properties of gingko, likely attributed to the 4′-methoxypyridoxine or B6 antivitamin [11]. There is a case report of fatal seizures when combined with valproate and phenytoin [75].

Ginseng has two active ingredients: ginsenosides and eleutherosides, known for its antioxidant and anti-inflammatory effects. It is well tolerated with low side-effect profile; however, with prolonged use, hypertension, nervousness, sleeplessness, skin eruptions, and morning diarrhea may occur; euphoric and agitated states have been reported. Early reports of decreased warfarin efficacy and manic-like episodes when used with MAO-inhibitors like phenelzine [76] have not been confirmed in later studies [39].

Saw palmetto is marketed as a herbal remedy for benign prostate hypertrophy. It is considered to be a relatively safe herbal medicine; however, case reports of pancreatitis and heart block suggest caution when used in megadoses [77, 78]. Early reports of coagulopathy associated with saw palmetto [79] have not been confirmed in larger clinical studies [39].

False-Positive Urine Drug Testing

Urine drug screening (UDS) is commonly used in a variety of settings, including the workplace, in athletics, criminal settings, and healthcare. Easy access to urine samples makes them ideal for UDS – usually via immunoassay. However, false positives and negatives can occur – often resulting in adverse consequences. For definitive results, gas chromatography-mass spectrometry needs to be utilized.

The Department of Health and Human Services' Guidelines for UDS in the workplace include testing for five substances: amphetamines, cannabinoids, cocaine, opiates, and phencyclidine [80]. In the healthcare settings, UDS for benzodiazepines, alcohol, and tricyclic antidepressants is also common. UDS may be confounded by substituting, diluting, or adulterating urine [81, 82].

Examples of "false positives" in UDS include:

- Using "hemp milk" (sold at health food stores) as a cause of false-positive UDS for cannabinoids.
- Consuming poppy seed pastries may give positive UDS for opiates.
- Dextromethorphan (in OTC cough syrup) may be false positive for opiates.
- Venlafaxine may result in false positive for methamphetamine [83].

Conclusion

People crave autonomy in healthcare and will often reach for the pharmacy aisle before calling a doctor. Patients may be putting themselves at risk for toxicity and drug interactions with the expanding use of herbal medications, OTCs, and dietary supplements. Clinicians need to be aware of potential drug interactions between prescribed and nonprescribed substances. It is important to take a thorough medication history that includes dietary habits, OTCs, supplements, and herbal remedies to predict and prevent potential interactions.

References

1. Cvetanovich GL, Ramakrishnan P, Klein JP, Rao VR, Ropper AH. Reversible cerebral vaso-constriction syndrome in a patient taking citalopram and Hydroxycut: a case report. J Med Case Rep. 2011;5(1):34. https://doi.org/10.1186/1752-1947-5-548.
2. Center for Food Safety, Nutrition A. Dietary Supplements. http://www.fda.gov/Food/DietarySupplements/.
3. Brown AC. An overview of herb and dietary supplement efficacy, safety and government regulations in the United States with suggested improvements. Part 1 of 5 series. Food Chem Toxicol. 2017;107(Pt A):449–71. https://doi.org/10.1016/j.fct.2016.11.001.
4. Qato DM, Alexander GC, Conti RM, Johnson M, Schumm P, Lindau ST. Use of prescription and over-the-counter medications and dietary supplements among older adults in the United States. JAMA. 2008;300(24):2867–78. https://doi.org/10.1001/jama.2008.892.
5. Espinoza EO, Mann MJ, Bleasdell B. Arsenic and mercury in traditional Chinese herbal balls. N Engl J Med. 2009;333(12):803–4. https://doi.org/10.1056/NEJM199509213331217.
6. Bent S, Ko R. Commonly used herbal medicines in the United States: a review. Am J Med. 2004;116(7):478–85. https://doi.org/10.1016/j.amjmed.2003.10.036.
7. Peng CC, Glassman PA, Trilli LE, Hayes-Hunter J, Good CB. Incidence and severity of potential drug–dietary supplement interactions in primary care patients: an exploratory study of 2 outpatient practices. Arch Intern Med. 2004;164(6):630–6. https://doi.org/10.1001/archinte.164.6.630.
8. Zhou S, Chan E, Pan S-Q, Huang M, Lee EJD. Pharmacokinetic interactions of drugs with St John's wort. J Psychopharmacol. 2016;18(2):262–76. https://doi.org/10.1177/0269881104042632.
9. Sheikh HU, Mathew PG. Reversible cerebral vasoconstriction syndrome: updates and new perspectives. Curr Pain Headache Rep. 2014;18(5):414. https://doi.org/10.1007/s11916-014-0414-7.
10. Thundiyil JG, Kearney TE, Olson KR. Evolving epidemiology of drug-induced seizures reported to a poison control center system. J Med Toxicol. 2007;3(1):15–9. https://doi.org/10.1007/BF03161033.
11. Jang H-S, Roh SY, Jeong EH, Kim B-S, Sunwoo MK. Ginkgotoxin induced seizure caused by vitamin B6 deficiency. J Epilepsy Res. 2015;5(2):104–6. https://doi.org/10.14581/jer.15018.
12. Boyer EW, Shannon M. The Serotonin syndrome. N Engl J Med. 2009;352(11):1112–20. https://doi.org/10.1056/NEJMra041867.
13. Parry GJ, Bredesen DE. Sensory neuropathy with low-dose pyridoxine. Neurology. 1985;35(10):1466. https://doi.org/10.1212/WNL.35.10.1466.
14. Schaumburg H, Kaplan J, Windebank A, et al. Sensory neuropathy from pyridoxine abuse. N Engl J Med. 1983;309(8):445–8. https://doi.org/10.1056/NEJM198308253090801.
15. Carol ML. Hydroxycut weight loss dietary supplements: a contributing factor in the development of exertional rhabdomyolysis in three U.S. Army soldiers. Mil Med. 2013;178(9):e1039–42. https://doi.org/10.7205/MILMED-D-13-00133.
16. Karamadoukis L, Shivashankar GH, Ludeman L, Williams AJ. An unusual complication of treatment with orlistat. Clin Nephrol. 2009;71(04):430–2. https://doi.org/10.5414/CNP71430.
17. Mangi MA, Rehman H, Rafique M, Illovsky M. Energy drinks and the risk of cardiovascular disease: a review of current literature. Cureus. 2017;9(6):e1322. https://doi.org/10.7759/cureus.1322.
18. Husain Z, Hussain K, Nair R. Diphenhydramine induced QT prolongation and torsade de pointes: an uncommon effect of a common drug. Cardiol J. 2010;17(5):509–11.
19. Saw JT, Bahari MB, Ang HH, Lim YH. Potential drug? herb interaction with antiplatelet/anti-coagulant drugs. Complement Ther Clin Pract. 2006;12(4):236–41. https://doi.org/10.1016/j.ctcp.2006.06.002.
20. Fakhar H, Hashemi TA. Effect of the garlic pill in comparison with Plavix on platelet aggregation and bleeding time. Iran J Ped Hematol Oncol. 2012;2(4):146–52.

21. Pedroso JL, Henriques Aquino CC, Escórcio Bezerra ML, et al. Ginkgo biloba and cerebral bleeding: a case report and critical review. Neurologist. 2011;17(2):89–90. https://doi.org/10.1097/NRL.0b013e3181f097b4.
22. Finkelstein Y, Goel G, Hutson JR. Drug misuse in adolescents presenting to the emergency department. Pediatr Emerg Care. 2017;33(7):451–6.
23. Palamar J. How ephedrine escaped regulation in the United States: a historical review of misuse and associated policy. Health Policy. 2011;99(1):1–9. https://doi.org/10.1016/j.healthpol.2010.07.007.
24. Costa I, Mendonça MD, Silva VE, Calado S. Herbal supplements association with reversible cerebral vasoconstriction syndrome: a case report. J Stroke Cerebrovasc Dis. 2017 Mar;26(3):673–6.
25. Baharith H, Zarrin A. Khat ? A new precipitating factor for reversible cerebral vasoconstriction syndrome: a case report. J Med Case Rep. 2016;10(1):1159. https://doi.org/10.1186/s13256-016-1155-5.
26. Tuladhar AM, Boogaarts HD, de Leeuw F-E, van Dijk E. Reversible cerebral vasoconstriction syndrome after chewing khat leaves. Cerebrovasc Dis. 2013;36(2):158–9. https://doi.org/10.1159/000353664.
27. Vrolijk MF, Opperhuizen A, Jansen EHJM, Hageman GJ, Bast A, Haenen GRMM. The vitamin B6 paradox: supplementation with high concentrations of pyridoxine leads to decreased vitamin B6 function. Toxicol in Vitro. 2017;44:206–12. https://doi.org/10.1016/j.tiv.2017.07.009.
28. Bacharach R, Lowden M, Ahmed A. Pyridoxine toxicity small fiber neuropathy with dysautonomia. J Clin Neuromuscul Dis. 2017;19(1):43–6. https://doi.org/10.1097/CND.0000000000000172.
29. Chan H, Billmeier GJ, Evans WE. Lead poisoning from ingestion of Chinese herbal medicine. Clin Toxicol. 1977;10(3):273–81. https://doi.org/10.3109/15563657708992423.
30. Gurley BJ, Steelman SC, Thomas SL. Multi-ingredient, caffeine-containing dietary supplements: history, safety, and efficacy. Clin Ther. 2015;37(2):275–301. https://doi.org/10.1016/j.clinthera.2014.08.012.
31. Lheureux P, Penaloza A, Gris M. Pyridoxine in clinical toxicology: a review. Eur J Emerg Med. 2005 Apr;12(2):78–85.
32. Lee Y-P, Liao J-T, Cheng Y-W, et al. Inhibition of human alcohol and aldehyde dehydrogenases by acetaminophen: assessment of the effects on first-pass metabolism of ethanol. Alcohol. 2013;47(7):559–65. https://doi.org/10.1016/j.alcohol.2013.09.001.
33. Haas DA. Adverse drug interactions in dental practice: interactions associated with analgesics, part III in a series. J Am Dent Assoc. 1999;130(3):397–407.
34. Honig PK, Gillespie BK. Drug interactions between prescribed and over-the-counter medication 1. Drug Saf. 1995;13(5):296–303. https://doi.org/10.2165/00002018-199513050-00003.
35. Marchetti S, Mazzanti R, Beijnen JH, Schellens JHM. Concise review: clinical relevance of drug drug and herb drug interactions mediated by the ABC transporter ABCB1 (MDR1, P-glycoprotein). Oncologist. 2007;12(8):927–41. https://doi.org/10.1634/theoncologist.12-8-927.
36. Taylor CP, Traynelis SF, Siffert J, Pope LE, Matsumoto RR. Pharmacology of dextromethorphan: relevance to dextromethorphan/quinidine (Nuedexta®) clinical use. Pharmacol Ther. 2016;164:170–82. https://doi.org/10.1016/j.pharmthera.2016.04.010.
37. Sadeque AJ, Wandel C, He H, Shah S, Wood AJ. Increased drug delivery to the brain by P-glycoprotein inhibition. Clin Pharmacol Ther. 2000;68(3):231–7. https://doi.org/10.1067/mcp.2000.109156.
38. Carrillo JA, Benitez J. Clinically significant pharmacokinetic interactions between dietary caffeine and medications. Clin Pharmacokinet. 2000;39(2):127–53. https://doi.org/10.2165/00003088-200039020-00004.
39. Izzo AA, Ernst E. Interactions between herbal medicines and prescribed drugs. Drugs. 2009;69(13):1777–98. https://doi.org/10.2165/11317010-000000000-00000.

40. Wilkinson GR. Drug metabolism and variability among patients in drug response. N Engl J Med. 2005;352(21):2211–21. https://doi.org/10.1056/NEJMra032424.
41. Benotsch EG, Koester S, Martin AM, Cejka A, Luckman D, Jeffers AJ. Intentional misuse of over-the-counter medications, mental health, and polysubstance use in young adults. J Community Health. 2013;39(4):688–95. https://doi.org/10.1007/s10900-013-9811-9.
42. Mowry JB, Spyker DA, Cantilena LR Jr, McMillan N, Ford M. 2013 annual report of the American Association of Poison Control Centers' National Poison Data System (NPDS): 31st annual report. Clin Toxicol. 2015;52(10):1032–283. https://doi.org/10.3109/15563650.2014.9 87397.
43. Weight loss supplements. Amazon. https://www.amazon.com/Weight-Loss-Products-Nutrition-Fitness/b?ie=UTF8&node=3774931. Published July 5, 2017. Accessed 7 May 2017.
44. Stevens T, Qadri A, Zein NN. Two patients with acute liver injury associated with use of the herbal weight-loss supplement hydroxycut. Ann Intern Med. 2005;142(6):477–8.
45. Araujo JL, Worman HJ. Acute liver injury associated with a newer formulation of the herbal weight loss supplement Hydroxycut. BMJ Case Reports 2015. https://doi.org/10.1136/bcr-2015-210303.
46. Kockler DR, McCarthy MW, Lawson CL. Seizure activity and unresponsiveness after hydroxycut ingestion. Pharmacotherapy. 2001;21(5):647–51.
47. Narasimha A, Shetty PH, Nanjundaswamy MH, Viswanath B, Bada Math S. Hydroxycut? Dietary supplements for weight loss: can they induce mania? Aust N Z J Psychiatry. 2013;47(12):1205–6. https://doi.org/10.1177/0004867413493522.
48. Dehoney S, Wellein M. Rhabdomyolysis associated with the nutritional supplement Hydroxycut. Am J Health Syst Pharm. 2009;66(2):142–8. https://doi.org/10.2146/ajhp070640.
49. Hendrickson BP, Shaikh N, Occhiogrosso M, Penzner JB. Mania induced by Garcinia cambogia. Prim Care Companion CNS Disord. 2016. https://doi.org/10.4088/PCC.15l01890.
50. Lopez AM, Kornegay J, Hendrickson RG. Serotonin toxicity associated with Garcinia cambogia over-the-counter supplement. J Med Toxicol. 2014;10(4):399–401. https://doi.org/10.1007/s13181-014-0390-7.
51. Umemura T, Ichijo T, Matsumoto A. Severe hepatic injury caused by orlistat. Am J Med. 2006;119(8):e7.
52. Harrison SA, Fecht W, Brunt EM, Neuschwander Tetri BA. Orlistat for overweight subjects with nonalcoholic steatohepatitis: a randomized, prospective trial. Hepatology. 2009;49(1):80–6. https://doi.org/10.1002/hep.22575.
53. Earnshaw I, Thachil J. Example of the drug interaction between ciclosporin and orlistat, resulting in relapse of Evan's syndrome. BMJ Case Rep. 2016:bcr2016217246. https://doi.org/10.1136/bcr-2016-217246.
54. de Moraes C, de Oliveira CA, Amaral MECD, Landini GA, Catisti R. Liver metabolic changes induced by conjugated linoleic acid in calorie-restricted rats. Arch Endocrinol Metab. 2017;61(1):45–53. https://doi.org/10.1590/2359-3997000000186.
55. FDA warns consumers to stop using hydroxycut products risk of liver injury. http://www.fda.govdownloadsNewsEventsPublicHealthFocusUCM.pdf.
56. Semwal RB, Semwal DK, Vermaak I, Viljoen A. A comprehensive scientific overview of Garcinia cambogia. Fitoterapia. 2015;102:134–48. https://doi.org/10.1016/j.fitote.2015.02.012.
57. Guerciolini R. Mode of action of orlistat. Int J Obes Relat Metab Disord. 1997;21(Suppl 3):S12–23.
58. Asher GN, Corbett AH, Hawke RL. Common herbal dietary supplement-drug interactions. Am Fam Physician. 2017;96(2):101–7.
59. Izzo AA. Interactions between herbs and conventional drugs: overview of the clinical data. Med Princ Pract. 2012;21(5):404–28. https://doi.org/10.1159/000334488.
60. Yuan C-S, Wei G, Dey L, et al. Brief communication: American ginseng reduces warfarin's effect in healthy patients: a randomized, controlled trial. Ann Intern Med. 2004;141(1):23–7.

61. Gurley BJ, Gardner SF, Hubbard MA, et al. In vivo effects of goldenseal, kava kava, black cohosh, and valerian on human cytochrome P450 1A2, 2D6, 2E1, and 3A4/5 phenotypes. Clin Pharmacol Ther. 2005;77(5):415–26. https://doi.org/10.1016/j.clpt.2005.01.009.
62. Yue QY, Jansson K. Herbal drug curbicin and anticoagulant effect with and without warfarin: possibly related to the vitamin E component. J Am Geriatr Soc. 2001;49(6):838.
63. Shike M, Doane AS, Russo L, et al. The effects of soy supplementation on gene expression in breast cancer: a randomized placebo-controlled study. J Natl Cancer Inst. 2014;106(9):dju189. https://doi.org/10.1093/jnci/dju189.
64. Izzo AA. Drug interactions with St. John's Wort (Hypericum perforatum): a review of the clinical evidence. Int J Clin Pharmacol Ther. 2004;42(03):139–48. https://doi.org/10.5414/CPP42139.
65. Shirasaka Y, Mori T, Murata Y, Nakanishi T, Tamai I. Substrate- and dose-dependent drug interactions with grapefruit juice caused by multiple binding sites on OATP2B1. Pharm Res. 2014;31(8):2035–43. https://doi.org/10.1007/s11095-014-1305-7.
66. Apaydin EA, Maher AR, Shanman R, et al. A systematic review of St. John's wort for major depressive disorder. Syst Rev. 2016;5(1):3135. https://doi.org/10.1186/s13643-016-0325-2.
67. Khawaja IS, Marotta RF, Lippmann S. Herbal medicines as a factor in delirium. Psychiatr Serv. 1999;50(7):969–70. https://doi.org/10.1176/ps.50.7.969a.
68. Dalwood J, Dhillon R, Tibrewal P, Gupta N, Bastiampillai T. St John's wort – is it safe in bipolar disorder? Aust N Z J Psychiatry. 2015;49(12):1226–7. https://doi.org/10.1177/0004867415585856.
69. Stevinson C, Ernst E. Can St. John's wort trigger psychoses? Int J Clin Pharmacol Ther. 2004;42(9):473–80.
70. Tattelman E. Health effects of garlic. Am Fam Physician. 2005;72:103–6.
71. Ried K, Travica N, Sali A. The effect of aged garlic extract on blood pressure and other cardiovascular risk factors in uncontrolled hypertensives: the AGE at heart trial. Integr Blood Press Control. 2016;9:9–21. https://doi.org/10.2147/IBPC.S93335.
72. Shafiekhani M, Faridi P, Kojuri J, Namazi S. Comparison of antiplatelet activity of garlic tablets with cardio-protective dose of aspirin in healthy volunteers: a randomized clinical trial. Avicenna J Phytomed. 2016;6(5):550–7.
73. Bone KM. Potential interaction of Ginkgo biloba leaf with antiplatelet or anticoagulant drugs: what is the evidence? In: Cott JM, Eisenbrand G, editors. Mol Nutr Food Res 2008;52(7):764–71. https://doi.org/10.1002/mnfr.200700098.
74. Jiang X, Williams KM, Liauw WS, et al. Effect of ginkgo and ginger on the pharmacokinetics and pharmacodynamics of warfarin in healthy subjects. Br J Clin Pharmacol. 2005;59(4):425–32. https://doi.org/10.1111/j.1365-2125.2005.02322.x.
75. Kupiec T, Raj V. Fatal seizures due to potential herb-drug interactions with Ginkgo biloba. J Anal Toxicol. 2005;29(7):755–8.
76. Kiefer D, Pantuso T. Panax ginseng. Am Fam Physician. 2003;68(8):1539–42.
77. Bruminhent J, Carrera P, Li Z, Amankona R, Roberts IM. Acute pancreatitis with saw palmetto use: a case report. J Med Case Rep. 2011;5(1):219. https://doi.org/10.1186/1752-1947-5-414.
78. Jipescu D, Patel A, Bohra H, Pientka A. Rare case of saw palmetto induced complete heart block. J Am Coll Cardiol. 2017;69(11):2310. https://doi.org/10.1016/S0735-1097(17)35699-1.
79. Villanueva S, González J. Coagulopathy induced by saw palmetto: a case report. Bol Asoc Med P R. 2009;101(3):48–50.
80. Federal register: mandatory guidelines for federal workplace drug testing programs. 2017. https://www.federalregister.gov/d/2017-00979/p-4.
81. Moeller KE, Lee KC, Kissack JC. Urine drug screening: practical guide for clinicians. Mayo Clin Proc. 2008;83(1):66–76. https://doi.org/10.4065/83.1.66.
82. Clinical drug testing in primary care. Substance Abuse and Mental Health Services Adminstration. samhsa.gov/shin/content/SMA12-4668/SMA12-4668.pdf. Published 2012. Accessed 25 Oct 2017.
83. Brahm NC, Yeager LL, Fox MD, Farmer KC, Palmer TA. Commonly prescribed medications and potential false-positive urine drug screens. Am J Health Syst Pharm. 2010;67(16):1344–50. https://doi.org/10.2146/ajhp090477.

Index

Printed in the United States
By Bookmasters